Assisted Living

Assisted Living

Needs, Practices, and Policies in Residential Care for the Elderly

Edited by Sheryl Zimmerman, Ph.D.
Philip D. Sloane, M.D., M.P.H.
J. Kevin Eckert, Ph.D.

Foreword by M. Powell Lawton, Ph.D.

The Johns Hopkins University Press
Baltimore and London

© 2001 The Johns Hopkins University Press
All rights reserved. Published 2001
Printed in the United States of America on acid-free paper
9 8 7 6 5 4 3 2 1

The Johns Hopkins University Press
2715 North Charles Street
Baltimore, Maryland 21218-4363
www.press.jhu.edu

Library of Congress Cataloging-in-Publication Data
Assisted living : needs, practices, and policies in residential care
for the elderly / edited by Sheryl Zimmerman, Philip D. Sloane,
and J. Kevin Eckert; with a foreword by M. Powell Lawton.
  p. ; cm.
Includes bibliographical references and index.
ISBN 0-8018-6705-3 (alk. paper)
   1. Congregate housing—United States.   2. Aged—Housing—
United States.   3. Aged—Care—United States.   4. Life care
communities—United States—Management.
   [DNLM: 1. Housing for the Elderly.   1. Long-Term Care—Aged.
WT 30 A8473 2001]   I. Zimmerman, Sheryl, 1957–   II. Sloane,
Philip D.   III. Eckert, J. Kevin.
   HD7287.92U6.x +

00-012114

A catalog record for this book is available from the British Library.

Contents

Foreword

My age peers and I experienced the beginning of age-targeted housing for older people. It was a time for excitement over the idea that a new form of community had been created to fill a niche of need that fell between the healthy elder able to live in the community and the frail elder who required an institution. The new housing form, often referred to as independent senior citizen housing, though targeted to the independent older person, in fact provided a "silent buffer" for people who aged in place in terms of declining health. That is, even though most builders and administrators of independent housing were careful to avoid the look of an institution and emphasized the vigor of its resident population, the fact was that all such housing provided safety nets. Friends were easy to make, if one wished. Near neighbors were available to help or to notice new signs of frailty. Every administrator either actively or passively picked up knowledge about growing signs of frailty and local referral resources. Even though administrators and residents fought the idea that residents were in a social service environment, they did have access to some of that expertise when in need.

This covert knowledge on both sides that some protection was available may be thought of as a first-level assurance of security in time of need. "Congregate housing" began almost as early as did independent housing, in recognition of the need of some sectors of the older population for more than a minimal degree of support. Congregate housing was always in short supply because of its additional cost, coupled with its all-or-nothing service mode—that is, the philosophy that services had to be supplied for and bought by all residents, to make it cost effective. Even when HUD, in its Congregate Housing Services Program (CHSP), attempted to target services to only those most needy, costs became so great that the CHSP remained tiny. Congregate housing thus remained a scarce commodity.

Assisted living in some ways seems like a reconstitution of congregate housing. I see an essential difference, however, one that ought to ensure that assisted living flourishes. Congregate housing was a graft to independent housing, with the intent to extend the independent housing model another notch in the direction of support. In contrast, assisted living is a graft to the nursing home, with the intent to extend this high-support model in the direction of greater independence. In other words, assisted living recognizes and addresses deficiencies of the nursing home, namely, frequent provision of excess care and independence-undermining features of everyday life. Along with the excess of care came many features of the physical and social environment whose primary purpose was to protect the physically ill patient. The medical model on which the nursing home is based is particularly inappropriate for many people with dementia, specifically for those with stable medical conditions. In its earlier history and up to the present, the nursing home has been overused in this respect because there was no other alternative. The social model of care that is possible when the major reason for nursing home residence is not health care allows much easier introduction of humanistic concerns for higher-order needs such as dignity, autonomy, self-growth, and privacy. Assisted living is growing because there was such a large segment of people needing an enhanced sense of security but not needing to relinquish total control over their lives.

From society's perspective, the graft away from the excess care of the nursing home has the potential for reducing the burden of care on the taxpayer. As of the beginning of the new century, this consideration is only a goal, not an achievement. The excitement of the early days of age-targeted housing was also enhanced because of these programs' intent to serve the poor. The sad fact is that an unfortunate proportion of the growth in assisted living comes from its appeal to the most solvent sector of the older population. Right now, assisted living is less expensive than nursing home care primarily for the aging family who might be subject to full-pay nursing home care. Some states are moving toward subsidy programs that can open assisted living to low-income and lower-middle-income elders. This deficit in the financial aspects of the current assisted living scene should be viewed as the impetus for private sponsors, researchers, and governmental policymakers to identify those especially appealing and effective features in today's assisted living environment and to devote major resources toward making them available to the large segment of the older population. The assisted living being built for the affluent will test the consumer appeal and the outcomes associated with pace-setting design and program innovations. Many such positive aspects of the assisted living context are not intrinsically expensive. It takes determination to differentiate quality-of-life innovations that may be duplicated at a lower cost from those that either are irrelevant to quality of life or are luxuries. The research and policy contributions by the authors represented in this book constitute an excellent beginning to the process of achieving broad usership with minimal sacrifice of quality.

M. Powell Lawton, Ph.D.
Philadelphia Geriatric Center

Preface

Assisted Living is composed of three parts. Part 1 focuses on broad, substantive matters in residential care/assisted living (RC/AL) as they have evolved in today's long-term health care environment. Nationally recognized experts from a variety of disciplines have contributed these chapters. Part 2 addresses the basic components of these care settings: residents and the structure and process of care. Data from the Collaborative Studies of Long-Term Care, a comprehensive multistate study of 193 RC/AL facilities (2,078 residents) and 40 nursing homes (761 residents), funded by the National Institute on Aging, inform these matters. Part 3 examines future directions in the field and presents implications of the information provided in parts 1 and 2.

The information reported in this book can help define the types of RC/AL that should be encouraged, through regulation, financing, and public payments. Similarly, it can help consumers and their families determine whether RC/AL can meet their needs and select an appropriate type of facility. The information also will be of significant interest to persons concerned with the health care and quality of life of the elderly population, including policymakers; practitioners; owners, operators and investors; home health planners; and researchers and students in a variety of disciplines.

The effort involved in the development of this book extends beyond the list of authors; without the help of many others, a work of this scope would not be possible. Initial thanks must go to the National Institute on Aging (NIA), one of the National Institutes of Health, for providing the funding that enabled us to conduct the Collaborative Studies of Long-Term Care (CS-LTC) and to elicit the contribution of national experts. Marcia Ory of the NIA deserves special thanks. Marcia's support and vision have guided the work of numerous investigators across the nation, and she thus plays a key role in the evolution of quality long-term care for our elderly. We also thank Gordon H. Defriese, previous director of the Cecil G. Sheps Center for Health Services Research at the University of North Carolina, Chapel Hill. Gordon has had a central role in improving the practice of long-term care across the state of North Carolina, and he has recognized and supported the contributions of the CS-LTC to this effort.

Next in line for appreciation are the residents and staff of the 233 long-term care facilities that participated in the CS-LTC. The staff often began their workday early or ended it late to make time to meet with our interviewers. They explained to us how long-term care is provided in their facility, sensitive to the special needs of their residents; with resident consent, they spoke to us over the course of two years so that we could learn how these individuals change over time. The participation of these generous caregivers bespeaks their own commitment to bettering the quality of long-term care. Having the welfare of our elderly in the hands of such dedicated people is a positive sign for the future.

We also thank the members and associates of the state departments that supported our study, including Jose Diez-Arguelles, Executive Director, Florida Assisted Living Association; Mary Ellen Early, Director of Public Policy, Florida Association of Homes for the Aging; LuMarie Polivka-West, Senior Director of Policy, Florida Health Care Association; Diane Dorlester, Executive Director, Maryland Assisted Living Association; Isabella Firth, President, Maryland Association of Non-Profit Homes for the Aging; William Abrams, President, New Jersey Association of Health Care Facilities; J. Craig Souza, President, North Carolina Health Care Facilities Association; Barbara Vaughn, Executive Director, North Carolina Assisted Living Association; and Lou Wilson, Executive Director, North Carolina Association of Long-Term Care Facilities.

The wealth of information from residents and staff was collected by a team of truly expert research interviewers. Betty Concha traveled throughout the four states of study, overseeing issues of subject consent and coordinating field arrangements at every level. She supervised twelve exceptionally agreeable and thoughtful evaluators, to whose insights we dedicated an entire chapter: Ida Altman, Joan Bassler, Susan Baxter, Shirley Carter, Betty Dorsey, Diane Eagle, Susan Fallen, David Fallen, Jo Magness, Connie Nunamaker, Ronald Nunamaker, and Barbara Smith. We make special mention of Mary Alice McGurrin and Christine Schmitt, two extremely dedicated women, who were solely responsible for collecting data for more than two thousand residents every quarter during the two years of study follow-up.

Finally, we would like to recognize the staff and investigators of the CS-LTC, who are colleagues in every sense of the word. In Maryland, we make particular mention of Verita Custis Buie for expert project coordination; there is no challenge that Verita cannot meet. Suzanne Miller was the primary editorial assistant for this book, and her attention to detail we knew to trust. She was helped by Stefanie Dansicker, with oversight by Cindy Geppi; Lori Gorschboth assisted in data management. We are grateful for the efforts of all of these individuals, as well as the investigative involvement of Drs. Ann Gruber-Baldini, J. Richard Hebel, Jay Magaziner, and Leslie Morgan. In North Carolina, we recognize the excellent research assistance provided by Anne Scott, C. Madeline Mitchell, April Points, and Andrea Shiffman Tuttle; data entry by Jane Darter; data management by Carol Porter; and administration by Cathy Rogers and Nancy Jenkins; investigators include Drs. Shulamit Bernard, William Kalsbeek, Gary Koch, Robert Konrad, Sally Stearns, Joan Walsh, and Judith Wildfire. We also extend thanks for the efforts of our student assistants: Wayne Anderson, R. Tamara Hodlewsky, Nan Sook Park, Maria Phillips, and Jacob Sloane.

We are grateful to have on our list of contributors many of the most notable national experts in the field of long-term care: our consultants, Drs. M. Powell Lawton and Catherine Hawes; Drs. Robert Mollica, Elizabeth Mutran, and Victor Regnier; and Mr. Michael Nolin. We are proud to highlight the contributions of these scholars to this text.

Contributors

Shulamit L. Bernard, Ph.D., R.N., Research Health Policy Analyst, Research Triangle Institute, Research Triangle Park, North Carolina

Verita Custis Buie, M.S., Project Coordinator, Division of Gerontology, Department of Epidemiology and Preventive Medicine, School of Medicine, University of Maryland, Baltimore, Maryland

Tejas Desai, M.S., doctoral candidate, Department of Biostatistics, School of Public Health, University of North Carolina at Chapel Hill, Chapel Hill, North Carolina

J. Kevin Eckert, Ph.D., Professor, Department of Sociology and Anthropology, University of Maryland, Baltimore County, Baltimore, Maryland

Ann L. Gruber-Baldini, Ph.D., Assistant Professor, Division of Gerontology, Department of Epidemiology and Preventive Medicine, School of Medicine, University of Maryland, Baltimore, Maryland

Catherine Hawes, Ph.D., Professor, Department of Health Policy and Administration, School of Rural Public Health, Texas A&M University, College Station, Texas

J. Richard Hebel, Ph.D., Professor, Department of Epidemiology and Preventive Medicine, School of Medicine, University of Maryland, Baltimore, Maryland

R. Tamara Hodlewsky, M.S., M.A., Ph.D. candidate, Department of Health Policy and Administration, University of North Carolina at Chapel Hill, Chapel Hill, North Carolina

Gary Grove Koch, Ph.D., Professor, Department of Biostatistics, School of Public Health, University of North Carolina at Chapel Hill, Chapel Hill, North Carolina

Jay Magaziner, Ph.D., M.S.Hyg., Professor and Director, Division of Gerontology, Department of Epidemiology and Preventive Medicine, School of Medicine, University of Maryland, Baltimore, Maryland

Manoj Menon, M.P.H., medical degree candidate, School of Medicine, University of North Carolina at Chapel Hill, Chapel Hill, North Carolina

Robert L. Mollica, Ed.D., Deputy Director, National Academy for State Health Policy, Portland, Maine

Leslie A. Morgan, Ph.D., Professor, Department of Sociology and Anthropology, University of Maryland, Baltimore County, Baltimore, Maryland

Elizabeth J. Mutran, Ph.D., Professor, Department of Health Behavior and Health Education, School of Public Health, and Director, Center on Minority Aging, University of North Carolina at Chapel Hill, Chapel Hill, North Carolina; and Senior Research Health Analyst, Research Triangle Institute, Research Triangle Park, North Carolina

Michael A. Nolin, M.A., Deputy Director, Center for Health Program Development, University of Maryland, Baltimore County, Baltimore, Maryland

Marcia G. Ory, Ph.D., M.P.H., Chief, Social Science Research on Aging, Behavioral and Social Research, National Institute on Aging, Bethesda, Maryland

Peter S. Reed, M.P.H., doctoral student, School of Public Health, University of North Carolina at Chapel Hill, Chapel Hill, North Carolina

Victor A. Regnier, F.A.I.A., Professor, School of Architecture, University of Southern California, Los Angeles, California

Anne Copeland Scott, M.S., Research Assistant, Program on Aging, Disability, and Long-Term Care, Cecil G. Sheps Center for Health Services Research, University of North Carolina at Chapel Hill, Chapel Hill, North Carolina

Philip D. Sloane, M.D., M.P.H., Elizabeth and Oscar Goodwin Distinguished Professor, Department of Family Medicine, School of Medicine, University of North Carolina at Chapel Hill, Chapel Hill, North Carolina

Sally C. Stearns, Ph.D., Associate Professor, Department of Health Policy and Administration, University of North Carolina at Chapel Hill, Chapel Hill, North Carolina

S. Sudha, Ph.D., Codirector, Investigator Development Core, Center on Minority Aging, University of North Carolina at Chapel Hill, Chapel Hill, North Carolina

Joan F. Walsh, Ph.D, Research Associate, Program on Aging, Disability and Long-Term Care, Cecil G. Sheps Center for Health Services Research, University of North Carolina at Chapel Hill, Chapel Hill, North Carolina

Judith B. Wildfire, M.P.H., Clinical Instructor, Jordan Institute for Families, School of Social Work, University of North Carolina at Chapel Hill, Chapel Hill, North Carolina

Sheryl Zimmerman, Ph.D., Associate Professor, School of Social Work, University of North Carolina at Chapel Hill, Chapel Hill, North Carolina

Assisted Living

Introduction

Catherine Hawes, Ph.D.

The past decade has seen the emergence and growth of a new industry known as assisted living. Consumer demand, concerns about nursing home quality, and pressure from providers have combined with state interest in containing long-term-care costs to produce dramatic growth in this industry. Initially, its development was largely a market response to both demographic trends and consumer preferences. More recently, however, state involvement in setting standards and developing Medicaid payment policies has expanded exponentially.

The "graying" of the U.S. population represents a major public policy challenge, particularly given estimates that the number of elderly persons needing long-term care will double to 14 million over the next two decades (US GAO, 1999). As a result there have been a number of private- and public-sector responses to meeting this growing need for long-term care. The initial response among state policymakers was to expand the role of residential care facilities. Other than nursing homes, the most common form of residential setting with long-term-care services is the entity generically known as board-and-care or residential-care homes. Such facilities are known by more than thirty different names across the country, including personal care homes, adult-care homes, adult congregate living facilities, and homes for the aged. As of the early 1990s, there were an estimated 40,000 such facilities, licensed and unlicensed, with an estimated 750,000 beds nationwide (Clark et al., 1994; Hawes et al., 1995; Hawes, Wildfire & Lux, 1993).

Recently the field of residential care has expanded with the development and rapid growth of a new and overlapping form of care, termed *assisted living* (ASHA, 1998; ALFA, 1998; Citro & Hermanson, 1999; Gulyas, 1997; Mollica, 1998). One-third of facilities that call themselves assisted living have been in business for five or fewer years, and 60 percent have been in operation for ten or fewer years (Hawes, Rose &

Phillips, 1999). Part of this growth can be attributed to increased state involvement. During the past decade, many states expanded their definition of residential care to include a specific licensure category known as "assisted living"; other states simply incorporated these facilities into their traditional concept of residential care (Hawes, Wildfire & Lux, 1993; Mollica, 1998). Further, more than half the states provided some type of Medicaid funding for services in assisted living facilities by 1998 (Mollica, 1998). However, the real impetus for growth has been from private investment, including both lenders and the stock market (ASHA, 1998; Conway, MacPherson & Sfiroudis, 1997; PVG, 1997; SeniorCare, 1998).

In the view of many observers, assisted living represents a promising new model of long-term care that blurs the sharp and invidious distinction between nursing homes and community-based care and reduces the chasm between receiving long-term care in one's own home and in an "institution." In addition, assisted living facilities are thought to provide (or be capable of providing) a range of services that makes them a viable but less institutional alternative to nursing homes (Kane & Wilson, 1993; Leon, Cheng & Neumann, 1998; Wilson, 1993). Despite such optimism, there is a general lack of knowledge about the assisted living industry. First, there is disagreement about the size of the industry. Second, there is tremendous variation among those facilities that call themselves assisted living. Third, there are questions about the performance of the industry and the quality of care. Finally, there is confusion about the role that assisted living plays in meeting the long-term-care needs of the elderly population and the interaction of assisted living with other segments of the health and long-term-care systems. This dearth of information is a serious matter, given the rapid growth of the industry, its increasingly prominent role in providing long-term care for frail elderly persons, and the largely uncritical enthusiasm that has dominated its emergence and growth.

The key philosophical tenets of assisted living are based on the goals of meeting customers' needs, promoting independence and dignity, and allowing residents to age in place in a homelike environment. As defined by the Assisted Living Quality Coalition,[1] an assisted living setting is "a congregate residential setting that provides or coordinates personal services, 24-hour supervision and assistance (scheduled and unscheduled), activities, and health related services; designed to minimize the need to move; designed to accommodate individual residents' changing needs and preferences; designed to maximize residents' dignity, autonomy, privacy, independence, and safety; and designed to encourage family and community involvement" (1998: 65). According to all three of the major industry trade associations, privacy and flexible services that will meet residents' scheduled and unscheduled needs and will allow residents to age in place are key elements of the philosophy of assisted living (ALFA, 1998; Gulyas, 1997; Hodlewsky, 1998).

Despite agreement on the philosophical underpinnings of assisted living, there is no consensus about which facilities are and which are not assisted living. As the National Center on Assisted Living observed, "Assisted living . . . is known by dozens of different terms throughout the country. . . . The multitude of names for assisted living reflects the diversity of services offered in the cloudy nexus between retirement housing and skilled nursing care" (Hodlewsky, 1998: 3). As a result there are widely divergent perceptions about the total number of assisted living facilities, with estimates that range from 10,000 to 40,000, providing services to between 350,000 and 1 million residents (ALFA, 1998; Citro & Hermanson, 1999; Hawes, Rose & Phillips, 1999; Hodlewsky, 1998; Mullen, 1997; Mollica, 1998). Probably the best estimate comes from a study by the U.S. Department of Health and Human Services (DHHS); it used a survey of a national probability sample of facilities to arrive at an estimate of the number of assisted living facilities nationwide that met a generally agreed-on definition of assisted living.[2] This study found that as of the beginning of 1998, there were an estimated 11,500 assisted living facilities with a total of just over 600,000 beds housing more than one-half million residents (Hawes, Rose & Phillips, 1999).

Even among these facilities, the DHHS study found tremendous variation. Most (57%) offered rooms, but many (43%) offered apartments. The vast majority of resident accommodations were private (73%), but a sizable proportion of rooms and apartments were shared by two or more unrelated individuals. Moreover, more than one-third of the residents shared a bathroom (Hawes, Rose & Phillips, 1999). More than half (58%) of the facilities that described themselves as assisted living had low-privacy environments in which most rooms were shared by at least two unrelated individuals and offered low services as well. That is, they did not offer residents assistance with at least two of the basic activities of daily living (ADLs) or medications. Only 11 percent of the assisted living facilities were estimated to offer both high privacy (mostly private rooms or apartments) and high services (offered a range of services, including ADL assistance, and would arrange or provide at least temporary nursing care and had a registered nurse on staff). In short, the name *assisted living* does not appear to provide a uniform definition of either the environment or the services offered by a facility.

In addition to variability among places calling themselves assisted living, there are growing concerns about quality, particularly given what many expect will be rising acuity among residents. States have sought to capitalize on the potential of assisted living and other forms of residential long-term care to reduce the use of nursing homes. Besides creating new licensure categories and expanding Medicaid waiver programs, many states are allowing higher levels of care to be provided in assisted living and other residential care facilities. Many (although not all) states are (1) permitting the provision of daily or intermittent nursing care (including skilled care) and hospice care in these facilities, (2) allowing retention of residents with greater levels of impairment, and (3) modifying their nurse practice acts (Hawes, Wildfire & Lux, 1993; Kane & Wilson, 1993; Mollica, 1998; Mollica & Snow, 1996). In theory, assisted living facilities are allowed to provide or arrange a much broader array of services and to allow residents to age in place; this may contribute to higher acuity levels among residents.

Despite the promise of assisted living, there is little systematic, empirical information about the actual performance of assisted living facilities. Moreover, there is some indication from a recent study by the General Accounting Office that there are troubling quality problems and that some of the marketing practices make it difficult for consumers to make intelligent and informed decisions when selecting such a facility (US GAO, 1999; see also US GAO, 1997). Because of these factors, the information provided in this book is crucial. Assisted living has been greeted by the public and by policymakers with largely uncritical enthusiasm, despite the variation among places calling themselves assisted living and despite the lack of information about their performance. Moreover, little is known about how quality may differ across various types of assisted living facilities (US GAO, 1999). The fact that this book provides data on the entire range of licensed residential care/assisted living (RC/AL) facilities, rather than a more limited (and probably artificial) definition of *assisted living*, adds to the policy relevance of this work.

While appreciating the similarities and differences between settings across the spectrum of RC/AL, one must keep in mind that no claims can yet be made regarding whether one setting is superior to the others. It is also important to understand that all of the settings are currently playing an important role in our nation's system of long-term care. Their role has changed over time, and whether it will be similar for the next generation of users remains speculation.

Notes

1. The Coalition is a group representing the Alzheimer's Association, the AARP, the American Association of Homes and Services for the Aging, the Assisted Living Federation of America, the American Seniors Housing Association, and the American Health Care Association–National Center for Assisted Living.

2. The study was done for the DHHS Office of the Assistant Secretary for Planning and Evaluation (ASPE) and excluded small homes (two to ten beds) that were mostly adult-care homes or other types of board-and-care facilities. It included only those facilities that served the elderly and called themselves assisted living or provided twenty-four-hour oversight, at least two meals a day, housekeeping, and assistance with at least two of the following: medications, bathing, dressing.

References

American Seniors Housing Association. 1998. *Seniors Housing Construction Report, 1998.* Washington, DC: American Seniors Housing Association.

Assisted Living Federation of America. 1998. *The Assisted Living Industry: An Overview, 1998.* Fairfax, VA: Price Waterhouse.

Assisted Living Quality Coalition. 1998. *Assisted Living Quality Initiative: Building a Structure That Promotes Quality.* Washington, DC: Assisted Living Quality Coalition.

Citro, J., & Hermanson, S. 1999. *Assisted Living in the United States.* Washington, DC: Public Policy Institute, American Association of Retired Persons.

Clark, R., Turek-Brezina, J., Hawes, C., & Chu, C. 1994. The supply of board and care homes: Results from the 1990 national health provider inventory. Presentation at the Annual Meeting of the Gerontological Society of America, Atlanta, GA, November.

Conway, M., MacPherson, A., & Sfiroudis, J. 1997. *The Assisted Living Sector: The Evolution Continues.* Global Equity Research, Health Services. New York: Salomon Brothers.

Gulyas, R. 1997. *The Not-for-Profit Assisted Living Industry: 1997 Profile.* Washington, DC: American Association of Homes and Services for the Aging.

Hawes, C., Mor, V., Wildfire, J., Lux, L., Green, R., Iannacchione, V., & Phillips, C. D. 1995. *Executive Summary: Analysis of the Effects of Regulation on the Quality of Care in Board and Care Homes.* Research Triangle Park, NC: Research Triangle Institute.

Hawes, C., Rose, M., & Phillips, C. D. 1999. A national study of assisted living for the frail elderly: Results of a national survey of facilities. Meyers Research Institute, Beachwood, OH.

Hawes, C., Wildfire, J., & Lux, L. 1993. *The Regulation of Board and Care Homes: Results of a Survey in the 50 States and the District of Columbia: National Summary.* Washington, DC: American Association of Retired Persons.

Hodlewsky, R. T. 1998. *Facts and Trends, 1998: The Assisted Living Source book.* Washington, DC: National Center for Assisted Living, American Health Care Association.

Kane, R. A., & Wilson, K. B. 1993. *Assisted Living in the United States: A New Paradigm for Residential Care for Frail Older Persons?* Washington, DC: American Association of Retired Persons.

Leon, J., Cheng, C-K., & Neumann, P. J. 1998. Alzheimer's Disease Care: Costs and Potential Savings. *Health Affairs* 17:206–16.

Mollica, R. 1998. *State Assisted Living Policy, 1998.* Portland, ME: National Academy for State Health Policy.

Mollica, R., & Snow, K. 1996. *State Assisted Living Policy, 1996.* Portland, ME: National Academy for State Health Policy.

Mullen, A. 1997. The assisted living industry: A critical assessment from 1997 forward. Presentation at the Assisted Living Market Research and Feasibility Summit sponsored by the National Investment Conference.

Province Valuation Group. 1997. *National Assisted Living Demand: A Bed-Need Assessment Using the Most Recently Published National Estimates and Projections.* [Special issue, summer]. Prognosis.

SeniorCare. January 1998. *SeniorCare Investor.* New Canaan, CT: Irving Levin Associates.

U.S. Congress, General Accounting Office. 1997. *Consumer Protection and Quality of Care Issues in Assisted Living.* Washington, DC: Government Printing Office.

———. 1999. *Assisted Living: Quality-of-Care and Consumer Protection Issues in Four States.* Washington, DC: Government Printing Office.

Wilson, K. B. 1993. Developing a viable model of assisted living. In P. Katz, R. L. Kane, & M. Myosotis (eds.), *Advances in Long-Term Care.* New York: Springer.

I Key Topics in Assisted Living

1 State Policy and Regulations

Robert L. Mollica, Ed.D.

Assisted living is both a generic concept and a specific model. In many states, there is considerable overlap between board-and-care and assisted living rules. Facilities and state regulators often use the terms *assisted living* and *board and care* interchangeably.

Defining assisted living and differentiating it from other forms of residential care, always a challenging undertaking, grows more difficult as state policymakers, regulators, legislators, consumers, and providers respond to the interests of local stakeholders. Twenty-nine states use the term *assisted living* as their licensing category. Some observers conclude therefore that assisted living is licensed only in states with a licensing category using that term. In fact, all fifty states license facilities that may be marketed as assisted living. Further blurring the picture, a license may not be required in some states when residents, rather than the facility, are responsible for arranging to obtain services from an outside agency.

Several states have created a separate assisted living licensing category while retaining older categories (e.g., residential-care facilities, personal care homes) that also allow shared bedrooms and limited services. Other states have consolidated the categories into one general set of rules that might cover assisted living, board and care, multiunit elderly housing, congregate housing, and sometimes adult family or foster care (e.g., Arizona, Maine, Maryland, and North Carolina). Still others set core requirements for licensed facilities and require an additional license to offer limited nursing services or a higher level of care (e.g., Florida and Louisiana).

As states update their rules, they often expand residents' ability to age in place and receive higher levels of care under their board-and-care rules. Although there are exceptions, there are three common differences between assisted living and board and care: assisted living statutes or regulations often contain a statement of philosophy that emphasizes privacy, independence, decision making, and autonomy; assisted living is more likely than board and care to emphasize apartment settings shared by choice of the residents; and assisted living allows facilities to provide or arrange nursing or health-related services and to admit or retain residents who may meet the level-of-care criteria for admission to a nursing facility.

State regulations set parameters for what facilities may offer. Admission and retention criteria establish the maximum boundaries for tenants, and the services allowed define the maximum allowable package that may be delivered. Within these limits, operators set policies for their facilities that determine which tenants may be admitted or retained and what services are provided. Although state regulations typically specify that the residence must develop written policies concerning whom it will serve and what services it will provide, the policies often are not clear and may lead to confusion among consumers (US GAO, 1999). Many consumers or family members have expectations of aging in place and receiving higher levels of services as the resident's needs change. They may be surprised when the facility points to their policy and asks a resident to move when the service need exceeds the facility's policy.

This chapter is based on a study of state assisted-living statutes and regulations conducted by the National Academy for State Health Policy under a grant from the U.S. Department of Health and Human Services, Office of the Assistant Secretary for Planning and Evaluation (Mollica, 1998), and a grant from the Retirement Research Foundation (Mollica, 2000). Information was obtained from surveys of state licensing and Medicaid agencies and an analysis of state laws, regulations, and proposed regulations in 1998 and 2000 and updated through telephone interviews with selected states since the survey.

State Approaches to Regulation

Policy Developments

The late 1990s were active years for developing state licensing and Medicaid reimbursement policy. In 1997–99 alone, eighteen states finalized new regulations (Arizona, Delaware, Hawaii, Idaho, Iowa, Kansas, Kentucky, Louisiana, Maine, Maryland, Minnesota, Nebraska, New Mexico, Oklahoma, Tennessee, Texas, West Virginia, and Wisconsin). Draft regulations were pending in Vermont, and other states were studying or planning to develop new regulations.

Thirty-nine states covered services in assisted living or board and care through their Medicaid program by October 2000. Four states (Connecticut, Illinois, Pennsylvania, and Rhode Island) were implementing demonstration programs, some in conjunction with their state housing finance agency, to test the impact of covering assisted living. A fifth demonstration was pending in Louisiana. Table 1.1 summarizes state activity. The first column lists each state and the District of Columbia; the second column indicates states that now have regulations using the term *assisted living*. The column "Drafting or Revising Regulations" identifies states that are drafting or revising assisted living or general board-and-care rules. The next column lists states that currently provide, or plan to provide, Medicaid funding to cover services in assisted living and board-and-care settings. States that have formed a task force or work group to study the regulation of assisted living are identified next.

Regulatory Models

Assisted living has multiple meanings. Often the variations reflect different approaches to regulation across states; each approach falls into one of four categories: board-and-care or institutional model, new housing and service model, service model, and umbrella model.

Institutional models (usually older board-and-care regulations) allow shared bedrooms without attached baths and either do not allow nursing-home-eligible residents to be admitted or do not allow facilities to provide nursing services. Two states, Alabama and Rhode Island, adopted *assisted living* as the name for their board-and-care licensing category. South Dakota and Wyoming renamed an existing category *assisted living* but allowed a higher level of service to be provided without changing the unit requirements. Arkansas and Illinois do not allow anyone requiring nursing home services to be served in a board-and-care facility; new legislation in Illinois will change this prohibition, however. Some states allow skilled nursing services to be provided for limited periods by a certified home health agency. The upgraded board-and-care approach recognizes that residents are aging in place and need more care to prevent a move to a nursing home. State policies have allowed these facilities to admit and retain people who need assistance with activities of daily living and some nursing services. Mutually exclusive level-of-care criteria have been revised to allow people who would qualify for admission to a nursing home to remain. This model retains the minimum requirements for the build-

Table 1.1. Summary of State Assisted Living and Board-and-Care Activity

State	Licensing Regulations/ Statutes Use *Term* Assisted Living	Regulations Revised Since June 1998	Drafting or Revising Assisted Living or Board-and-Care Regulations	Medicaid Funding	Studying Assisted Living/ Task Force
AL	✓		✓	Planned	
AK	✓		✓	✓	
AZ	✓	✓		✓	
AR			✓	✓	✓
CA			✓	Planned	✓
CO				✓[a]	
CT	✓			✓[b]	
DC	Pending		✓	Planned	
DE	✓		✓	✓	✓
FL	✓	✓	✓	✓	✓
GA				✓[a]	
HI	✓	✓		✓	
ID	✓	✓		✓	
IL	✓		✓	✓[c]	
IN				Planned	✓
IA	✓		✓	✓	✓
KS	✓	✓		✓	
KY	✓[d]		✓		
LA	✓	✓		Planned[b]	
ME	✓		✓	✓	
MD	✓			✓	
MA	✓		✓	✓	
MI				✓	✓
MN	✓	✓		✓	
MS		✓		Pending	
MO			✓	✓[a]	
MT				✓[a]	
NE	✓			✓	
NV		✓		✓[a]	
NH		✓	✓	✓[e]	✓
NJ	✓	✓		✓	

(*continued*)

Table 1.1. (*Continued*)

State	Licensing Regulations/ Statutes Use Term Assisted Living	Regulations Revised Since June 1998	Drafting or Revising Assisted Living or Board-and- Care Regulations	Medicaid Funding	Studying Assisted Living/ Task Force
NM			✓	✓	
NY				✓	✓
NC	✓	✓		✓	
ND				✓	✓
OH			✓		✓
OK	✓				✓
OR	✓	✓		✓	
PA				Pilot[f]	✓
RI	✓	✓	✓	✓	✓
SC			✓	✓	✓
SD	✓	✓		✓	
TN	✓			Planned	
TX	✓	✓	✓	✓	
UT	✓	✓	✓	✓	
VA	✓		✓		✓
VT			✓	✓[a]	
WA			✓	✓	✓
WV[g]		✓	✓		✓
WI[h]			✓	✓	
WY	✓		✓		✓

[a]Medicaid covers services in board-and-care settings through a waiver or under the state plan. (Vermont will cover services in assisted living facilities when its regulations are finalized.)
[b]Pilot projects authorized but the waiver has not been submitted to HCFA and they have not begun to enroll beneficiaries.
[c]Waiver services can be provided to residents living in unlicensed facilities. These facilities provide housing, and residents arrange services with an outside agency.
[d]Kentucky will convert from a voluntary to a mandatory certification program.
[e]New Hampshire will use the term when its regulations are final.
[f]This pilot will provide case management to residents in a limited number of personal-care homes in Philadelphia. Other services are not included.
[g]West Virginia has developed rules for residential-care apartments.
[h]Wisconsin changed the name of its category from assisted living to residential-care apartment complexes.

ing and units, usually multiple-occupancy bedrooms with shared bathrooms and tub-shower areas.

The new housing and service model licenses or certifies facilities providing assisted living services that are defined by law or regulation. These models require apartment settings and allow facilities to admit and retain nursing-home-eligible tenants. Depending on the state, rules may allow some or all of the needs met in a nursing home to also be met in assisted living. Policies in states with this approach have a statement of philosophy that emphasizes resident autonomy and creates a prominent role for residents in developing and delivering services. By licensing the setting and services, states distinguish these facilities from board and care and have attempted to develop more flexible regulations. Examples of this approach to licensing can be found in Hawaii, Kansas, Oregon, and Vermont (draft), and in Medicaid waiver standards in North Dakota and Washington.

The service model focuses on the provider of service, whether it is the residence itself or an outside agency, and allows existing building codes and requirements—rather than new licensing standards—to address the housing structure. This model simplifies the regulatory environment by focusing on the services delivered rather than the architecture. Service regulation approaches may include requirements that define which buildings (apartment units, minimum living space) may qualify as assisted living, but the licensing agency's staff do not otherwise apply their standards to the building's characteristics. The service model can be developed for apartment settings (Connecticut) or multiple settings (Texas Medicaid waiver program).

States using an umbrella model issue regulations for assisted living that cover two or more types of housing and services: residential care facilities, congregate housing, multiunit or conventional elderly housing, adult family care, and assisted living. States representing this approach include Florida, Louisiana, Maine, Maryland, New Jersey, New York, North Carolina, and Utah.

Key Domains Covered by State Regulations
The Assisted Living Philosophy

Several regulatory approaches have developed assisted living as a consumer-focused residential model with a clear philosophy that attempts to differentiate assisted living from board and care. This model organizes the setting and the delivery of service around the resident rather than the facility. States that emphasize consumers use terms such as *independence, dignity, privacy, decision making,* and *autonomy* as a foundation for their policy. Statutes, licensing regulations, and Medicaid requirements in twenty-eight states, up from twenty-two in 1998 and fifteen states in 1996, contain a statement of their philosophy of assisted living. States that have adopted or proposed this philosophy are Arizona, Delaware, Florida, Hawaii, Idaho, Illinois (demonstration program), Iowa, Kansas, Kentucky, Louisiana, Maine, Maryland, Massachusetts, Montana, Nebraska, New Jersey, New Mexico, Oregon, Rhode Island, South Carolina, Texas, Utah, Vermont (draft), Virginia, Washington, West Virginia, Wisconsin, and Wyoming. Massachusetts includes its language in a section that allows the secretary of elder affairs to waive certain requirements for bathrooms as long as the residences meet the stated principles.

Oregon's definition says that "assisted living promotes resident self-direction and participation in decisions that emphasize choice, dignity, privacy, individuality, independence and home-like surroundings" (Oregon Administration Rules: 411-056-0005). Florida's statute states the purpose of assisted living as "to promote availability of appropriate services for elderly and disabled persons in the least restrictive and most home-like environment, to encourage the development of facilities which promote the dignity, individuality, privacy and decision-making ability" (Florida Statutes: chaps. 400, 401). The Florida law also states that facilities should be operated and regulated as residential environments and not as medical or nursing facilities. The regulations require facilities to develop policies that allow residents to age in place and that maximize independence, dignity, choice, and decision making of residents. New Jersey amended its rules to emphasize the values of assisted living and introduce managed risk. Facilities must provide and coordinate services "in a manner which promotes and encourages assisted living values." These values are concerned with the organization, development, and implementation of services and other facility or program features so as to promote and encourage each resident's choice, dignity, independence, individuality, and privacy in a homelike environment. The values promote aging in place and shared responsibility.

By itself, stating an assisted living philosophy may not change practice. Specific steps are necessary to put the philosophy into practice, such as specifying that single-occupancy living units are required, or perhaps that living units may be shared only by choice, or that a shared-risk process is to be used to develop a service plan and training for facility staff based on the principles of assisted living. Apartment units are required in seven of the twenty-eight states with a statement of the philosophy. Five states have mixed requirements that allow bedrooms in some arrangements but require apartments in all newly constructed facilities. Sixteen states allow sharing (apartments or bedrooms) only by choice of the residents. Eighteen states use a shared-risk process for developing tenant service agreements or service plans. Connecticut, which licenses assisted living service agencies and not facilities, does not have a statement of philosophy but specifies that sharing is allowed only by choice. Ohio and Oklahoma use a shared-risk provision but have no statement of philosophy. Nine states include a philosophy of assisted living but do not address the remaining areas that would objectify the philosophy. Training that covers the principles of assisted living is specified by thirteen states.

Living Unit Options

Regulations that include a philosophy set the context for other provisions. The design of the living unit is an important feature of residential, non-institutional settings. Single-occupancy apartments or rooms dominate the private market. When required by regulation, this issue often creates conflict. Older board-and-care rules allow shared rooms, toilets, and bathing facilities; existing facilities that seek to be licensed for assisted living oppose rules requiring apartment-style units and single occupancy. Some states grandfathered existing buildings when assisted living rules were promulgated, or they maintained separate board-and-care categories that allow shared rooms. To some extent, market forces rather than minimum licensing standards will define the type of units built for and occupied by the private market. As the upper-income market becomes saturated and more companies seek to serve low- and moderate-income elders, efforts to develop "affordable" models may compromise on single occupancy.

Medicaid policy will play a critical role in shaping the market over time. Some operators contend that shared occupancy is the only way to develop affordable units. Thus far, Medicaid policy in several states has recognized the importance of single occupancy in fulfilling the principles stated in their policy and has developed a reimbursement level that allows facilities to contract with Medicaid at the market rate. Other states have required apartments but do not specify that apartment units can be shared only by choice. Whether Medicaid's role continues in maintaining the apartment and single-occupancy threshold for low-income residents remains to be seen.

The design of the living unit affects privacy, which is measured primarily by the type of unit, the ability of residents to lock their doors, and the behavior of staff. States that have based their policy on privacy have emphasized apartments with an attached bath. Autonomy is promoted by the availability of cooking facilities within the unit. Of the states that have established or proposed assisted living policy in this area, the following require apartments: Connecticut, Hawaii, Kansas, Louisiana, Minnesota, New Jersey, North Dakota, Oregon, Vermont (draft), Wisconsin, and Washington. (New Jersey's rules require apartment settings for all new construction but allow existing Personal Care Homes with shared rooms to convert to assisted living. North Dakota and Washington require apartments under the Medicaid program rather than the state's licensing requirements.)

Thirty-one states have rules that allow two people to share a unit or bedroom. Several of these states have multiple licensing categories, and the two-person limit may apply to only one of the categories. Fifteen states have licensing categories that allow four people to share a room; five states allow three people to share a unit, and one state allows up to five people to share a room.

Table 1.2 presents state policy concerning living units. States that allow shared units generally have developed policy that broadens the scope of residential options and may create two or more types of buildings, each with different requirements (e.g., Florida, New York, Texas, Utah). The table may also be understood as a continuum. On one end are residences that offer single-occupancy units with kitchenette and skilled services to residents. On the other end are residences that provide shared units without cooking capacity to residents who cannot receive skilled services in an assisted living setting. Though a state's policy sets the parameters for what may be offered and provided, the actual practice may be more narrow. Shared units may be allowed, but the market may produce very few or no settings that offer shared units. Further, facilities constructed prior to the development of assisted living may offer shared units, whereas most, if not all, newly constructed buildings have private units.

Table 1.2. State Policy Concerning Living Units

| Assisted Living Rules | | Shared Rooms | |
Apartment Units	Multiple Settings	Assisted Living Rules	Board and Care
Connecticut	Arizona[a]	Alabama	Arkansas
Hawaii	Alaska	Nebraska	California
Illinois (pilot)	Delaware	Rhode Island	Colorado
Kansas	Florida	South Dakota	Georgia
Louisiana	Iowa	Virginia	Idaho
Minnesota (Medicaid)	Kentucky	Wyoming	Indiana
New Jersey	Maine		Michigan
North Dakota (Medicaid)	Maryland		Mississippi
Oregon	Massachusetts		Missouri
Vermont (draft)	New Mexico (Medicaid)		Montana
Washington (Medicaid)	New York (Medicaid)		Nevada
Wisconsin	North Carolina		New Hampshire
	Oklahoma		Ohio
	Utah		Pennsylvania
	Texas (Medicaid)		South Carolina
			West Virginia

Notes: The first two columns indicate the policy of existing or draft assisted living regulations that require apartments or license multiple settings (apartment units and rooms). The last two columns list states whose policy addresses only bedrooms through assisted living or board-and-care regulations.

[a]Arizona's new regulations require apartments in assisted living centers (facilities with eleven or more units) and allow shared rooms in assisted living homes (fewer than ten units).

Resident Agreements

Consumer satisfaction with assisted living depends to some extent on the resident's knowledge of the facility's obligations and the conditions of tenancy. Consumer expectations are shaped by marketing materials and resident agreements, and clear and understandable agreements promote satisfaction with and understanding of assisted living. State rules often require these agreements, which typically cover provisions dealing with available services, fees, resident rights and responsibilities, occupancy, and move-out or discharge issues. The agreements include a description of the fee or charges to be paid, the basis of the fee or what is covered, other services available at additional costs, who will be responsible for payment, and the method and timing of payment. Refund policy is also covered by agreements in many states. Other issues addressed include the amount of advance notice for rate changes and the management of resident funds. If prospective residents or family members are not aware of these provisions at the outset, they are likely to be disappointed if the facility later makes changes that were not clearly explained in the agreement and during the marketing process.

The content of resident agreements varies by state. Maryland's rules require disclosure of the level of care that the facility is licensed to provide and the level of care needed by the resident at the time of admission. Wisconsin requires that the agreement indicate the qualifications of staff who will provide services and specify whether services are provided directly or by contract. The resident agreement in Colorado must set forth a care plan that outlines functional capacity and needs. Statements setting forth resident rights and the provisions that allow staff to inspect living quarters, with the resident's permission, are also required by some states. Other states require that a list of residents' rights be provided to each resident, without including it as part of the resident agreement. Grievance procedures may also be covered in the agreement or provided separately to residents.

Terms of occupancy may be addressed; they may include the provision of furnishings, the policy concerning pets, admissions, and descriptions of the reasons for which a resident may be involuntarily moved, as well as the time frame and process for informing the resident and arranging for the move. In Maryland the terms must specify procedures to be followed when a resident's accommodations are changed. Agreements may also include the facility's "bed hold" policy for times when residents temporarily move to a hospital, a nursing home, or some other location. Other issues addressed by states include the size of the type and the language used in the agreement and how often the agreement must be updated.

Tenant Policy or Admission-and-Retention Criteria

The most consistent and significant trends among states have been broadening the level of service that may be offered and the acuity level of residents who may be served in assisted living. Some states use very general criteria, whereas others are very specific. The criteria found in state regulations can be grouped into five areas: general, health-related, functional, Alzheimer disease and dementia, and behavioral.

Eighteen states use general criteria stating that the facility must be able to meet the resident's needs. Regulations in Hawaii and draft regulations in Vermont rely primarily on these criteria. Wisconsin also uses a general threshold but limits the amount of services any resident can receive to twenty-eight hours a week. Other states allow facilities to admit and retain residents whose needs can be met but include other limits. In effect, the requirement is used in combination with others that screen out residents with certain conditions and set expectations that any facility admitting residents with allowable service needs must be capable of meeting those needs.

Some states use health criteria such as requiring that a resident must have stable health conditions or must not need twenty-four-hour nursing care. These criteria may be interpreted to mean that anyone needing a feeding tube, sterile wound care, or ventilator care could not be served. Several states identify the specific types of care that may not be provided. Twenty-six states specify that residents must not need twenty-four-hour nursing care. Four states (Arizona, Kansas, New Jersey, and Vermont) allow twenty-four-hour care if the facility meets certain criteria (e.g., it is licensed to provide that level of care, or a care plan has been approved by the licensing agency). Nine states do not allow residents who need hospital or nursing home care to be served, and rules in eight states specify that facilities may provide part-time or intermittent nursing care. States may specifically exclude certain conditions or services. For example, ten states prohibit serving anyone with Stage III or IV ulcers. Eight do not allow anyone who is ventilator dependent to be served or anyone needing a nasogastric tube. Fourteen states specify that persons with a communicable disease may not be admitted or retained.

Criteria dealing with functional status/capacity and Alzheimer disease are less frequent. Six states require that residents be ambulatory, and five require that they be able to evacuate without assistance. Four states specify that residents may not be totally bedfast; other states allow this level of care under specified conditions. Four states say that facilities can admit people with mild dementia; however, most states allow people with dementia to be served without specifying it in their regulations. Facilities in twenty states may not admit or retain people who are a danger to themselves or others, and people who need restraints are specifically excluded by regulations in nine states.

Vermont will soon join Arizona, Hawaii, Kansas, Maine, New Jersey, and Oregon as one of the states with the broadest policies. Oregon's regulations do not limit who may be served as long as the facility can meet their needs. The rules contain move-out criteria that allow residents to choose to remain in their living environment despite functional decline. Facilities may ask residents to leave if the resident's behavior poses an imminent danger to self or others, if the facility cannot meet the resident's needs, if services are not available, if the resident has a documented pattern of noncompliance with agreements necessary for assisted living, or for nonpayment.

Regulations in Arizona, Kansas, Maine, and New Jersey are flexible and encourage aging in place. Arizona sets requirements for different supplemental licensing levels. Facilities providing supervisory care services may serve residents needing health or health-related services that are provided by a home health agency or a licensed hospice agency. Additional requirements allow facilities in Arizona providing personal care services to serve residents who require continuous nursing services, are bedfast, or have Stage III or IV pressure sores. Residents requiring continuous nursing services may be served if nursing services are provided by a private duty nurse or a hospice agency or if the facility is a foster-care home operated by a licensed nurse. These facilities may serve someone who is bedfast or has Stage III or IV pressure sores if a physician authorizes residency and if nursing services are provided by a private duty nurse, a hospice agency, a licensed nurse, or a home health agency and the facility is meeting the resident's needs. These facilities may not admit residents unable to direct their care. Facilities in Arizona must have a supplemental license to provide directed care services in order to serve people with Alzheimer disease who are not able to direct their care. This license requires policies that ensure the safety of residents who may wander, that control access and egress, and that provide appropriate training for staff. Maine's rules require that facilities describe in their licensing application who will be admitted and the types of services to be provided. The rules also require facilities to permit reasonable modifications at the expense of the tenant or other willing payer to allow persons with disabilities to reside in licensed facilities.

Negotiated Risk

The negotiated-risk process has developed as a means of implementing the consumer-focused philosophy of assisted living. Seventeen states have adopted or proposed a negotiated-risk process to involve residents in care planning and to respect resident preferences that may pose risk to the resident or other residents. The negotiated-risk process allows residents to identify a need and determine the help they receive from staff. For example, if the resident has difficulty bathing, the resident may require help getting to the bathroom and unfastening clothing. Yet a resident may prefer to undress and get into the tub and bathe herself or himself even though the staff member and perhaps a family member feel the resident may be placed at risk of falling. The risk is expressed, but the final decision to bathe rests with the resident.

Values assume a prominent role in shaping policy in several states. Many states use values language developed in Oregon, which reads: "Assisted living promotes resident self direction and participation in decisions that emphasize choice, dignity, privacy, individuality, independence and home-like surroundings" (Oregon Administration Rules: 411-056-0005). Each facility must have written policies and procedures that incorporate such principles. Service plans are reviewed for the extent to which the resident has been involved and the extent to which the resident's choices as well as the principles of assisted living are reflected.

Washington provides for a negotiated-risk agreement that is developed as a joint effort between the resident, family members (when appropriate), the case manager, and facility staff. The purpose of the agreement is to define the services that will be provided to the resident with consideration for preferences of the resident as to how services are to be delivered. The agreement lists needs and preferences for a range of services and specific areas of activity under each service. A separate form is provided to document amendments to the original agreement. Signature space is provided for the resident, a family member, the facility staff, and the case manager. If assistance with bathing is needed, the process allows the resident to determine and choose what assistance will be provided, how often, and when. It allows residents to preserve traditional patterns for eating and preparing meals and engaging in social activities. The negotiated-service agreement puts into practice a philosophy that stresses consumer choice, autonomy, and independence over a facility-determined regimen with fixed schedules of activities and tasks that might be more convenient for staff and for the management of an efficient facility. It places residents ahead of the staff and administrators and helps turn a facility into a home.

New Jersey defines managed risk as the process of balancing resident choice and independence with the health and safety of the resident and other persons in the facility. If a resident's preference or decision places the resident or others at risk or is likely to lead to adverse consequences, such risks or consequences are discussed with the resident and, if the resident agrees, a resident representative. A formal plan to avoid or reduce negative or adverse outcomes is negotiated. The rules provide that choice and independence may need to be limited when the resident's individual choice, preference, or actions place the resident or others at risk. The managed-risk process requires that staff identify the cause for concern, discuss the concern with the resident, seek to negotiate a managed-risk agreement that minimizes risk and adverse consequences and offers possible alternatives while respecting resident preferences, and document the process of negotiation or lack of agreement and the decisions reached.

Allowable Services

Regulations defining the services that may be offered or arranged by assisted living facilities reflect the admission and retention criteria. States seeking to facilitate aging in place and to offer consumers more long-term-care options allow more extensive services. These states view assisted living as a person's home. In a single-family home or apartment in an elderly housing complex, older people can receive a high level of care from home health agencies and in-home service programs. Several states extend that level of care to assisted living facilities and allow services to be provided or arranged so that residents can remain in a setting. Mutually exclusive resident policies, which prohibit anyone needing nursing home level of services from being served in a board-and-care facility, have been replaced by aging-in-place provisions. However, drawing the line regarding the amount and intensity of allowable services has been controversial. During the rule-making process in many states, some nursing home operators see assisted living as competition for their residents and oppose rules that allow skilled nursing services to be delivered outside the home or nursing home setting.

Provisions for Residents with Alzheimer Disease and Dementia

Thirty states reported that they have specific requirements for facilities serving people with dementia or Alzheimer disease. Requirements address one or more of the following: disclosure requirements, admission or retention criteria, staffing patterns and staff training, activities, and environmental provisions. Staff training accounts for the special provisions in the majority of these states.

Disclosure provisions typically require facilities that advertise themselves as operating special-care facilities or units or as caring for people with Alzheimer disease to describe in writing how they are different. The regulations may require a description of the philosophy of care, admission and discharge criteria, the process for arranging a discharge, services covered, the cost of care, special activities available, and differences in the environment. A voluntary disclosure process has been adopted in California under which facilities offering special services for people with Alzheimer disease disclose information concerning their program. A consumer's guide has been developed to alert family members to several key questions that should be asked. The recommended areas include the philosophy of the program and how it meets the needs of people with Alzheimer disease, the preadmission assessment process used by the facility, the transition to admission, the care and activities that will be provided, staffing patterns and the special training received by staff, the physical environment, and indicators of success used by the facility.

Eight states have admission or retention criteria that directly refer to people with Alzheimer disease. Tennessee does not allow people in the later stages of the disease to be served. People with Alzheimer disease may be served only after a multidisciplinary team determines that care can be provided safely. The determination must be reviewed quarterly. Florida allows people with Alzheimer disease to be retained in facilities with an extended congregate-care license if they do not have a medical condition requiring nursing services. Georgia requires that residents must be able to make simple decisions. California's criteria allow the admission of people with Alzheimer disease who are not able to respond to verbal instructions. Vermont's draft rules allow, but do not require, facilities to serve people who cannot make simple decisions.

Training is regulated, as well. In Maine all new employees in facilities with Alzheimer's or dementia care units must receive a minimum of eight hours of classroom orientation and eight hours of clinical orientation. The trainer must have experience and knowledge in the care of individuals with Alzheimer disease or other dementias. Florida's rules require four hours of initial training in areas of the disease related to the normal aging process: diagnosing Alzheimer disease; characteristics of the disease process; psychological issues, including resident abuse; stress management and burnout for staff, families, and residents; and ethical issues. An additional four hours is required on medical information, behavior management, and therapeutic approaches. Direct-care staff must participate in four hours of continuing education each year.

Regulations in Arizona will require a special license to service people who are unable to direct their own care. These facilities are required to have services that are appropriate to people with Alzheimer disease, including cognitive stimulation, encouragement to eat meals and snacks, and supervision to ensure personal safety. Staff must receive twelve hours of additional training or demonstrate skills in communicating with residents, managing difficult behaviors, and developing and providing social, recreational, and rehabilitative activities.

Requirements for Assisted Living Facility Administrators

Two other important areas of regulation address the requirements for administrators and for staff orientation and training. Regulations in five states do not describe any requirements for the administrators of assisted living facilities or assisted living service agencies. One-half of the states require that administrators must be at least 21 years of age; six states specify 18 as the age requirement, one state 19, and one 25. Seventeen states do not have an age requirement.

In addition to age, state rules typically set standards for education and training. Eighteen states require a high school diploma or G.E.D., and seven include advanced degree requirements, which sometimes vary with the level of care offered by the facility. Ten states have experience requirements; thirteen identify specific abilities or knowledge that an administrator must have. Licensing or certification of administrators is required by seventeen states. Twenty-two states have an annual requirement for continuing education or hours of in-service training, with the number of hours ranging from six to forty per year. Twenty-five states include criminal background checks in their requirements for administrators.

Staff Training Requirements

State regulations typically require an orientation for new staff and annual in-service training. Training requirements can be very general or specific. Ten states require direct-care staff to successfully complete an approved course. Other states specify the areas to be covered during training, some specify the number of hours to be spent in training, and many states include requirements for both topic areas and the number of hours. Training requirements can be grouped into five domains: direct care, health-related matters, knowledge, safety and emergency issues, and process.

Direct care includes tasks performed by staff directly with residents, such as personal care. Health-related tasks include basic nursing skills, preventive and restorative services, observation and reporting skills, and medication administration and assistance. Required knowledge tends to address the aging process, death and dying, psychosocial needs, assessment skills, care-plan development, communication skills, and community resources. The safety issues most often mentioned are cardiopulmonary resuscitation, first aid, fire safety and emergency procedures, and infection control. Process issues covered by training requirements include agency practices, regulations and laws, legal and ethical issues, complaint procedures, record keeping, reporting of abuse and neglect, and confidentiality.

Thirty-five states require training on resident rights, the most common of all issues described in state rules. Direct-care skills are covered as training in personal care or direct-care skills (26 states), as areas that are appropriate or related to the tasks or duties of staff (17 states), and more generally as tasks necessary to meet the needs of consumers (13 states). There is considerable overlap between these areas, as fifteen states require training in two or all three of the areas. Other direct-care areas include nutrition and food preparation (18 states), dementia or Alzheimer's care (15), mental health and emotional needs (16), general requirements (13), principles of assisted living (12), housekeeping and sanitation (14), hygiene (11), and training related to the use of restraints (7).

The most common health-related topics are medication administration and assistance (23 states) and observation or reporting skills (14 states). Preventive or restorative nursing services and basic nursing skills are required in three states. Safety and emergency issues are also important components of training in these facilities. Thirty-three states require training in fire, safety, and emergency procedures. Twenty-three cover first aid, with fifteen requiring CPR training. Infection prevention and control is also required in twenty-four states. Fewer states address the aging process (11), communication skills (9), assessment skills (8), psychosocial needs (6), care plan development (5), and death and dying (4).

Public Subsidies

Public policy concerning subsidies for elders in residential settings has paralleled the emergence of new residential long-term-care models. Subsidies for low-income older persons may be provided through the federal Supplemental Security Income program (SSI), through state supplements to the federal SSI program, or through Medicaid. Many states have created living arrangements under a state supplement to the federal SSI payment for residential settings. These supplemental payments cover room and board and sometimes personal care. The payment standards typically were created years ago, before the emergence of assisted living and the higher level of care provided in assisted living and, more frequently, in board-and-care settings. SSI payments developed primarily for board rather than care are quite low in relation to the fees in assisted living facilities. Many observers contend that they are low in relation to the actual cost of meeting the increasing needs of low-income board-and-care residents. States are now developing policies that combine SSI and Medicaid to provide an appropriate level of service and to encourage aging in place.

The Social Security Administration publishes an annual report describing each state's living arrangements and the amount of the state supplement. Individual states may use a specific term to refer to their supplement, and some use the term SSI to refer to both the federal payment and any state supplement. The federal payment in 2000 was $512 a month; it is adjusted each January based on the cost of living. A 3–5 percent increase took effect January 1, 2001.

Medicaid Reimbursement

States may fund services in assisted living or board-and-care settings through Medicaid 2176 Home and Community-Based Care Waivers or as a regular state plan service. States most often use the Home and Community-Based Care Waiver (1915 [c]). However, a few states use Medic-

Table 1.3. Differences in Medicaid Coverage

Issue	State Plan Service	1915 (c) Waivers
Functional criteria	Beneficiaries must need the service covered	Must meet the state's nursing home level-of-care criteria
Entitlement	States must provide services to all beneficiaries who qualify for Medicaid	States limit spending for waiver services
Income	Beneficiaries must be on SSI or otherwise eligible for Medicaid	State may set eligibility up to 300% ($1,536) of the federal SSI payment standard ($512)

Note: SSI = Supplemental Security Income.

aid state plan services, typically personal care. The two forms of coverage differ in three important ways; they are summarized in table 1.3.

First, waiver services are available only to beneficiaries who meet the state's nursing home level-of-care criteria; that is, they would be eligible to enter a nursing home if they applied. Nursing home eligibility is not required for beneficiaries using state plan services. Second, states set limits on the number of beneficiaries who can be served through waiver programs. The limits are defined as expenditure caps that are part of the cost-neutrality formula required for approval. Waivers are approved only if the state demonstrates that Medicaid long-term-care expenditures under the waiver will not exceed expenditures that would have been made in the absence of the waiver. States do not receive federal reimbursements for any waiver expenditures that exceed the amount stated in the cost-neutrality calculation. In contrast, state plan services are an entitlement, meaning that all beneficiaries who meet the eligibility criteria must be served. Federal funding continues to match state expenditures without any cap.

Finally, under Home and Community-Based Care Waiver programs, states may use an eligibility category that allows beneficiaries with incomes less than 300 percent of the federal SSI benefit ($530 a month in 2001) to be eligible and receive all Medicaid services. In the absence of this provision, people who live at home and have too much income to qualify for Medicaid would be forced to spend down their income and assets to qualify, often by needlessly entering an expensive nursing home. Using this eligibility approach, states can pay for assisted living and other services to give people alternatives to nursing home admission. Tenants who meet the nursing home criteria can become eligible for Medicaid without spending their excess income. They may retain the income to pay the room and board costs while Medicaid covers the services. In contrast to the more generous eligibility option available under Home and Community-Based Care Waivers, beneficiaries are eligible under the regular Medicaid state plan if they receive SSI or meet the state's medically needy standards. However, community beneficiaries are unlikely to incur sufficient expenses to qualify for Medicaid unless they enter a nursing facility. The 300 percent eligibility option addresses this limitation.

Current State Activity: The Use of Waivers and State Plan Services

Thirty-nine states covered services in assisted living and board-and- care facilities in 2000, up from thirty-two in June 1998, and six more planned to do so. Participation rose from 40,000 in 1998 to over 60,000 in 2000. States using personal care under the state plan have higher participation rates than states using the waiver. For example, roughly a third of all Medicaid beneficiaries nationwide in assisted living or other residential-care settings are in North Carolina, and another 20 percent are in Missouri and New York. Waiver participation is much lower. Participation in Nevada rose from approximately 52 recipients in 1998 to 125 in 2000. New Jersey saw participation grow from 119 to 700 in two years. Oregon and Washington served 1,400–1,500 in 1998 and 2,572 and 2,919, respectively in 2000. Enrollment rose in New York from 2,100 to 3,150 participants. Though still small, enrollment has risen because programs have matured in several states; facilities, state managers, and local agencies are more familiar with the model. The supply of assisted living has grown dramatically; and as facilities struggle to maintain occupancy rates, they may be more likely to contract with Medicaid to retain residents who have spent their resources and cannot afford the monthly fee. Despite the growth, rates in many states are too low to allow facilities to serve residents who meet the waiver requirements; that is, residents must meet the state's criteria for entering a nursing home.

Paying for the Housing Costs

As in any reimbursement system, the amount of the payment and the approach to reimbursement create incentives for provider behavior. Five primary approaches are used by states in setting rates for assisted living and board-and-care services: flat rates, flat rates that vary by type of setting, tiered rates, case-mix rate systems, and rates based on care plan or fee for service. Flat rates provide a monthly payment regardless of the nature and extent of health and functional impairments and service needs. Rates that vary by setting provide different payment levels for apartment units than for bedrooms and different levels for shared versus single occupancy. Tiered rates create three to five levels based on the type and extent of impairments in activities of daily living. Case-mix payment systems are based on similar systems for varying payments for residents in nursing facilities. These systems usually have eight or more levels of payment. Finally, fee-for-service systems base the payment on the number of units of service and a rate set for each unit of service.

One of the critical issues facing the expansion of assisted living for Medicaid beneficiaries is room and board. Under section 1915 (c), Medicaid cannot pay for room and board outside a hospital or a nursing home, except in limited circumstances such as respite care and meals that are served as part of a day care program. The part of the monthly fee for assisted living that is attributable to room and board costs must be paid by the beneficiary. However, Medicaid policy has a further critical impact on access to assisted living through its payment decisions. Medicaid's historical approach to setting rates for nursing homes has carried over to assisted living. Nursing home rates include the costs of services, meals, and housing. As states develop assisted living rates, they tend to set rates that include services, meals, and housing costs, even though Medicaid pays only for the services. Medicaid programs typically limit how much facilities may charge for room and board, and the amount is usually tied to the state's SSI payment for a single elderly beneficiary living in the community. This policy may create disincentives for facilities to serve Medicaid beneficiaries since the SSI payment, and therefore the maximum amount beneficiaries may be charged for housing costs, may be well below the facility's actual housing and meal costs.

As states set rates for assisted living, there are two separate areas for decisions. The first relates to whether the Medicaid rate should address housing costs. There is historical precedent for states to cover housing costs, but there are significant differences between nursing homes and assisted living. Medicaid pays the costs of housing in nursing homes. Medicaid sets the payment rate; residents apply their income to the rate and Medicaid pays any remaining balance. Since Medicaid cannot cover housing costs in assisted living, there is no need for Medicaid to address this area, particularly if it does so in a way that limits access to care. The amount paid for the housing costs could be left to the resident and the facility to determine. Wisconsin is an example of a state that sets only the service rate.

The second area deals with the needs of two different groups, SSI beneficiaries and noncash beneficiaries. States that do set a rate that includes housing costs paid by the resident usually limit the housing component to the state's SSI payment (the federal SSI payment plus the state supplement, if any). This payment may be below the actual cost of housing. Massachusetts has recognized the difference between the community benefit standard and the cost of housing in assisted living. The state has created a separate living arrangement for assisted living with a higher payment standard ($948).

Most Medicaid nursing home residents are not SSI recipients. They have too much income to qualify for SSI and are eligible under medically needy spend-down rules or meet the state's optional eligibility category based on a percentage of the federal SSI payment. Many of these beneficiaries have sufficient income from Social Security or pensions, or both, to pay the housing costs. How much of the income is actually available depends on the state's policy. States that limit the housing costs to the SSI payment apply any excess income to reduce the Medicaid service payment. Using section 1915 (c), states can apply institutional income rules to waiver eligibility. That is, states can serve beneficiaries with incomes up to 300 percent ($1,590 in 2001) of the federal SSI payment. Beneficiaries with income below that level are eligible for Medicaid. Once they become eligible, separate rules apply to the treatment of income. Under those rules, states decide how much of the beneficiary's income can be retained as a maintenance allowance. This provision allows beneficiaries living in the community to keep enough money to pay their rent, utilities, food, clothing, and other costs. Similarly in assisted living, residents need to retain sufficient income to pay the housing costs and other items that are not covered by the monthly fee. If states set the maintenance allowance above the SSI level, facilities whose housing costs are greater than the amount of the state SSI supplement would be able to serve low-income beneficiaries. In the absence of an adequate maintenance allowance, the resident will likely be forced to move to a nursing home. Setting a higher maintenance allowance may allow more beneficiaries to be served in assisted living settings; however, it will increase Medicaid's service payment since it reduces the "excess income" that is applied to the cost of services. Despite the higher service payment, Medicaid will still pay less for services in assisted living than it would for nursing home care.

Regulatory Challenges

As states develop regulations to keep pace with and to shape a changing market, new challenges await them. As assisted living expands, people who need personal care and some nursing care have more options. Medicare's Diagnosis Related Group (DRG) payment system creates incentives for hospitals to discharge people to nursing homes for rehabilitation. Increasing Medicare enrollment in managed care also encourages the use of lower settings. Nursing homes tend to serve people with higher medical needs; people with lower needs are using assisted living and home care services. Though the national supply of nursing homes is declining, occupancy rates are also declining. Regulators believe that assisted living has contributed to these trends.

As state regulations allow higher levels of care, concerns about quality and safety follow close behind. States that have several years' experience with assisted living rules are now reviewing and revising the rules to consider new approaches to quality and standards for facilities serving residents with Alzheimer disease. States seek to encourage residential, consumer-centered service options, but they are eager to avoid repeating the heavy regulatory approach governing nursing homes. Approaches that focus on outcomes and consumer satisfaction are still evolving. The main challenge to states, the assisted living industry, and advocates is to develop new models of oversight and quality before widespread instances of poor quality force regulators to use prescriptive approaches to staffing standards, level of care, medication administration, and oversight.

Affordability is another major challenge facing states. As private-pay residents have migrated to assisted living from nursing homes, subsidies for low-income beneficiaries have lagged behind. Although over one-half of the states cover services in assisted living under Medicaid, participation is low. Unless participation expands, low-income residents may be left with more limited options such as nursing homes or older, board-and-care type facilities that offer shared rooms. The opportunity to develop more affordable options is available to state policymakers. Industry surveys show that about one-half of the assisted living facilities have monthly fees below $2,200, which is considerably lower than Medicaid payments to a nursing home. There are a number of reasons why Medicaid occupancy rates in assisted living have been slow to expand, but states have the tools to support further expansion. Their ability to use those tools is affected by pressures to reduce public spending in general and Medicaid spending in particular and by opposition from special-interest groups that enjoy preferential treatment under Medicaid reimbursement policy.

States face conflicting pressures from stakeholder groups and taxpayers and will be challenged to develop policies that create high-quality services in residential settings offering affordable choices for low-income beneficiaries. These pressures make expansion difficult for services that offer beneficiaries more choice unless savings can be achieved to pay for them. Payments to nursing homes are the most likely source of savings, but faced with declining occupancy, tighter rate regulations, and an evolving Medicare Prospective Payment System, nursing home owners often oppose expanding coverage of other service options. States are attempting to create more balanced long-term-care systems, which means shifting resources from a historical overreliance on institutional care to a blend of institutional, residential, community, and in-home services.

References

Mollica, R. L. 1998. *State Assisted Living Policy, 1998.* Portland, ME: National Academy for State Health Policy.

———. 2000. *State Assisted Living Policy, 2000.* Portland, ME: National Academy for State Health Policy.

U.S. Congress, General Accounting Office. 1999. *Assisted Living: Quality-of-Care and Consumer Protection Issues in Four States.* GAO-HEHS-99-27. Washington, DC: General Accounting Office.

2 Residential Care/Assisted Living in the Changing Health Care Environment

Michael A. Nolin, M.A., and Robert L. Mollica, Ed.D.

The most significant trends in the health care environment over the 1980s and 1990s were the rise of managed care and the development of integrated provider or delivery systems. Some view these two changes as having transformed the health care system itself and as linked indicators for assessing the evolution of health care market forces in any given metropolitan region (Burns et al., 1997). There is little doubt that these trends have had considerable interaction and effect on each other. Together and separately, they are major determinants in shaping the health care environment and thus hold considerable importance for the residential care/ assisted living (RC/AL) industry.

The growing interest in private financing alternatives for long-term care is a third health care change that merits consideration, because it has particular significance for RC/AL. This growing interest is a result of the realization among policymakers and consumers that the ability of public systems to meet the long-term-care needs of an aging population has its limits. There is a concurrent realization that with increased longevity and chronic disabling conditions, personal resources can be quickly exhausted in the absence of thoughtful planning and preparation. Though not yet dramatically changing current policy and consumer practice, there are indications that significant shifts in consumer behavior may be under way. These changes would have implications for the current and future growth of RC/AL.

This chapter examines these major trends and emerging factors regarding the private financing of long-term-care services. The modest impact of managed health care and integrated delivery systems on RC/AL is explained, as well as the potential importance of the shift toward private financing of long-term care.

Managed Care

Medicare

In the past twenty years, the managed care movement has engulfed, with remarkable alacrity and thoroughness, all insured populations and almost all geographic areas of the United States. During this period, the vast majority of insured Americans have gone from fee-for-service insurance coverage to some form of managed care program. *Managed care* has been defined in a variety of ways, often identifying the increased alignment of provider and payer as a defining characteristic. An operational, and perhaps overly friendly, definition views managed care as a "method of providing care and services through financing mechanisms which coordinate care across time, place and provider, emphasizing prevention, risk/reward sharing and appropriate utilization of services based on consumer and community needs for an outcome of maximum health and well-being at lower overall costs" (AAHSA, 1996). The paradigmatic but by no means exclusive embodiment of managed care has been the health maintenance organization (HMO). An HMO is an entity that, for a fixed premium, provides or arranges the provision of designated health services needed by voluntarily enrolled members. The dramatic growth of managed care is reflected in the rise in stock value of the HMO industry from $3 billion in 1987 to almost $39 billion in 1997 (Kaiser, 1999).

Since the RC/AL industry is largely dedicated to serving the senior population, it is particularly important to study the growth of managed care in the Medicare program. Medicare, the federal health insurance program for the elderly and the disabled, has experienced an increase in the number of managed care plans and a steady increase in managed care enrollment among its beneficiaries. In December 1998, the number of managed care plans with Medicare contracts increased to 346, with a total enrollment of over 6 million, compared with 95 plans and an enrollment of 1.5 million in 1992.

The Congressional Budget Office in 1997 projected a Medicare HMO enrollment of almost 15 million by 2007 (Kaiser, 1999) (fig. 2.1). However, the growth may be more modest because the Balanced Budget Act of 1997 effectively limited the increases in capitation rates in many larger markets in an effort to correct for overpayments and a payment formula bias unfavorable to rural areas. By October 1999, plan participation had dropped to 310, and actual enrollment grew to 6.3 million beneficiaries.

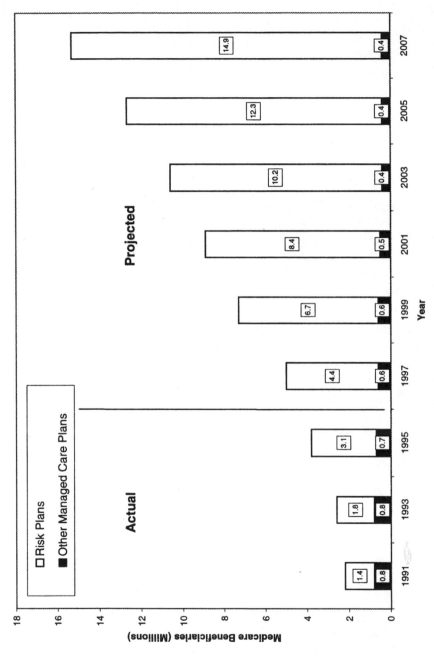

Fig. 2.1. The 1997 Congressional Budget Office projection of Medicare managed care enrollment, 1991–2007. Historical data from Kaiser Family Foundation, 1999. Used with permission of the Henry J. Kaiser Family Foundation of Menlo Park, CA. The Kaiser Family Foundation is an independent health care philanthropy and is not associated with Kaiser Permanente or Kaiser Industries.

HMOs contracting with Medicare receive a monthly payment of 95 percent of the fee-for-service expenditures in the county in which the beneficiary resides. The fee-for-service expenditure level for all Medicare Part A and Part B benefits is established for each county in the nation through a formula that establishes the average adjusted per capita cost (AAPCC). The capitation payments to Medicare HMOs are adjusted by age, gender, welfare, and institutional status. Rates for people in an institution are significantly higher than rates for people in the community. Before 1997 the federal Health Care Financing Administration (HCFA), which administers the Medicare and Medicaid programs, considered residents in RC/AL as institutionalized in the same manner as nursing home residents. Consequently, Medicare HMOs received a higher capitation payment for the medical care (Medicare benefits) of individuals residing in certain RC/AL facilities. Since 1997, however, HCFA determined that the medical costs associated with RC/AL did not warrant an enhanced payment, and individuals residing in RC/AL facilities no longer generate a higher Medicare HMO payment.

The enhanced capitation for nursing home residents has prompted the development of managed care products targeting this population. In collaborative arrangements with individual nursing facilities or nursing home networks, managed care products have emerged that incorporate more responsive nursing facility on-site medical management techniques. Such changes are positive, as there is evidence that expanded on-site medical management in the nursing facility reduces hospital inpatient and emergency room utilization and the associated Medicare costs. The enhanced Medicare capitation for nursing home residents constitutes a significant incentive for the creation of managed care products specifically designed to meet the needs of institutionalized Medicare beneficiaries. Unfortunately, the absence of this enhanced capitation incentive diminishes the likelihood of specialized Medicare managed care products designed for RC/AL residents.

Analysts and senior housing entrepreneurs, including those associated with RC/AL and independent-living and continuing-care retirement communities (CCRCs), have routinely highlighted opportunities associated with the growth of managed care. Senior housing providers are frequently challenged to demonstrate cost savings to "managed care professionals" through effective service pricing policies in order to prepare for a capitated environment (Miceli, 1997). Some even see consolidation within the seniors housing and long-term-care industries in response to the emergence of "health networks, with integrated delivery systems" that emphasize the "cost and service advantages necessary to succeed in the era of managed care" (ASHA, 1998: 72).

In contrast, HMOs view RC/AL as a long-term-care service setting that is not covered by Medicare or managed care plans with Medicare contracts. Although managed care plans have the flexibility to provide services that meet the needs of their members and to substitute with non-Medicare covered services that are more cost-effective, the prospects for developing relationships between RC/AL facilities and HMOs are largely conceptual and offer a number of barriers (Mollica, 1998). For example, The Medicare+Choice program, created by the Balanced Budget Act of 1997, authorized federal contracting with a variety of managed care and fee-for-service entities that are not licensed HMOs; HMOs and most other Medicare contractors under Medicare+Choice are not responsible for long-term-care services and are not likely to routinely provide financial reimbursement for those residential service settings that provide low-level support for individuals with some limitations in activities of daily living.

A convergence of interest between Medicare managed care and service-enriched senior housing is more likely to occur in the area of health plan marketing and on-site health services. The presence of health plan primary-care providers or physician extenders in a senior housing facility or campus can be advantageous to the managed care plan as a marketing opportunity. Some larger senior housing facilities and CCRCs have entered into exclusive arrangements with managed care plans, providing a financial benefit to the owners and a marketing and enrollment opportunity for the managed care provider. One continuing-care retirement community in Maryland, with twenty-five hundred residents on a campus offering independent apartments, assisted living facilities, and nursing facilities, also includes medical clinics and physician offices. This CCRC, which also operates a limited home health agency for campus residents and has contracted with local hospitals, has entered into a full-risk contract with a Medicare HMO for care of residents who have voluntarily enrolled in the HMO. Larger RC/AL facilities could structure similar service and financial contracts (with or without full-risk arrangements) with managed Medicare care plans.

Medicaid

Medicare is a public insurance program providing coverage for most acute and primary care needs. Medicaid, in contrast, can be best understood as a health and long-term-care purchasing program for low-income beneficiaries. Unlike traditional insurance, which protects people against financial catastrophe, Medicaid is designed to protect people after financial catastrophe has occurred (Moon, 1996), even though many Medicaid recipients have low utilization rates.

It is especially important to understand the dynamics of the Medicaid program because seniors with limitations in functional status living in the community are disproportionately characterized by low income (Komisar, Lambrew & Feder, 1996) (fig. 2.2). State Medical Assistance (Medicaid) programs provide health coverage to certain low-income and indigent, uninsured individuals of all ages. State-appropriated funds are matched by federal funds in these state-operated programs. States may add specified optional services to a federally mandated core package that includes most primary, acute, behavioral, rehabilitative, and long-term-care services. In 1995 elderly Medicaid recipients accounted for 11 percent of total recipients and 30 percent of all Medicaid patient care costs. Long-term-care services constitute one-third of the Medicaid service expenditures, most of which (64%) is payment for nursing home care (Kaiser, 1999) (fig. 2.3).

Almost all states have transferred at least a portion of their Medicaid recipients from fee-for-service to managed care organizations. These managed care programs have generally been designed for poor families and not the elderly poor, although welfare reform enacted by Congress in 1996 uncoupled Medicaid and welfare eligibility. Medicaid recipients who are elderly or disabled have generally been less likely to be moved into state Medicaid managed care plans (US GAO, 1996), because of special service needs and other obstacles such as coordinating with Medicare, which remains the primary payer for overlapping coverage when individuals are dually eligible for Medicaid and Medicare.

In 1997 twenty-four states enrolled elderly Medicaid beneficiaries in managed care plans (Mollica, 1998). Enrollment in the majority of these plans was voluntary. Unlike Medicare, the Medicaid program presents real and not merely theoretical opportunities for the use of RC/AL for a lower level of care and as an aging-in-place alternative. RC/AL is more frequently being used as substitute service coverage in state programs, ei-

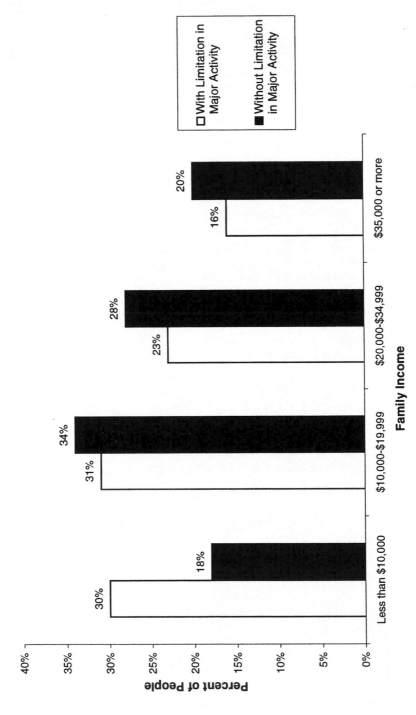

Fig. 2.2. Income distribution of community residents age 70 and over and functional status, 1994. Historical data from Komisar, Lambrew & Feder, 1996. "Limitation in major activity" indicates people with limitations in their capacity for independent living (e.g., the ability to bathe, dress, shop, etc.) because of a chronic condition. Used with permission of The Commonwealth Fund.

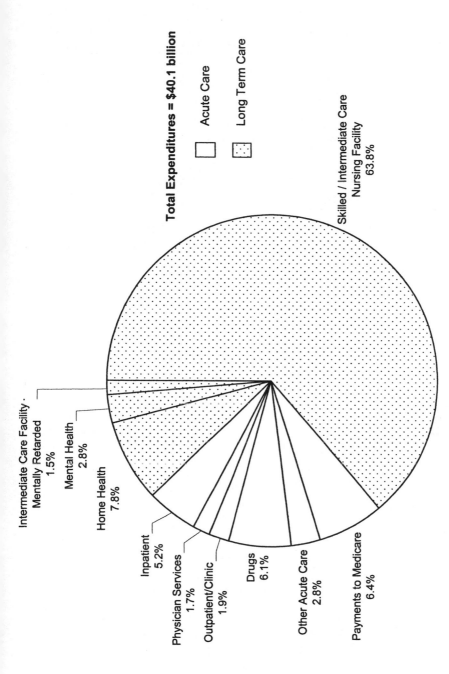

Total Expenditures = \$40.1 billion

□ Acute Care

⊡ Long Term Care

Skilled / Intermediate Care
Nursing Facility
63.8%

Intermediate Care Facility -
Mentally Retarded
1.5%

Mental Health
2.8%

Home Health
7.8%

Inpatient
5.2%

Physician Services
1.7%

Outpatient/Clinic
1.9%

Drugs
6.1%

Other Acute Care
2.8%

Payments to Medicare
6.4%

Fig. 2.3. Medicaid expenditures for elderly beneficiaries, by type of service, 1995. Historical data from Kaiser Family Foundation, 1999. Used with permission of the Henry J. Kaiser Family Foundation of Menlo Park, CA. The Kaiser Family Foundation is an independent health care philanthropy and is not associated with Kaiser Permanente or Kaiser Industries.

ther in fee-for-service or Medicaid managed care plans. By November 1999, thirty-nine state Medicaid programs reimbursed for services in RC/AL settings, either through a waiver program or state plan coverage, although the actual number of people benefiting from this coverage was very low (approximately 40,000 individuals out of a total Medicaid aged and disabled population of over 10 million). Approximately 30,000 of the 40,000 individuals are in the states of North Carolina, Missouri, and New York. Low participation in Medicaid-supported RC/AL may be attributable to the state waiver requirement that makes RC/AL available only to those who are certified for a nursing home level of care (Mollica, 1998) and to the low Medicaid reimbursement available in some states for RC/AL providers.

The Arizona Long Term Care System (ALTCS) presents a useful illustration of the context in which state policymakers have extended coverage for RC/AL. ALTCS is the state's Medicaid managed long-term-care program. ALTCS operates through capitated, at-risk, public and private program contractors. Program contractors (or plans) receive capitated payments to provide institutional care as well as community- and home-based care for those individuals certified as needing long-term care. In 1996 the Arizona legislature approved an assisted living pilot program following a persistent effort by one ALTCS program contractor to demonstrate the cost-effectiveness of including this setting as an option for its ALTCS enrollees. The project, called the Supportive Residential Living (SRL) Pilot, authorized RC/AL as an alternative for those who have been otherwise determined to be in need of a nursing home level of care. The pilot program, limited to 100 participants for the initial two years, demonstrated significant savings when the total costs of the SRL center and the nursing facility were compared (*SRL Pilot Report*, 1995). The cost savings to the Medicaid program averaged $1,141 per member per month, derived from the per diem payment differential between nursing facilities and the SRL facility. Cost savings of approximately 30 percent were recorded for Medicare covered services such as inpatient hospitalization, emergency room usage, and physician services. Based on the results of this pilot program, the assisted living coverage was expanded from pilot status to permanent state plan coverage. The pilot period extended from 1993 to 1996. With almost three additional years of experience as a permanent feature of the ALTCS program, the current participation is approximately 250 individuals. This modest participation is for the most part due to the restricted use of supportive residential living as a high-end service substitution for nursing facilities, as distinct from using it for the needs of those who are less impaired and require an aging-in-place supportive environment. Generally, the targeting of more severely impaired nursing-home-eligible clients and other restrictions on the utilization of RC/AL by Medicaid recipients are attributable to budget-sensitive state legislatures; they are reluctant to expand Medicaid programs since new benefits, even if demonstrated to be cost-saving for some, are likely to represent additional aggregate spending because of increased participation (Wiener, 1996).

On a national level, the failed Clinton health care reform initiative sought to expand home- and community-based service programs outside of Medicaid. In the absence of comprehensive reform through the Clinton or any other initiative, and in light of the continuing reluctance of states to expand Medicaid benefits, there is a sobering expectation that even if serious debate on proposals to expand long-term care occurs again in the next few years, it is not likely that any long-term-care piece will more than be modest, at least initially (Moon, 1996). The dim prospect of significant federal reform initiatives or state budget expansions leading to expanded home- and community-based services must be preeminent in any discussion that suggests Medicaid as a key contributor to the growth of RC/AL for low- and middle-income populations.

Medicare-Medicaid Coordinated Programs

The preceding sections have highlighted how the coverage restrictions of Medicare, the budget constraints of Medicaid, and the bifurcated coverage provided by both present obstacles to the development of RC/AL alternatives for individuals who are elderly, disabled, and low-income. Federal and state governments, as health care payers, have attempted through a variety of demonstration and waiver programs to integrate acute, primary, and long-term-care funding for individuals who qualify for both Medicare and Medicaid. Integrated care and financing projects hold more promise for the use of RC/AL as a preferred alternative for both nursing home substitution and for aging-in-place opportunities. For example, the Program of All-Inclusive Care for the Elderly (PACE) is a federal demonstration program authorized by the Omnibus Budget Reconciliation Act of 1986 and based on the experience of On Lok Senior Health Services. On Lok was established in 1972 as an adult day care program serving the Chinatown area of San Francisco. Building on the On Lok program, the PACE demonstrations are provider-based organizations operating as risk-bearing managed care entities that enroll frail (nursing-home-eligible) elderly persons and provide comprehensive medical and long-term-care services. The care management is built on a geriatric team approach and the use of adult day center services (Kane, Illston & Miller, 1992). The PACE organizations assume risk under capitation payments from both Medicare and Medicaid. The Medicare PACE capitation is a formularized enhancement of the AAPCC to adjust for the higher disability level of the PACE enrollees. The care philosophy and financial incentive for the PACE agency is to provide those preventive and supportive services that will result in reduced hospital and nursing facility usage. The combined Medicare and Medicaid capitation allows for the creative use of alternative settings, including RC/AL, which achieve the financial and care-plan goals. As previously noted, this incentive is not as forcefully engaged when care is managed separately under Medicaid and Medicare.

One PACE program in Denver has significantly invested in RC/AL as a logical expansion of its health care interests. Total Longterm Care, Inc. (TLC) is a Colorado PACE agency with an enrollment of 280 frail, elderly individuals. TLC has contracted with a variety of RC/AL providers that are classified as personal care boarding homes under Colorado licensing regulations (Reyes, 1999). These facilities may also be certified as "alternative care facilities" for the Colorado Medicaid program. In one arrangement, TLC has contracted for a block of thirty-two units in a facility. Most of the units are occupied by individuals who permanently require a more supportive environment because of changes in their functional status. A few units are reserved for transitional residence following hospital or nursing home discharge. The remainder of the facility's residents are a mix of private pays and Medicaid waiver individuals who are not enrolled in the PACE program.

An integrated-care system furnishes a unique environment characterized by a financial incentive to manage care at lowest levels, service flexibility through capitated payment systems, and coordinated Medicare-Medicaid benefit coverage. These characteristics are key ingredients in forging a productive and organic link between health care delivery and RC/AL. The Balanced Budget Act of 1997 authorized the mainstreaming of PACE programs by removing the restrictions related to achieving demonstration status. Even with the increased growth of PACE sites as a result of the removal of demonstration status, PACE programs will continue to serve small numbers of people; the number of individuals enrolled in PACE programs in September 1999 was approximately fifty-five hundred. The importance of PACE to RC/AL is the implication that when provider systems whose mission it is to serve the frail are afforded coverage flexibility, full risk, and coordinated payment (Medicare and Medicaid), there is a strong likelihood that assisted living and other supported residential environments will be used. PACE-type programs are in a nascent stage, but future health care reform and public financing will likely support the continued expansion of integrated-care delivery approaches.

In conclusion, using managed care as a vehicle to integrate care and financing for individuals who are eligible for both Medicare and Medicaid provides an environment for collaborative efforts between public payers of services for elderly persons and RC/AL. As a payer of medical care services, traditional Medicare plans are rather weak potential payer sources for RC/AL. Theoretically at least, managed Medicare plans have a financial incentive to place functionally permanently impaired individuals in nursing facilities since the Medicare capitation payment is enhanced for nursing facility residents but not for those who are receiving community-based long-term-care services, including RC/AL. In addition, nursing facility coverage under Medicare is limited. Medicaid alone has great potential but may be a limited financing partner for RC/AL. Though incentives are strong to use lower and less costly levels of care, state legislatures need to review RC/AL as a substitute for higher levels of care and as part of a restructuring of a long-term-care system that offers beneficiaries more choices. Total costs can be controlled by changing the supply of services, such as by reducing the number of nursing facilities and increasing the number of residential and in-home services. Obtaining funding from state legislatures, however, is not always easy. RC/AL as a "waivered" service limits financial exposure by allowing states to establish numerical limits on service expenditures and therefore on the number of participants, restricting usage to individuals who would otherwise qualify for nursing home placement. Integrated Medicare-Medicaid systems that incorporate primary, acute, and long-term care for the frail, such as the PACE program and a few state-based programs, hold greater promise for the creative and flexible use of RC/AL.

Integrated Delivery Systems

The other major change in the current health care environment is the emergence of Integrated Delivery Systems (IDSs), which are also referred to as Organized Delivery Systems or Integrated Service Networks. Without entering into the discussion of whether the nature of IDSs' interaction with managed care organizations is discontinuous, anticipatory, or spurious (Burns et al., 1997), one can agree that these "two forces . . . are separate but closely linked developments that have emerged in response to several conditions in the health care environment . . . and the trend toward greater integration is due in part to the growth of managed care" (Shortell & Hull, 1996). The integration phenomenon is frequently categorized as "horizontal" among similar provider types and "vertical" among various types of providers and provider systems along a continuum of care. The dynamics of vertical integration within IDSs are of interest to RC/AL since this health integration is a driving force behind the nursing home efforts to consolidate with senior housing and RC/AL enterprises. According to the American Seniors Housing Association, much of this consolidation, development, and acquisition among nursing homes and senior housing–residential care reflects an effort to provide a continuum of care that will "build critical mass" as the nursing home industry faces "increased managed care influence and decreasing entitlement funding" (ASHA, 1998: 72). Vertically integrated systems can be configured according to many ownership, equity partnership, affiliation, and contractual arrangements and can be led by a variety of network integrators, as represented in figure 2.4 (Shortell, Gillies & Anderson, 1994).

RC/AL facilities are participating in integrated or organized delivery systems through diverse arrangements ranging from hospital ownership to broader affiliation via service alliances. Georgia Baptist Health Care System in Atlanta has added, through a joint venture, several RC/AL facilities to its integrated system, which already includes three long-term-care facilities and a home health agency (Ngeo, 1998). Multistate hospital corporations have also developed systems involving scores of RC/AL facilities (AHA, 1998). Establishing a continuum of care may not always be the primary reason for the addition of RC/AL to health service systems, however. Increasing market visibility and other financial considerations sometimes represent greater appeal. The American Hospital Association's 1998 Multi-Unit Providers' Survey indicates a continuing robust

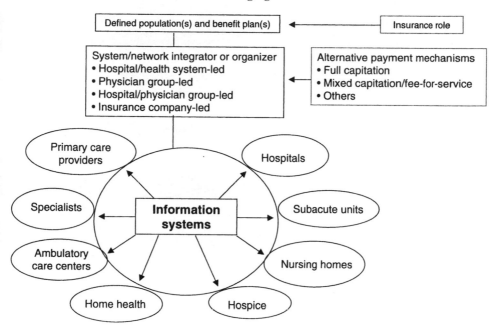

Fig. 2.4. Model of integrated service delivery. Historical data from Shortell & Hull, 1996. Used with permission of Health Administration Press.

growth in the number of RC/AL units owned or managed by hospitals (Ngeo, 1998). Further growth and evolution in these hospital-affiliated RC/AL facilities should be expected.

Long-Term-Care Insurance

Almost 6 million long-term-care insurance policies had been sold from 1987 to June 1998; the number of policies sold in 1997 alone was approximately 600,000 (fig. 2.5). It is likely that the number and rate of both individual- and employer-based long-term-care policies will continue to grow rapidly in the coming years. The demise of comprehensive health care reform in 1994, a growing lack of confidence about the future of Social Security and Medicare (AARP, 1999), and increased marketing activity may have contributed to the increased demand for long-term-care insurance. The Health Insurance Portability and Accountability Act of 1996 (HIPAA) stimulated further growth through the introduction of tax ben-

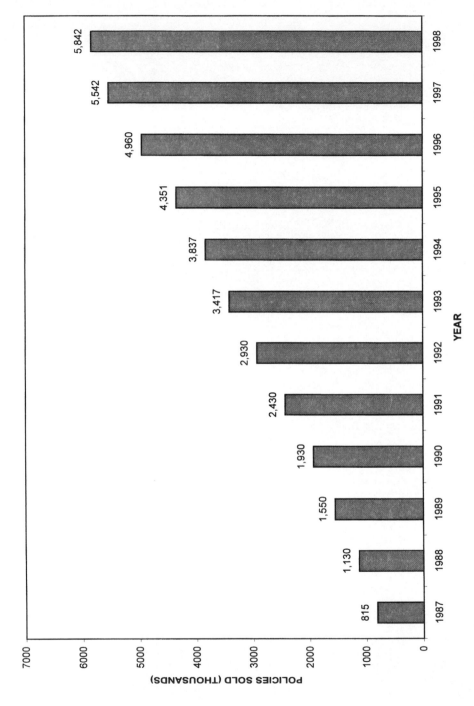

Fig. 2.5. Number of long-term-insurance policies sold cumulatively, 1987–98. Historical data from HIAA, 2000. Used with permission of the Health Insurance Association of America.

efits linked to the purchase of certain long-term-care policies. HIPAA led the way for many states to adopt the federal tax clarifications and benefits into their tax laws. A number of states continue to wrestle with developing incentives that encourage people to purchase long-term-care insurance. For example, Maine has a direct tax deduction for premiums paid for state-qualified long-term-care insurance policies. The HIPAA momentum is likely to be sustained through legislation enacted as a result of President Clinton's FY 2000 budget, which contains specific provisions for a national consumer education program regarding long-term-care financing options. The budget proposal also includes conducting long-term-care public forums as well as the offering of long-term-care insurance group purchasing by federal employees (H.R. 110, 106th Congress).

States have also adopted Medicaid program modifications to stimulate the purchase of private long-term-care insurance. Four states participate in the Partnership for Long Term Care, which provides long-term-care insurance through a cooperative public-private initiative. In this partnership, Medicaid acts as a reinsurer for private health insurance, providing Medicaid financing care when insurance coverage is exhausted and allowing the policyholder to protect assets to the level of premium payouts (McCall et al., 1998).

The structure is in place for accelerated growth in long-term-care insurance coverage arising from HIPAA or through innovative programs such as the Partnership. In 1997 there were 119 companies that sold long-term-care insurance. This figure includes companies that sold life insurance policies with an accelerated death-benefit rider specific to long-term care (HIAA, 1997b). Unlike policies sold in the past, which generally limited coverage to nursing facilities and were triggered by "medical necessity" criteria, most of these policies include some level of RC/AL coverage. All of the eleven sellers responsible for 80 percent of the individual policies sold in 1997 included a RC/AL facility benefit and home health care, and none included "medical necessity only" restrictions (HIAA, 1997b).

The growth potential for the private long-term-care insurance market is a factor of perceived need and affordability. The insurance industry considers education to be of primary concern, since the vast majority (upward of 70% to age 60) of the baby boomers could afford the premium costs of long-term-care insurance when affordability is defined as less than 2 percent of income (Mulvey & Stucki, 1998). Affordability for elderly persons, however, is vastly reduced.

The Future

The transformation of health care with the advent of managed care and integrated delivery systems provides an inviting platform for the emergence of a vibrant business and service nexus with RC/AL. But this relationship will remain limited to pilot ventures and special programs (e.g., PACE) until there is a significant expansion and reform of long-term-care coverage. It is too early to draw conclusions regarding the surge in long-term-care insurance activity and its continued growth and effect on the future financing of care, including RC/AL. However, the growing numbers and influence of the elderly population with disabling conditions may yet provide the stimulant needed to address the pressing long-term-care policy considerations. The frustrations associated with securing and financing supportive services and residential environments may yet "engender broader and deeper public support than there is today for government financing of long-term care" (Binstock, 1996).

References

American Association of Homes and Services for the Aging. 1996. *Strategic Work Place for AAHSA's Initiative on Managed Care.* Washington, DC: American Association of Homes and Services for the Aging.

American Association of Retired Persons. 1999. Baby boomers envision their retirement: An AARP segmentation analysis. Conducted for the AARP by Roper Starch Worldwide. American Association of Retired Persons, Washington, DC.

American Hospital Association. 1998. Multi-systems provider survey. *Modern Healthcare,* May 25.

American Seniors Housing Association and Capital Research Group. 1998. 1996 acquisition markets seniors housing and long-term care. In M. Anikeeff and G. R. Mueller (eds.), *Seniors Housing.* Boston: Kluwer Academic Publishers.

Binstock, R. H. 1996. The politics of enacting long-term care insurance. In R. H. Binstock, L. E. Cluff, & O. von Mering (eds.), *The Future of Long-Term Care: Social and Policy Issues.* Baltimore: Johns Hopkins University Press.

Burns, L. R., Bazzoli, G. J., Dynan, L., & Wholey, D. R. 1997. Managed care, market stages, and integrated delivery systems: Is there a relationship? *Health Affairs* 16 (6): 204–18.

Health Insurance Association of America. 1997a. *LTC Survey.* Washington, DC: Health Insurance Association of America.

———. 1997b. *Research Findings: Long-Term Care Insurance in 1997.* Washington, DC: Health Insurance Association of America.

———. 2000. *Research Findings: Long-Term Care Insurance in 1987–1998.* Washington, DC: Health Insurance Association of America.

Kaiser Family Foundation. 1999. *A Financial Overview of the Managed Care Industry.* March 1999. Washington, DC: Henry J. Kaiser Family Foundation.

Kane, R. L., Illston, L. H., & Miller, N. A. 1992. Qualitative analysis of the Program of All-Inclusive Care for the Elderly (PACE). *Gerontologist* 32 (6): 771–80.

Komisar, H. L., Lambrew, J. M., & Feder, J. 1996. *Long-Term Care for the Elderly: A Chart Book.* Washington, DC: Institute for Health Care Research and Policy, Georgetown University.

Managed Medicare and Medicaid. 1999. Vol. 5, no. 12. Washington, D.C.: Atlantic Information Service. March 29.

McCall, N., Mangle, S., Bauer, E., & Knickman, J. 1998. Factors important in the purchase of partnership long-term care insurance. *Health Services Research* 33 (2, pt. 1): 187–203.

Miceli, M. K. 1997. *Pricing Health Related Services in Senior Housing.* NIC, vol. 5. Annapolis, MD: National Investment Conference for the Senior Living and Long Term Care Industries.

Mollica, R. L. 1998. *State Assisted Living Policy: 1998.* Portland, ME: National Academy for State Health Policy.

Moon, M. 1996. The special health care needs of the elderly. In S. H. Altman & U. E. Reinhardt (eds.), *Strategic Choices for a Changing Health Care System.* Chicago: Health Administration Press.

Mulvey, J., & Stucki, B. 1998. *Who Will Pay for the Baby Boomers' Long-Term Care Needs?* Washington, DC: Policy Research, American Council of Life Insurance.

Ngeo, C. 1998. Growing like wild: Hospitals enter booming assisted-living business. *Modern Healthcare* 28 (31): 26–28, 30, 32.

Reyes, David. 1999. Telephone interview by author, March.

Shortell, S. M., Gillies, R. R., & Anderson, D. A. 1994. The new world of managed care: Creating organized delivery systems. *Health Affairs* 13 (4): 49.

Shortell, S. M., & Hull, K. E. 1996. The new organization of the health care delivery system. In S. H. Altman and U. E. Reinhardt (eds.), *Strategic Choices for a Changing Health Care System.* Chicago: Health Administration Press.

Supportive Residential Living Pilot Report. 1995. Phoenix, AZ: Maricopa Managed Care Systems, December.

U.S. Congress, General Accounting Office. 1996. *Medicaid Managed Care: Serving the Disabled Challenges State Programs* (GAO/HEHS-967-136). Washington, DC: Government Printing Office.

Wiener, J. M. 1996. *Can Medicaid Long-Term Care Expenditures for the Elderly Be Reduced?* New York: Commonwealth Fund.

3 Creating a Therapeutic Environment
Lessons from Northern European Models

Victor A. Regnier, F.A.I.A., and Anne Copeland Scott, M.S.

Assisted living provides long-term-care services in a setting that is residential in both character and appearance. Design professionals have been instrumental in leading the orientation toward assisted living and away from the traditional institutional setting of skilled nursing facilities. The design of the environment plays an important role by providing a supportive and humane setting for the evolution of this housing and service type. All assisted living projects should strive to

- Appear residential
- Be perceived by residents as small in size
- Provide privacy and completeness in residential units
- Recognize each resident's uniqueness
- Foster independence, interdependence, and individuality
- Focus on health maintenance, physical movement, and mental stimulation
- Support family involvement
- Maintain connections with the surrounding community
- Serve frail persons

Although few facilities meet all of these criteria, the list provides a standard for the development of highly supportive, humane residential housing for the mentally and physically frail. In this chapter, after offering a conceptual overview of therapeutic environments, we discuss each component in reference to northern European models of assisted living.

Therapeutic Environments

Creating an innovative and attractive assisted living environment requires careful thought about how the building will serve the needs of the residents, promote therapeutic goals, operate efficiently, encourage social ex-

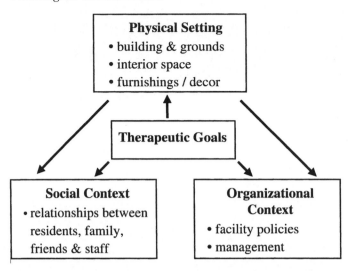

Fig. 3.1. Design and service goals must be implemented within the physical, social, and organizational context of a facility. The physical environment influences both the social context (relationships between residents and their family, friends, and staff) and the organizational context (facility policies and management interaction).

change, and support stimulating activities. Objectives and project design principles should guide the development process by employing methods that remind decision-makers of the potential side effects of various decisions. Such consideration is especially important in a housing type like assisted living, where operational objectives, therapeutic considerations, and the enhancement of social exchange are at stake. Cohen and Weisman (1991) developed a conceptual model to understand the key relationships between the elements of long-term-care facilities (see fig. 3.1). Although the model was developed to describe relationships in dementia units, it is relevant to assisted living as well. The conceptual framework suggests that facility goals must be implemented by examining their relationship to the physical (building and grounds, interior space, and furnishings), organizational (facility policies and management), and social (residents, family, friends, and staff) contexts of a facility and that the physical environment affects both the social and the organizational domains. Cohen and Weisman suggest that these three domains must be coordinated with one another in an effort to facilitate therapeutic goals. In this regard it is important to have a clear understanding of what constitutes therapeutic goals.

Assisted living should be viewed as a therapeutic environment where caregiving assistance and competence-building interventions encourage the highest level of independence. *Therapeutic* in this context should be broadly defined, including as its primary aims concern for physical activity, mental stimulation, and opportunities for social exchange. The literature contrasts environments that are "prosthetic" (i.e., aim to overcome problems by providing the older person with a device that substitutes for a disability) with those that are "therapeutic" (i.e., provide a measure of challenge along with the goal of renewing lost abilities or building new competencies). Lawton's competence-press theory, which suggests that the best match between the environment and the individual is one that engages ability rather than passively supports need, is consistent with this idea (Lawton & Nahemow, 1973; Lawton, 1980). Examples of prosthetic interventions are grab bars adjacent to a toilet and a pair of eyeglasses. A small kitchenette where a resident can prepare a meal or a snack could be considered a therapeutic feature.

Assisted living is a housing type that serves both the physically and the mentally impaired. In most facilities these two groups are viewed, at least in part, as having separate needs to which the environment must respond in different ways. A major difference between nursing homes and assisted living is the attitude toward programs that merely support and those that challenge and thus keep residents at a higher level of functioning and independence.

The ultimate success of an assisted living program geared toward keeping older frail residents out of a nursing home is the management's commitment to a therapeutic philosophy. The physical environment should be an active contributor to this goal, by setting the stage for a therapeutic focus of mental stimulation, physical exercise, and social exchange. Making these experiences more convenient or central to the life of residents has important physical and social ramifications.

Medical versus Residential Model

The nursing home is modeled physically and operationally on the hospital (i.e., a medical model). Its building codes specify wide unit doors and corridors for the exiting of patients in beds. Regulations that specify staffing levels are tied to the number of beds served and the location of the nurses' stations used to monitor those beds. Efficiency dictates highly centralized plans, which, in turn, result in dense, double-loaded corridor configurations with relatively narrow unit widths. Nurses and aides are also trained in the medical model, meaning that autonomy, mobility, and self-care are tolerated rather than encouraged and that privacy, freedom, and dignity are secondary to efficiency and safety.

In contrast, assisted living in America has emerged as a type of residential housing rather than a medical institution. It has grown out of the desire to keep older people living independently in a comfortable residential setting for as long as possible. It emulates in character and style a large, comfortable manor house. Other models for the physical layout of common spaces are country villas and bed-and-breakfast pensions.

Northern Europeans and Americans have taken different approaches to the design of assisted living. Medically minded nursing home providers in America who are concerned with serving this population often remodel conventional nursing home wards and call them assisted living. In these settings, conventional two-bed nursing home rooms often have merely been renamed, carpeted, and converted to single-occupancy use. Such facilities still conform to the rigid nursing home model of wide doors and extruded double-loaded corridors, and they have nurses' stations just as institutional skilled care settings do.

When sponsors approach assisted living as a health care environment by placing it in the same building as the nursing home and referring to the entire facility as a "health center," the outcome is often disappointing. In these models, assisted living, often located on a separate floor, is stacked above or below a traditional skilled nursing unit. The regulatory standards for the nursing unit layout also affect the assisted living portion of the building. The result is a narrow, long unit with poor access to daylight and inadequate square footage. This commingling of nursing units and so-called assisted living presents assisted living as an institutional health care environment, irreparably damaging the therapeutic philosophy of the setting. A few cosmetic adjustments to this "medical model" of assisted living cannot overcome the effect of its appearance as an institution. Ideally, residential assisted living models recognize through their design that the size, scale, and configuration of a building create the feeling of a home-like environment. In these models, residential housing rather than the hospital is the pattern for design and operation. The facility's identity as housing and not an institutional building must be reinforced by its architectural character, organization, and management philosophy. When assisted living is no more than a decorated nursing home, it loses its potential as a viable alternative to institutionalization.

Northern Europe as a Model to Achieve Goals of Assisted Living

Europe experienced an early demographic shift toward an aging society and had postwar governments with progressive social policies. Consequently, housing programs for the elderly were introduced about fifteen to twenty years earlier there than in the United States. These programs emphasized noninstitutional alternatives for the frail, which were reflected in building codes, experimental programs, attitudes toward independence, and financial commitments (ASVVO, 1991; Bull, 1987; Husbanken, 1987; Lindstrom, 1989).

In northern Europe, social service, health care, and housing agencies recognize the influence of new architectural forms in challenging conventional thinking about social problems. These facilities provide useful models incorporating social, organizational, and physical factors to create a therapeutic environment for residents in assisted living. Whereas punitive regulations in the United States have forced patients to relocate as their health care needs increase, the absence of such regulations in Europe has promoted an enlightened societal attitude about aging in place and caring for people in a range of community contexts. Within northern European countries, a diversity of assisted living solutions are available to meet varied geographic and cultural circumstances. One key concept is the service house, which Sweden, Norway, Denmark, Finland, and the Netherlands have all used to provide housing and services to the frail elderly. It is a model that varies in size depending on the surrounding catchment area and in scale depending on its urban, suburban, or small-town location.

Europeans tend to conceptualize the physical building, community, and services provided as a single entity. They develop a system of social and community connections by overlapping retail, service, and residential functions on a single site. Housing is only one component of the service house. Home-delivered services are also centered here for people living in conventional housing in the surrounding neighborhood. It is common for a service house to combine the community aspects of a senior citizen center, the residential attributes of housing for the frail, and the service support capability of a home care agency or a community health center. A noteworthy aspect of the European approach is its commitment to keeping older people independent for as long as possible. This commitment starts with a broad-based home care system and is backed up by service housing for those with the most intense needs (Soderstrom and Viklund, 1986). Clearly, Europeans treat housing as one component of a continuum of services offered to frail older people in the community. Older people move to a service house when it is considered the best combination of service supports needed to enhance the well-being and independence of the individual. Only severely impaired dementia victims with behavioral problems and complicated medical cases are candidates for institutionalization.

Another major difference between systems of care in the United States and northern Europe is the financial commitment northern Europeans have made to providing high-quality housing and services for middle- to lower-income populations. Funding is obtained from a combination of national health insurance and housing subsidies. Even though there is a range of income groups living in assisted living, everyone receives the same quality of care and housing. Therefore, the overall standard of housing for the frail elderly is higher than in comparable housing in the United States. Furthermore, in Europe, the strategy is to deliver health and personal care services to all needy elderly, whether they reside in housing built for the frail or in private homes. In the United States, assisted living is primarily provided as private-pay housing and services. When assisted living residents spend down their savings, they can be offered only nursing home care as an alternative housing and service arrangement. The key difference is that in Europe, housing is conceptualized as a service to older people.

Northern Europe provides specific mechanisms through which to achieve the nine goals listed at the beginning of this chapter for the physical, organizational, and social environment of assisted living housing. We address each of these goals here, with related recommendations.

Creating Environments That Appear Residential

The character, appearance, imagery, and precedent of assisted living should be related to residential housing. Associations with residential housing can be explored through the appearance and configuration of the building and the furnishing of interior space. The outward appearance of the building should employ residential elements such as sloped roofs, gables, attached porches, and dormers for scale purposes. Residential materials, finishes, and treatments should be used. Interior rooms should have varied character and purpose, just as in a house. Larger spaces, such as dining and living areas, can be broken into several smaller spaces. Ideally, open stairs should connect floors, and units should be clustered in small groups to stimulate the development of informal friendships and helping behaviors. And the building should fit into a comfortable community context of residential properties and light commercial uses.

Architecture that looks and feels residential communicates to prospective and current residents that an assisted living building is designed as housing. If it looks like housing, feels like housing, and smells like housing, then it acts like housing. Housing must be infused with services to allow residents with significant disabilities to live there. The image of housing is important not only to the older person but also to the family members who visit and to the staff. If the staff feel that they are working in a housing environment rather than an institution, their actions and attitudes are different. For example, it is easier for staff to grasp the need for privacy and autonomy in a *housing* context than in a medical context.

A sloping roof, the hearth, and the front door are basic symbolic residential elements (Rybczynski, 1989). The roof provides shelter; the hearth provides warmth and togetherness; and the entry sequence and the front door establish expectations for a friendly setting (Alexander, Ishikawa, and Silverstein, 1977). Figures 3.2 and 3.3 show examples of features that encourage a residential feel.

Creating the Perception That an Environment Is Small in Size

Overall, the setting should be as small as it can be without sacrificing economic stability and the capability to provide twenty-four-hour assistance. It is important to remember that the larger the building, the more easily it can both overwhelm its residents and lose its residential feel. When the building is small enough for residents to know one another and for the administrator to know each resident well, a sense of family develops. Such familiarity can enhance the emotional support system.

An assisted living project should have the minimum number of units possible to achieve an acceptable operational economy of scale. This number varies by region, state, and physical context. Most settings require a minimum of forty to fifty units to offer competitive rental rates and pro-

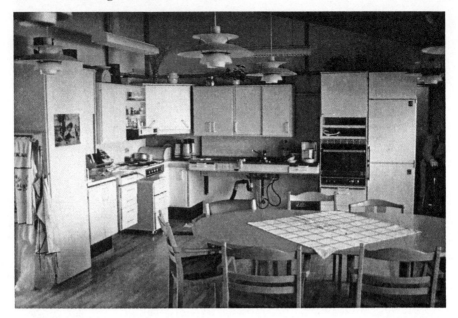

Fig. 3.2. Small-group spaces for dining adjacent to a residentially scaled serving kitchen represent a common pattern in Danish housing for mentally and physically impaired older people.

vide reliable twenty-four-hour care. The size needs to be large enough to accommodate the fixed costs of professional management; this factor is becoming ever more important as higher-acuity populations reside in these facilities. In Europe, projects are sized for the service needs of frail older residents in the immediate one-to-three-mile radius, a practice that achieves the economies of scale needed for efficient service production.

Clustering of residential units is one means through which the perception of small size can be achieved in larger facilities. Clustering units in small groups also appears to greatly benefit social interaction. If a seventy-unit project is broken into seven different ten-unit arrangements, it will look and feel different (and better) than it would if there were one monolithic seventy-unit setting. With unit clusters, the architecture of the building fosters opportunities for residents to get to know one another better. These informal contacts often lead to deeper, more substantial helping relationships that decrease reliance on formal care.

Another strategy to create an environment that feels smaller is reducing the perceived scale of the dining room. The dining room is important because residents spend more time there than in any other public space. If a large dining room is subdivided into smaller, more intimate spaces with three to four tables, the feeling of a pleasant, small dining area can be achieved. Another alternative is to have smaller dining areas located throughout the building. This can make it easier for less ambulatory residents to reach the dining room independently.

In nursing homes in Denmark, residents typically reside in single-occupancy units with a full bathroom. The organization, design, and management approach is based on clusters of eight units each. Residents from each cluster eat together in a small dining room rather than in a large-group setting. The decentralized nature of the facility allows clusters to be designed around naturally lighted, single-loaded corridors and landscaped courtyards. Swedish nursing homes and small-group homes base cluster sizes on the number of residents who can comfortably sit family-style around a large dining room table. This design enhances communication and the ability to motivate residents to engage in independent activities and behaviors.

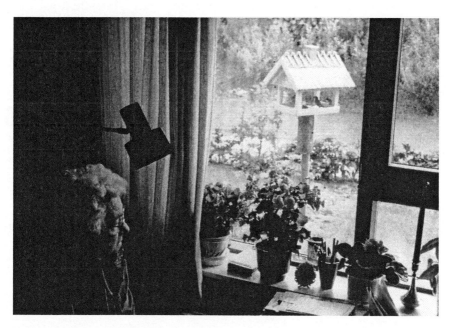

Fig. 3.3. Plants on the windowsill and a bird feeder near a window can greatly enhance the quality of life for a resident.

Providing Residential Privacy and Completeness

Privacy (physical, auditory, and visual) is often poorly addressed by long-term-care environments. Solutions to privacy problems do exist, but they are challenging to implement because of economic and regulatory factors. Although privacy is difficult to ensure in group living, it is important because it provides the older person with a sense of self and separateness from others. Designers should provide places for seclusion where residents can be free from unauthorized intrusion.

One of the most disturbing aspects of a nursing home reported by visitors is the public nature of care provision and treatment. Care is rarely provided behind closed doors. Furthermore, in nursing homes the boundaries between private and public domains are often blurred. In assisted living, the environment should be designed to encourage social interaction but also to assure privacy. Privacy should be achieved through a combination of efforts, including leasing policies that encourage single occupancy, design features such as locks on doors that residents can control, and management practices that require staff to identify themselves before they enter a room.

The individual resident room or apartment should be designed to look like a "normal" dwelling, not like a hospital room. It should be complete, with a full bathroom and at least a kitchenette. This design fosters both privacy and autonomy. Providing an extra space for an overnight visitor (perhaps a family member) is also desirable and can be achieved by adding a small alcove. Linking dwelling units to corridor spaces through windows and Dutch doors facilitates a social connection between residents while allowing privacy as an option. The unit edge can be further personalized through accessories like street numbers, plants, artwork, photographs, doorbells, and light fixtures that give each unit entry individuality and distinction.

Recognizing the Uniqueness of Each Resident

Each older person who enters assisted living has up to that time had a life of unique experiences. These different life experiences have nurtured diverse interests, abilities, values, and knowledge bases. Gerontologists argue that as we age, life's experiences and our own personal strengths and weaknesses make us more unique rather than more uniform in our beliefs and our understanding of daily life events. Capturing that diversity within a group setting is important. In fact, one route to better person-environment congruence is to recognize the diversity among residents and match this diversity through environmental programming (Lawton & Nahemow, 1973). Settings should not be dependent on large, preconceived group activities. Instead, small-group activities that are meaningful to a range of participants should be encouraged. They can make the social life of the place extraordinarily rich.

Numerous design elements can assist in creating a sense of individuality, including features that have their origin in the single-family house. Personalization of individual space is facilitated when furniture, accessories, photographs, artwork, and special collectibles can easily be displayed. On the exterior of the unit, creating an alcove by recessing the door is a common approach. Symbolically, this captures a portion of the semipublic corridor for display purposes and personalization.

The most common features used to define an entry are a mailbox, a shelf for resting packages or displaying items, a doorbell or door knocker, a street number, a wall-mounted light, a peephole for looking out, a welcome mat, and a planter. Dutch projects utilize features such as these more than other European cultures. Dutch projects often employ windows, alcoves, Dutch doors, and plant clusters to create a sense of personal expression at the unit edge. Dutch doors (half doors or farm doors) are a versatile element because they open the unit to the corridor while simultaneously protecting the resident's privacy and security. They also make it possible for residents to see what is happening outside of their unit.

Fostering Independence, Interdependence, and Individuality

The focus of care in assisted living should be on self-maintenance with assistance, and residents should be able to help themselves and one another. Fostering individuality requires an understanding of the unique attributes of each resident and a program that allows those unique qualities to be supported. Resident assessments should identify the individual capabilities and competencies of each person. This assessment should also clarify how the community can help the person and how the person can contribute to the community. One-sided caregiving without resident reciprocity builds dependence, not a sense of belonging or participation in a community.

Independence is often defined by the ability to make choices, control events, and be autonomous. Assessments should identify, preserve, and build on residents' strengths, while overcoming weaknesses through therapy and prosthetic intervention. Promoting opportunities for them to make choices and control events that influence significant outcomes makes older people feel more at home, more satisfied, and more task-independent than they do in settings that are highly restricted and regimented. Having a sense of mastery and control has been found to have pronounced positive effects on life satisfaction.

The Dutch and the Danes are particularly committed to a philosophy of caregiving that stresses self-maintenance and independence. They encourage older persons to exercise the maximum amount of personal control in normal daily activities by having them do as much for themselves as possible. Such a model of care is more difficult to implement than doing the work for the resident, but the benefits are great. Residents feel more confident, with a greater sense of self-esteem through practicing behaviors that increase their overall abilities. This therapeutic approach to providing care builds competence; it is referred to as providing care by "putting your hands in your pockets" or "sitting on your hands." The Dutch and the Danes believe that taking self-maintenance responsibilities away from older people makes them more passive and encourages disengagement. Over time, this can lead to learned helplessness behaviors as well as muscle strength decline and general health problems due to inactivity (Seligman, 1975).

Helping one another provides a sense of contribution that bolsters self-esteem and minimizes formal intervention. As residents adapt to the social environment of a group setting, they often create informal helping relationships that constitute another type of social network. Smaller facilities that encourage interdependent helping behaviors are the most likely to experience this bond of affiliation. Networks of interdependence occur when residents who know one another recognize opportunities for reciprocity. In general, these exchanges extend from friendships. They occur somewhat randomly, aided by propinquity and shared interests.

Creating spaces where residents can gather for spontaneous social exchange, helping activities, or scheduled social and recreational activities is necessary for a successful, well-formulated spatial layout. Observation and social exchange are two different but interrelated activities that must be accommodated in spaces that are appropriately designed and located. The most popular and heavily used social areas are those that make it easy for residents to join and leave the group and are situated in places with views of on- and off-site activities. Also, the building layout itself can generate circulation patterns that are interesting to watch.

Focusing on Health Maintenance, Physical Movement, and Mental Stimulation

Maximizing health and independence for as long as possible is a major goal of assisted living. Monitoring health through preventive checks, encouraging good nutritional habits, and careful attention to medications constructs a safety net of health oversight. Exercise therapy can build upper and lower body strength, increase aerobic capacity, and achieve muscle control over problems like incontinence. Activities that stimulate the mind, such as reading and discussion groups, create opportunities for friendship formation, informal social exchange, and the sharing of personal feelings. This contact counteracts depression while replacing friendships that have been lost through attrition and relocation.

The degree of focus on rehabilitation and therapeutic intervention is an area in which the United States and Europe differ markedly, and much can be learned from the European approach. As mentioned earlier, the northern European version of assisted living is viewed as a setting in which the mental and physical competency of a resident can be *strengthened, maintained, or restored.* Service houses in Denmark have created community attitudes that vest responsibility for occupational and physical therapy in older residents. They are expected to maintain their competency through rigorous programs that frequently include daily workouts on therapy equipment.

Physical therapy can involve special equipment set aside in specific rooms, or it can be designed into the building. Ideally, the design of the building should make physical therapy and exercise a normal aspect of life in the facility. Corridors, courtyards, and gardens can be designed to encourage physical therapy and exercise. Equipment can be decentralized and placed in hallways or atriums, making it accessible to residents whenever they feel like using it (see fig. 3.4). Walking for exercise can be promoted in corridors. Atrium projects, especially those with inside gardens, can allow residents to walk in a protected environment that has many outdoor attributes.

The most impressive therapeutic facilities are the ergotherapy (occupational therapy) and physical therapy rooms of the Danish *plegehem* (pronounced *play em*), equivalent to the skilled nursing facility in the United

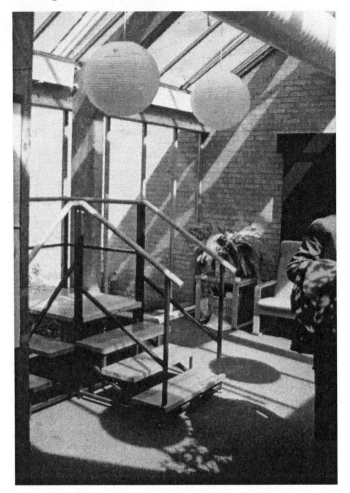

Fig. 3.4. Opportunities for physical therapy can be pursued in almost any location. This light-filled corridor space in a Danish nursing home is a wonderful informal place to exercise, using this stair-stepping equipment.

States. The Danish system is focused on making therapy a "normal" activity, similar in nature to the routinized responsibilities of working people or the housekeeping responsibilities of homemakers. Ergotherapy, like work, is a productive enterprise that gives residents a sense of satisfaction. The activities that are typically pursued involve weaving and small-motor manipulation tasks, and they often result in a product (e.g., place mats, rugs, napkins, jewelry) that has meaning and value. Another ergotherapy focus is the restoration of self-maintenance abilities through the use of training kitchens and the exercise of activities of daily living. Ergotherapy creatively pursues the notion that older residents have a responsibility to stay active and engaged.

Environments can support a range of therapeutic activities through the design of rooms and spaces that encourage physical and mental exercise. Artwork that represents familiar positive emotional relationships can stimulate memory by recalling positive past associations. Sitting areas where residents can observe off-site and on-site activities and outdoor garden areas that promote spirituality use the environment to stimulate vicarious engagement.

Design elements also can provide for the inclusion of children, animals, and plants in facility life. In Lonkoping, Sweden, city officials have pursued an aggressive plan of constructing family housing adjacent to elder-care facilities. In these arrangements, day care for children is often located in the same building used by the elderly. In one project, windows along a busy corridor allow residents to watch children playing in the day care center. Swedish homes also incorporate animals into the home's daily routine. Animal-assisted therapy facilitates emotional responses through the unconditional affection that pets provide. Europeans also seem to be more sensitive to the therapeutic potential of plants, although some U.S. facilities, following Edenization principles, are beginning to make more use of plants (see fig. 3.5). Resident rooms in Danish nursing homes frequently open onto outdoor patios, and raised planter beds are often incorporated to allow wheelchair-bound residents access to the color, texture, and aroma of plants. Swedish group homes for people with dementia often contain herb and vegetable gardens.

Supporting Family Involvement

Most institutions seem to be designed with the assumption that family responsibility ends when the resident moves into the building. Instead of being viewed as a significant source of information, affective support, and inspiration to the resident, family involvement is not maximized. Long-term care should not be managed in this way. Assessments that involve family members in caregiving partnerships allow family members to participate in making decisions and in managing care. The environment can support family gatherings, overnight stays, shared activities, and mean-

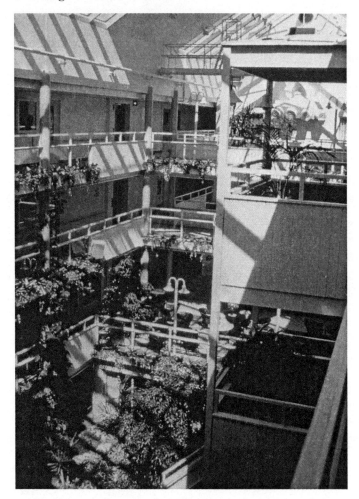

Fig. 3.5. The atrium in the Kuuselaan Palvelukoti in Tampere, Finland, is a beautiful space that brings in natural light and is suffused with plants. This project includes two small group homes for people with dementia. Residents can age in place and order more services as their needs increase.

ingful conversations between family members and residents. When family members become participating partners in the life of the place, they add vitality and energy, while saving money. They can also play a stimulating role in the lives of other residents. Furthermore, in the process of being made attractive to families and being designed to support social relationships, a facility can also come to serve as a community resource. Information, education, peer group discussion, adult day care, respite care, and home care referrals are services that can be developed to benefit families.

One way to reconceptualize the pattern of family involvement is to examine other models of social care, such as day care for children. Family participation is an important and integral aspect of the way these settings are operated. There are many regulations governing child day care, but the ability to accommodate family needs and desires is not compromised by them. Home-delivered care is another integrated family model, which coordinates formal and informal resources to keep the older person functioning independently outside an institution. The radical idea of giving the family shared responsibility to provide services within a setting where formal help can be efficiently ordered when necessary expands the parameters of how to design family-centered models of long-term care.

In some assisted living facilities, residents are assessed using a community care model. Significant resources from residents themselves, their families, and other residents are considered sources of support. Facilities for laundry are made available to family members, meals are offered to them at discount prices, and they are encouraged to help in any way they can. Care plans are devised by consulting the older person and the person's family in specifying needed services. Other models have managed to adapt a home care philosophy within a long-term-care environment. This type of caregiving is a true partnership, and care plans allow family members to share the burden of care. They can do laundry, organize and administer medications, supervise baths, and help their family member to the dining room. Care needs are assessed and monitored by a case manager, and residents pay only for the care they use. Case managers ensure that the appropriate level of care is provided either by a family member or a formal care attendant. These partnerships distribute work between formal and informal sources, but it must be noted that in some states this approach violates state statutes that consider providing care in this way as illegally operating a facility without a license.

Unfortunately, European systems seem less able to provide creative insights with regard to incorporating family involvement, partly as a result of their success in providing adequate financial support through nationalized health insurance. Northern Europeans pay the highest taxes in the world, and one benefit is a system of excellent care from cradle to grave. This system has seemingly preempted efforts to develop creative family care options. The family interaction that does occur in European models is largely social in nature. Family members visit, transport residents to the doctor, and occasionally help with light cleaning tasks; they offer little instrumental care because the system provides it. The system has established high expectations for services, without the need for significant family input.

That being said, there are still some things to be gained by examining northern European models. One particularly good model is the Swedish small-group home. In this alternative for dementia residents, the family can exert influence and take responsibility more easily. Its generally small size (usually limited to 6–8 residents) allows families to host events and take a very active role in setting policies and scheduling activities. In group homes, care attendants are trained to work with family members. The staff counsels relatives about general strategies that can make communication more effective, and family members provide specific information about the past lives of residents that make it easier for staff to communicate and connect with demented residents. When a staff member knows that a resident was a dog lover or an avid gardener or an accomplished musician or a world traveler, he or she can bridge the communication gap more easily.

One major impediment to family interaction in the United States is the small semiprivate room, which is the prevalent model most nursing homes follow. Private conversations and personalization of the environment suffer when a room is both small and semiprivate. Families also feel unwelcome and uncomfortable when there are few common spaces that accommodate family interaction; spaces like small cafés, intimate sitting areas, solarium greenhouses, picnic spaces, and enclosed porches are often absent. This lack of inviting common space gives families the feeling that they are not an important constituency, thus reinforcing the dominant nature of management's presence. Providing places within the building for family members to meet and socialize is a way to encourage visiting behaviors. European service houses provide many choices, because they are physically connected to a range of spaces that are open to the surrounding neighborhood, such as restaurants and activity spaces. In Finland, one facility has an atrium that is contiguous with an open-plan crafts and reading room. These rooms, in turn, open onto an exterior garden. Special events involving families utilize all three connected spaces, thereby facilitating larger groups. In American assisted living, the enclosed porch has become an attractive room for family visits. Some homes have focused on creating small-group social spaces in alcoves adjacent to major pedestrian thoroughfares. Others open their dining area to outside customers, encouraging family members to think of the facility as a restaurant where everyone can eat. Many facilities seek opportunities to host families for picnics, barbecues, and parties, especially on holidays historically associated with family events such as Thanksgiving, Labor Day, and Memorial Day.

Another way of helping families to become involved in the care of older relatives is to make services like respite and day care available to frail older people living with family caregivers in the community. European housing models almost universally adopt this community-oriented approach. They view their role as providing a range of services for residents and older people in the community, as well as those dwelling within the facility.

Maintaining Connections with the Surrounding Community

Settings should integrate residents with rather than isolate them from community resources and contacts. Housing projects that develop inventive ways to serve the surrounding community become less internally focused and better connected to the fabric of the community. Intergenerational exchange programs with preschools have been successful in forging exchange relationships between older people and children. Encouraging residents to visit their old neighborhood to attend church, have their hair styled, or visit the bank maintains linkages and connections with old friends and familiar places. These activities allow residents to draw on a wider range of interactions, rather than narrowing their choices.

In the United States, facilities that care for frail older people are often cognizant of the opportunity to serve such people living in the neighborhood but are rarely organized to pursue this idea. These neighborhood residents often require either home care services of a more sporadic nature or monitoring services such as emergency response. Housing projects that deliver community services to neighbors along with serving residents create a hybrid model that combines the continuity of care associated with assisted living, the service support system of a senior community center, and the outreach efforts of a home care agency. This is the foundation for northern European housing and service systems for the frail.

Three main approaches to providing community service exist in northern Europe. The first is the community-based center, which offers a range of services at a central site that neighborhood residents can visit. It can include services as diverse as occupational and physical therapy, meals, adult day care, medical checkups, recreational opportunities, and social activities. The second approach is one in which services are provided from this center and delivered to the neighborhood residents in their own homes. Home-delivered meals, homemaker services, home health care, emergency medical response, and transportation are some of the most common services provided to neighborhood residents. The desire to serve a community population gives the project a strong civic presence in the city. Third, housing co-located with other compatible land uses, like child-care services, outpatient clinics, pharmacies, restaurants, and grocery stores offers for all residents more support and better access to caregivers. These mixed-use models have the potential to connect housing with a range of compatible land uses, thereby further integrating the project into the surrounding context (see fig. 3.6).

The service house holds the greatest promise as a model for the inte-

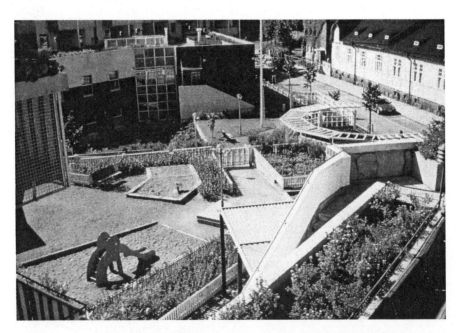

Fig. 3.6. Off the courtyard of this U-shaped, mixed-use Helsinki senior housing complex are a health clinic and a child-care center. The courtyard contains sitting areas for older people that overlook a children's playground.

gration of neighborhood-based housing and community services (Bull & Lise-Saglie, 1991). These mixed-use buildings are often located above or adjacent to shopping centers or town squares and are sited overlooking retail streets and sidewalks. In Europe, how a project fits, complements, and improves the urban context is an important indicator of how well it serves the broader community.

Adaptations to Increasing Frailty

The average resident of an assisted living setting is likely to be in the 82-to-87 age range and has an average length of stay of between 2.5 and 3.0 years. Assisted living facilities should assume that approximately 30 percent of the resident population are experiencing some problems with incontinence and that nearly 50 percent are having problems with cognitive impairment (ALFA, 1999).

Adaptability is important because resident needs change over time and because different people experience change at different rates and in different ways. Some have mental impairments, whereas others need greater assistance with activities of daily living and instrumental activities of daily living. The environment should be able to compensate for many deficits and to adapt to changing resident needs. Bathrooms and kitchens are the primary rooms in which adaptation is necessary. These two rooms are the most important spaces where "work" activities take place. For an assisted living population that is likely to take all meals in a congregate dining room, the kitchen is not so critical as the bathroom.

Bathing, toileting, and grooming continue to be some of the most important if not the most important tasks that establish a resident's level of independence. The most accommodating, safety-enhancing and supportive designs for the shower, the toilet and its surroundings, the lavatory, pharmaceutical storage, and the mirror are necessary for maintaining optimum independence. The design approach should be one that embraces the unique physiological qualities of the older person and allows adaptation as impairment increases. For example, the toilet grab bar should be designed and positioned to fit the height, reach, and strength limitations of a specific older resident. A one-size-fits-all attitude, which is often reinforced by rigid ADA (Americans with Disabilities Act) requirements, is precisely the wrong way to establish the best and most effective fit.

Bathrooms designed to facilitate a transfer from a wheelchair or walker should be large enough to allow attendants freedom of movement in assisting with toilet and shower transfers. European bathrooms are often arranged to accommodate an open shower in one corner of the bathroom. This type of design facilitates wheelchair access, making it easier for older residents and attendants to navigate inside the room. Danish units almost universally specify a wide sliding pocket or barn door to the bathroom, which eliminates the problem of dealing with an inconvenient door swing and facilitates the use of larger, wider openings that can accommodate transfers more easily. Clever ideas about how to increase storage space and create more flexible bathrooms are also common. In some service houses, large, wheelchair-accessible bathrooms are specified and filled with cabinetry that can be removed if a resident in a wheelchair needs more space for maneuvering.

Kitchens offer residents the opportunity to exercise many independent behaviors. Specifying a large, 500- to 600-square-foot unit with a full kitchen is common in Danish and Swedish service houses. The most common kitchen arrangements in Europe are open U- and L-shaped alcoves. Kitchen tables located on one side of an L-shaped configuration can be removed if the unit needs more space for wheelchair access. Most servicehouse kitchens are complete and offer a range of appliances, including microwave ovens. Stovetops are designed with timers and switches that can be used safely by residents. Systems that provide daily reassurance of resident well-being are common in appliances in Europe and the United States. Many European systems have wired these reassurance systems into the refrigerator, for example, or the toilet. When someone opens the refrigerator door or flushes the toilet in the morning, the mechanism automatically resets itself for the next day, assuring management that the resident is all right.

In summary, the dwelling unit, in particular, should be flexible enough to meet the changing needs of the frail older person, considerate enough to increase mastery and control, and complete enough to deliver privacy and a symbolic sense of home. Unit designs should make it easier for residents to age in place; manipulate and access appliances, fixtures, storage spaces, windows, and doors; preserve the privacy, sanctity, and autonomy of their unit; personalize and decorate their unit to suit their own needs and preferences; make the necessary bathroom transfers with assistance or by themselves; maintain the maximum amount of choice and independence within the setting; and safely call for help and assistance when necessary.

The Effect of Regulation on the Goals of Assisted Living

Rules and regulations are established to guide practice, ensure safety, and provide a reasonable level of quality assurance. In the United States, the regulation of group living environments has been generally overprescriptive and rigid. The design of environments for frail older people is a casebook example of how commonly held good intentions have been transformed into a nightmare of overlapping, contradictory, and counterintuitive constraints. The response to problems of abuse in nursing homes has led to the introduction of regulations that narrow flexibility, limit experimentation with promising therapies, and discourage creative approaches to care management. The system's prescriptive nature often assigns a standard response to a problem rather than encouraging a rational and balanced assessment of the situation as the basis for potential solutions.

Regulations affect both the physical and the operational environment. The most challenging regulations are those that place limitations on the family's involvement in providing care and those that discourage therapies involving residents in daily work activities such as setting the table, washing dishes, and preparing food. Staff are often required to carry out tasks such as feeding, toileting, and bathing, thus not challenging a person's self-maintenance capabilities. Keeping residents from practicing activities of daily living and taking away the option to make choices about the help they need or want is psychologically devastating.

Regulations often center on physical design and zoning considerations because they are tangible and controllable and because personnel problems are more time-consuming and difficult to identify and address. Fire safety regulations typically focus entirely on issues of safety to the exclusion of quality-of-life factors. Strict codes that limit the use of residential materials and features (such as open stairs and fireplaces), when combined with relatively low construction budgets, often result in stark, overly institutional settings. Also, zoning laws often specify separate land uses for institutions and hospitals, so that mixed-use programs are not possible. Environmental impacts such as increased neighborhood traffic and parking sometimes force sponsors to drop efforts to create age-integrated land uses. These situations result in a continuing trend toward isolation and segregation.

Zoning laws, state regulations, and building codes have combined to create a morass of overlapping restrictions that keep U.S. projects from emulating some of the most successful qualities of European developments. Our European neighbors have managed to create a long-term-care system that is not needlessly hamstrung by pointless and arbitrary rules that destroy opportunities for self-initiated resident activity and emphasize staff accountability over caregiving. With financial resources dwindling and the demand for present and future housing for our elderly increasing, there is much room for improvement and there are many identifiable directions toward which to strive.

Conclusion

Housing for frail elderly persons provides a useful lens through which a society's assumptions can be observed and examined. Foreign models are designed for people with the same mental and physical impairments as those in the United States, yet they are different from a physical, spiritual, and operational perspective. Examining these models can improve our understanding of how the physical environment can liberate or incarcerate its inhabitants. Denmark, Sweden, Finland, Norway, and the Netherlands have all developed unique, innovative models of long-term care. The liberal sharing of information between countries with related but different cultures has allowed ideas to be transplanted, refined, and improved. Many northern European ideas involving self-management, participatory governance, and therapy through normal activities of daily living run counter to laws and regulations initiated in the United States that purport to safeguard the elderly. Reflecting on these alternative models leads to the conclusion that the United States has much to do in addressing the diverse needs of older people, who must be understood as unique individuals and treated as such.

References

Alexander, C. S., Ishikawa, S., & Silverstein, M. 1977. *A Pattern Language.* New York: Oxford University Press.
Assisted Living Federation of America. 1999. *The Assisted Living Industry 1999: An Overview.* Fairfax, VA.
ASVVO. 1991. *Integratie ven verzorging en verpleging.* Amsterdam: ASVVO.
Bull, G. 1987. *Boliger for Eldre.* Oslo: Bolig for Livet.

Bull, G., & Lise-Saglie, I. 1991. *Service Flats: An Alternative to Institutions in the Care of the Elderly.* Oslo: Norwegian Building Research Institute.

Cohen, U., & Weisman, J. 1991. *Holding On to Home: Designing Environments for People with Dementia.* Baltimore: Johns Hopkins University Press.

Husbanken. 1987. *La oss bo midt i livet!* Oslo: Husbanken.

Lawton, M. P. 1980. *Environment and Aging.* Monterey: Brooks/Cole Publishing.

Lawton, M. P., & Nahemow, L. 1973. Ecology and the aging process. In C. Eisdorfer and M. P. Lawton (eds.), *Psychology of Adult Development and Aging.* Washington, DC: American Psychological Association.

Lindstrom, B. 1989. *Gode boliger til aeldre.* Copenhagen: Bybberiets Udviklingsrad.

Parmelee, P., & Lawton, M. P. 1990. The design of special environments for the aged. In J. E. Birren & K. W. Schaie (eds.), *Handbook of the Psychology of Aging,* 3d ed. New York: Academic Press.

Pynoos, J., & Regnier, V. 1991. Improving residential environments for the frail elderly: Bridging the gap between theory and application. In J. Birren, J. Lubben, J. Rowe, & D. Deutchman (eds.), *The Concept and Measurement of Quality of Life in the Frail Elderly.* New York: Academic Press.

Regnier, V. 1997. *Assisted Living Housing for the Elderly: Design Innovations from the United States and Europe.* New York: Wiley.

Regnier, V., Hamilton, J., & Yatabe, S. 1995. *Assisted Living for the Aged and Frail: Innovations in Design, Management, and Financing.* New York: Columbia University Press.

Regnier, V., & Pynoos, J. (eds). 1987. *Housing for the Aged: Design Directives and Policy Considerations.* New York: Elsevier.

Rybczynski, W. 1989. *The Most Beautiful House in the World.* New York: Penguin Books.

Seligman, M. 1975. *Helplessness: On Depression, Development, and Death.* San Francisco: Freeman.

Soderstrom, B., & Viklund, E. 1986. *Housing Care and Service for Elderly and Old People: The Situation in Sweden.* Stockholm: Swedish Ministry of Housing and Physical Planning.

Wilson, K. B. 1990. Assisted living: The merger of housing and long-term care services. *Long Term Care Advances* 1:208.

4 Staffing Problems and Strategies in Assisted Living

R. Tamara Hodlewsky, M.S., M.A.

Staffing is one of the most important challenges facing the residential care/assisted living (RC/AL) industry today. Clearly, direct-care staff are responsible for delivering many of the services that define RC/AL, and they play a key role in determining the quality of care that residents receive. As the demand for long-term-care services grows in years to come, the demand for nurse aides will grow dramatically; specifically, the U.S. Department of Labor predicts a 58 percent increase in the number of nurse aide jobs between 1998 and 2008 (U.S. Department of Labor, 2000). However, facilities are already having substantial trouble recruiting and retaining appropriate numbers of qualified direct-care staff, especially nurse aides.

The staffing problem has been attracting attention for a number of years and results in concerns about quality. Turnover rates in RC/AL range from 30 percent to more than 60 percent (NCAL, 1998), leading to high search and training costs—funds that could be used to improve the quality of care. A recent General Accounting Office report declared inadequate staffing to be one of the most commonly cited quality-of-care problems in the industry (US GAO, 1999). The Senate Special Committee on Aging held special hearings on the staffing problem in nursing facilities in late 1999, and interest in other segments of the long-term-care industry is usually not far behind. Unfortunately, the staffing shortage does not appear to be a temporary situation, and this leads to concerns among providers, regulators, and consumers that providing the high-quality care that is at the heart of the philosophy of assisted living will become more difficult.

The difficulty in finding sufficient numbers of qualified staff has several causes and no clear solution. Nurse aide jobs in long-term care generally offer low wages (minimum wage or slightly higher), few benefits, and the risk of injury while lifting or moving residents who need assistance. The currently low unemployment rates exacerbate the problem, forcing long-term-care settings to compete with other service sectors for an increasingly tight labor pool. Of course, there are thousands of dedicated and qualified nurses and nurse aides fulfilling the care needs of RC/AL residents today, despite the less-than-optimal tangible rewards. The challenge lies in attracting enough such individuals to care for a growing elderly population. This chapter overviews four perspectives (regulatory, economic, labor, and management) that offer four different—but not mutually exclusive—approaches to facing the staffing challenge in RC/AL.

The Regulatory Perspective

The regulatory approach to ensuring sufficient quantity and qualifications of staff focuses primarily on consumer protection. It places the responsibility for attracting and retaining quality staff on the facility, regardless of economic conditions and the adequacy of government reimbursement or other payment. Although the fundamental logic behind this approach is appealing, implementation is inherently difficult. How can regulators define the appropriate number of nurses and nurse aides per facility or per resident when facilities vary widely—both among states and within states—in the acuity level of residents? How do staffing requirements change when there are more residents with dementia in the facility or when residents are chair-bound or bedfast? Even assuming that regulators could determine appropriate staffing ratios for different acuity levels, it would be impossible to accommodate each potential combination of residents' needs in a meaningful way. Thus, most attempts at regulating staffing levels have focused on minimum staffing requirements that are binding constraints only for facilities with the lowest acuity levels.

Staff Levels

The challenge in regulating sufficient staffing levels or ratios is exacerbated by the complex organizational structures that exist in the industry today. Approximately 69 percent of RC/AL facilities nationwide contract, or allow residents to contract, with home health agencies to provide nursing care; two-thirds contract with hospice agencies (NCAL, 1998). Home health and hospice services are regulated separately. Therefore, staffing ratios dictated by RC/AL regulators should account for the probability that nonfacility staff may be contributing to resident care regularly or when called upon in case of need.

Since there is no federal regulation of RC/AL in general, there is no federal regulation of the number of staff required in these facilities. Most states address the issue of staffing in their RC/AL regulations, but those regulations vary widely in specificity. Three broadly defined and sometimes overlapping policies can be described as follows, from the most specific to the least specific:

Staffing Ratios. Fifteen states specify minimum staffing ratios for at least one level of care that can be classified as RC/AL (see table 4.1). The ratios range from one staff person per forty residents at all times in Missouri to one staff person per six residents at all times in Alabama. Most of the states with staffing ratios have separate requirements for waking hours and sleeping hours, sometimes dividing the day into several shifts with different ratios. Most do not differentiate among different types of direct-care staff. Some states, such as Pennsylvania and South Dakota, designate a minimum number of care hours per resident day (1 hour and 0.8 hours, respectively) rather than (or in addition to) the number of staff that need to be in the facility at any given time (NCAL, 2000).

Twenty-Four-Hour Availability. An additional fifteen states require the presence or the on-call availability of a direct-care staff person twenty-four hours a day, consistent with the philosophy of RC/AL. Two states (Connecticut and New Jersey) require twenty-four-hour RN availability, and several other states (Iowa, Ohio, and West Virginia) require the presence of an RN when medications are administered or certain other nursing tasks are performed.

Sufficient Staffing. The vast majority of states, including those that designate minimum staffing as described above, require that staffing be "sufficient to meet the needs of residents in the facility." Facilities are not allowed to accept or retain residents whose needs cannot be met by the staff. Recognizing that facilities have heterogeneous resident populations and offer a wide range of services, most states leave particular staffing decisions to the expertise of facility managers, with oversight through the complaint and survey processes. The assumption underlying this policy is that both facility managers and state surveyors are able to identify staffing needs when faced with a particular resident or resident population.

Though offering some guidance to facilities and some assurance to consumers, each of these policies is imperfect from a regulatory perspec-

Table 4.1. States with Minimum Staffing Ratios

State	Minimum Staffing Ratio
Alabama	One staff member on site per 6 residents at all times
Arkansas	One staff member on site per 1–16 residents; varies by day, evening, night
California	One staff member on site for up to 16 residents; one awake staff member on site for 16–100 residents; one awake staff member and one on call for 101–200 residents
Florida	Complex but depends on number of residents (e.g., 375 staff hours per week would be required for a facility with 46–55 residents)
Georgia	One staff member on site per 15 residents during waking hours; one staff member per 25 residents during sleeping hours
Maine	One staff member on site per 12 residents from 7:00 A.M. to 3:00 P.M.; one staff member on site per 18 residents from 3:00 P.M. to 11:00 P.M.; one staff member on site per 30 residents from 11:00 P.M. to 7:00 A.M.
Michigan	One staff member on site per 15 residents during waking hours; one staff member per 20 residents during sleeping hours
Mississippi	Varies by level of care and by time of day (e.g., in a Level 1 facility, one staff member on site per 10 residents from 7:00 A.M. to 3:00 P.M.)
Missouri	One staff member on site per 40 residents at all times
New Mexico	One staff member on site per 15 residents during waking hours; one staff member on site for up to 60 residents during sleeping hours; two staff members on site for 61–120 residents during sleeping hours; three staff members on site for more than 120 residents during sleeping hours
New York	One staff member on site per 1–40 residents; varies by day, evening, night
North Carolina	Complex but depends on total number of residents in the facility and varies by time of day and by task
Pennsylvania	Sufficient staff to provide one hour of personal care per resident per day
South Carolina	One staff member on site per 10 residents during waking hours; one staff member per 44 residents during sleeping hours
South Dakota	Sufficient staff to provide 0.8 hours of personal care per resident per day

Source: Adapted from NCAL, 2000.

tive. As noted earlier, appropriate staffing ratios are difficult to establish, and minimum ratios may be far from adequate in higher-acuity facilities. Facility management may indeed be best able to judge staffing needs of the facility; however, it is not clear that good intentions and market forces alone will guarantee appropriate staffing decisions. From a consumer-protection standpoint, consistent and credible oversight then becomes crucial. Yet at this time, states vary widely in processes for inspecting facilities and investigating complaints (US GAO, 1999).

Staff Qualifications

A second component of the regulatory approach concerns the quality rather than the quantity of staff. Quality can be screened during the hiring process and enhanced after hiring through orientation and training programs. Opinions seem to be mixed on the need for regulation of this aspect: some states include only one or two of the most basic requirements (e.g., staff should receive an orientation), whereas others prescribe specific content areas of training programs. In general, the regulations are intended to ensure minimum levels of staff competence and training in RC/AL, both for new entrants to long-term care and for staff who may have worked in other long-term-care settings and are unfamiliar with the philosophy of RC/AL. These regulations generally take one of several forms.

Criminal Background Checks. Regulations are in place in some states to prevent people with criminal backgrounds from running facilities or providing care. One-half of all states require some type of criminal background check for administrators applying for licensure. Only one-third of states require criminal background checks for direct-care staff, although many other states encourage (but do not require) the checks or disallow the hiring of anyone with a criminal background (Mollica, 1998). In almost all cases, the criminal background check is limited to searching a state registry or database, so applicants with criminal backgrounds in other states may fail to be identified. Industry representatives are currently working with the federal government to enable timely access to a national registry and to require criminal background checks for all long-term-care staff positions.

Certification. Many states require potential administrators to meet some minimal standards of age (most frequently 21 or older) and education (high school or G.E.D.; sometimes an advanced degree) and to have specific knowledge or experience in managing a long-term-care facility.

Seventeen states require administrators to have a license or certification (Mollica, 1998). Requirements are less defined for direct-care staff. Just three states (Connecticut, Oklahoma, and Utah) require personal care aides in RC/AL to be certified nursing assistants (CNAs). Several other states require either CNA status or completion of another acceptable training program (NCAL, 2000). Although certification does not guarantee quality of staff, it does ensure basic knowledge and training in caregiving and may reflect a longer-term commitment to the industry.

Orientation and Continuing Education. Many states also regulate the content of orientation and training programs and the number of hours of continuing education completed per year. The content of orientation programs required by various states includes direct-care issues, such as hygiene, nutrition, direct-care skills, and principles of RC/AL; health-related issues, such as observation and reporting and medication assistance; knowledge areas, such as resident rights, aging, psychosocial needs, death and dying, and care plan development; safety issues, such as cardiopulmonary resuscitation, first aid, fire safety, and emergency procedures; and facility processes, such as record-keeping and reporting abuse and neglect (Mollica, 1998). Twenty-two states specify the number of hours of continuing education required each year for administrators, ranging from eight to forty hours. Approximately one-third of all states specify continuing education hours for direct-care staff, ranging from six to twenty-four hours per year (NCAL, 2000).

The regulatory approach to staffing in RC/AL, as in other long-term-care settings, can be viewed as defining a lower bound for the quantity and quality of staff. It is a mechanism for identifying facilities with chronic problems and assuring consumers a minimal level. However, especially in an industry as heterogeneous as RC/AL, regulation is limited in its ability to provide positive incentives for facilities to improve staffing levels and quality beyond the minimum required. Furthermore, regulation cannot effectively address the major staffing issue facing the industry today: the staff shortage. Requiring facilities to hire more staff is not effective when there are no applicants to be hired.

The Economic Perspective

The economic approach to improving the quantity and quality of staff in long-term care is rooted in improving wages and benefits of staff posi-

tions, thereby increasing the ability of facility managers to attract and retain quality staff. Representatives of long-term-care industries have long
contended that Medicaid reimbursement rates are too low, leading to
wages that often fail to attract skilled and dedicated nurse aides. The recent economic boom and the accompanying low unemployment rates
have exacerbated the problem. Some states have implemented rate
increases that specifically target nurse aide wages in an attempt to address
the staffing shortage, and some policies under consideration strive to increase nurse aide job opportunities and satisfaction.

Wage and Benefit Pass-Throughs

Approximately one-third of all states have approved or implemented
Medicaid reimbursement increases to providers that are designated in
whole or in part for nurse aide salaries or benefits, or both. The designated portion may be an absolute dollar amount or a percentage. Dollar-
amount increases have ranged from $0.50 per hour to $2.14 per hour and
$4.93 per patient day; percentages of the increase dedicated to wages and
benefits were roughly in the 75–80 percent range. Some states have directed reimbursement increases to particular shifts or to incentive-based
wage differentials. However, many of the states with wage and benefit
pass-throughs limit the increases to home health or nursing facility staff,
excluding RC/AL (NCDFS, 1999).

Job Opportunity and Satisfaction

Some states (Mississippi, Maine, Alaska, and Delaware) are considering or
experimenting with programs to create career ladders for nurse aides and
thereby increase job satisfaction and performance incentives. Several levels within the nurse aide job category would be defined, each higher level
corresponding to more training and increased pay (NCDFS, 1999).

New Labor Sources

A number of states are viewing their welfare reform efforts as an opportunity to increase the labor pool for long-term care, but few states to date
have implemented plans to encourage nurse aide training among former
welfare recipients (NCDFS, 1999).

It is important to note that policies based on the economic perspective
are closely tied to government reimbursement, which may have only a
minimal direct effect on the RC/AL industry in many states. Although

the majority of states now allow Medicaid funding for RC/AL services through waivers or through a state plan, the number of actual Medicaid beneficiaries in RC/AL is still quite small—approximately forty thousand in all (Mollica, 1998). This figure accounts for less than 5 percent of RC/AL residents nationwide (NCAL, 1998), although a handful of states certainly have much higher percentages and would experience a stronger impact from changes in Medicaid reimbursement than other states.

If policies to improve staffing through reimbursement are aimed mainly at nursing facilities and home health care, there are still important indirect effects on the private-pay sector of the RC/AL industry. The indirect effects could be positive or negative. If the policies increase pay and job satisfaction for nurse aides in general and attract more people to the field, they could increase the labor pool available for all long-term-care industries, including RC/AL. However, if higher wages and benefits make nursing facility and home health jobs more attractive than jobs in RC/AL, the field may lose some of its share of that labor pool. The net effect will depend on the ability of the RC/AL industry to stay competitive with other segments of the long-term-care market in attracting and retaining quality staff.

The Labor Perspective

The labor approach to staffing problems in long-term-care facilities is based on improving working conditions for direct-care staff. The U.S. Department of Labor cited nursing and personal care facilities as among the workplaces with the highest injury rates, 13.8 injuries per 100 full-time workers in 1998 (U.S. Department of Labor, 2000). Although the rates have been declining in recent years as the industry and government work to make the industry safer, direct-care staff still face a serious risk of ergonomic injury when lifting or moving residents. Combined with generally low pay and few benefits, the risk of injury can be a serious impediment to attracting and retaining staff. Both organized labor and the federal government are actively seeking changes to the working environment in long-term care.

Traditionally, unions attracted mostly manufacturing workers and had little involvement in health care industries. That fact seems to be changing. The Service Employees International Union (SEIU), the largest union in the country representing service employees, now reports more than 700,000 members in health care facilities and more than 100,000 members in nursing facilities alone (SEIU, 2000). The SEIU is specifically targeting nursing facilities, contending that quality of care is inextricably linked with working conditions for direct-care staff and that unionization would ameliorate problems of understaffing, high turnover, and lack of training that lead to substandard quality. Facility owners often contend that unions interfere with the owners' ongoing efforts to improve management-staff relations and working conditions and may not even improve the situation of workers they represent. If unionization rates increase in nursing facilities, they will certainly increase in all segments of the long-term-care industry, and at least some growth seems likely. At this time it is unclear exactly what effect increased unionization would have on staffing and on long-term care in general, but it could have a noticeable impact on the nature of the staff recruitment and retention problem.

More directly related to working conditions, in November 1999, the Occupational Safety and Health Administration (OSHA) published a controversial proposed rule on ergonomics (OSHA, 2000) which could have a major impact on long-term-care facilities. The rule was under development for a number of years and has been delayed by contentions in Congress and in the industry that research was insufficient to support the rule and that the industry was making progress on its own. The rule covers all "manual handling jobs" in which a core element of the job requires forceful lifting or lowering, pushing, pulling, and carrying and explicitly includes patient-handling jobs such as those held by nurse aides in long-term-care settings. It requires facilities to set up a comprehensive ergonomics program for each job covered and specifies six elements that the program must contain, including special training and job hazard analysis and control. OSHA has estimated the costs of implementation at an average of $700 per establishment covered by the rule or $150 per job covered, but there are fears that the real cost to facilities will be significantly higher. Both the cost estimates and the potential effectiveness of the rule in reducing workplace injuries are controversial, but the potential for a significant impact exists in any case.

Advocates of the labor perspective on staffing in long-term care attempt to improve working conditions for direct-care staff, an endeavor that all would agree is worthwhile and necessary. However, as appealing as the idea may be, implementation is complex. It is unclear whether current efforts will actually succeed in improving the working environment for direct-care staff and what effect any improvements will have on the quantity and quality of staff available in RC/AL settings.

The Management Perspective

Although the challenges of identifying and maintaining quality staff cannot be overestimated, there are facilities that have successfully maintained a sufficient complement of competent staff. RC/AL providers who have successfully built a team of committed caregivers attribute much of their success to the groundwork involved in effective hiring and instilling a sense of value into staff positions.

Strategies to Identify Qualified Staff

The first problem facilities face is the recruitment of staff to fill personnel shortages. It is thought that long-term-care settings make this problem worse by underselling the nursing assistant job and the quality of the facility as a setting in which to work. Facilities do not highlight, for example, that workers will learn about health care—a benefit that is not common to other jobs open to applicants with the same level of education and skills. Therefore, a management strategy to recruit good staff is to market the facility as a place that offers opportunities for meaningful and caring work (ICLTC, 1997).

Hiring is further complicated because the importance of personnel selection to organizational performance is often overlooked, especially when the options for hiring good staff are few. Certain personality traits (such as flexibility, empathy, and warmth) are considered important for RC/AL workers, but little has been written regarding how to assess such characteristics or examine them against job performance. Instead, hiring decisions tend to be based on perceptions of these qualities, which offers no guarantee of hiring a quality employee. Because personality, intelligence, and communication skills are likely to affect job performance, staff-resident relations, overall satisfaction, and longevity, some administrators have taken to using situational tests during the hiring process. Applicants are asked to respond to standardized hypothetical incidents in critical performance areas. Questions such as "What would you do if a resident hit you? How do you bathe a resistive resident?" and "What do you do when a resident wanders?" are used to assist in determining an applicant's experience and ability to work in a setting embracing the philosophy of RC/AL.

Strategies to Retain Staff

No matter the field, an important contributor to staff retention is valuing the employee and communicating that worth to him or her. Traditionally, mechanisms to convey value are largely reliant on increased compensation or promotion, or both; RC/AL is handicapped in this regard by limited financial resources and limited upward mobility. Pay raises are few, and promotions and career paths are constricted unless the setting is operated by a large corporation. In RC/AL, social and other nonmonetary rewards (such as recognizing an "employee of the month") and ongoing worker education convey value and are associated with reduced staff turnover (ICLTC, 1997).

Nurse assistants' motivations for working in long-term care are usually humanitarian in nature; they value the chance to contribute and to gain a sense of meaning (ICLTC, 1997). Evidence exists that when aides are enabled to provide care with which they themselves are satisfied, they become committed caregivers and committed employees (Brannon & Smyer, 1994). Structural changes in lateral and vertical communication systems are often recommended to provide clarity about how one's work fits with the organizational mission and to provide a sense of empowerment; prominent among these changes are continuous quality-management programs, such as Total Quality Management (TQM). TQM uses the frontline expertise of aides to identify and correct problems; it empowers them to change the organization's system of providing care. Short-term gains are increased morale, higher staff retention, and happier residents (Ceol, 1993). In other areas, efforts have been made to improve the effectiveness of the nurse aide's role through adjustments in job design, including lateralization into skill or functional areas, and vertical specialization, creating career ladders. Evaluation of the vertical specialization strategies has been scarce but positive in terms of reduced turnover (Brannon & Smyer, 1994).

Nurse aides attribute job dissatisfaction to negative peer attitudes, lack of assistance with heavy-care residents, and not being valued by the professional nursing staff; a lack of proper equipment also hinders their ability to perform their duties in a timely fashion (ICLTC, 1998). Four factors are highlighted as relating to worker burnout: (1) lack of time to complete basic tasks, (2) staff shortages that increase the workload, (3) lack of training on how to deal with stressful situations such as aggressive residents or the death of a patient, and (4) lack of good supervision (Brannon & Smyer, 1994; ICLTC, 1997). Indeed, supervision of aides is frequently an ill-defined responsibility, and only a minority of long-term-care managers have been trained in the roles and skills of managing people and processes (Yee, 1994). Attending to all of these areas is likely to increase retention.

Despite the many recommendations to increase staff satisfaction and retention, and despite the fact that many facilities are successful in these areas, recommendations are far from a solution. Hiring qualified staff assumes a qualified pool of applicants, and retaining staff assumes the ability to provide real incentives (including financial) and reduce real problems (including the risk of injury). Thus, the success of the management perspective in addressing staffing needs is inextricably related to regulatory, economic, and labor strategies.

Conclusions

Clearly, there is no simple solution to the staffing problem in RC/AL. Regulations may define lower bounds for staffing ratios, staff qualifications, and staff training, but they are limited in their ability to promote quality beyond a minimal level. Efforts to increase direct-care staff wages through the reimbursement process may have a limited effect on the largely private-pay RC/AL industry. Plans to improve the working conditions of direct-care staff are difficult to implement and may be very costly. Management strategies to recruit and retain workers, such as restructuring personnel, are somewhat limited by the economic environment in which they operate. However, each of these approaches offers some progress, and perhaps in combination they can result in an amelioration of the staffing situation in RC/AL.

Regardless of government policies, the industry itself will have to continue to look for ways to ensure adequate staffing and guarantee the quality of care the residents expect and deserve. Even in this competitive economic environment, many facilities manage to attract and retain qualified and dedicated staff. Other facilities may learn from the staffing patterns and strategies of the highest-quality facilities; perhaps an industry-based exchange of staffing data and best practices could benefit the RC/AL industry and ultimately benefit the residents they serve. A combination of industry initiatives and government policies is clearly the best hope for solving the problem. The problem is complex, and staffing promises to remain one of the important challenges facing the RC/AL industry in years to come.

Acknowledgment

The author thanks Andrea Shiffman Tuttle, M.S.W., University of North Carolina at Chapel Hill, and Barbara Shoemaker, Marketing Director, ALFA University, for their contributions to the management perspective presented in this chapter.

References

Brannon, D., & Smyer, M. A. 1994. Good work and good care in nursing homes. *Generations* 18 (3): 34–39.

Ceol, D. W. 1993. Total quality management. *Provider* 19 (9): 34–38.

Illinois Council on Long-Term-Care. 1997. Addressing the challenge of retaining nursing aides. *Close Up.* <http://www.nursinghome.org/closeup/cupdocuments/cu218.htm>, December 29, 2000.

———. 1998. CNA recruitment and retention. *Close Up.* <http://www.nursinghome.org/closeup/cupdocuments/cu279.htm>, December 29, 2000.

Mollica, R. L. 1998. *State Assisted Living Policy, 1998.* Portland, ME: National Academy for State Health Policy.

National Center for Assisted Living. 1998. *Facts and Trends: The Assisted Living Sourcebook, 1998.* Washington, DC: American Health Care Association.

———. 2000. *Assisted Living State Regulatory Review, 2000.* Washington, DC: American Health Care Association.

North Carolina Division of Facility Services. 1999. *Comparing State Efforts to Address the Recruitment and Retention of Nurse Aide and Other Paraprofessional Aide Workers.* Raleigh: North Carolina Division of Facility Services.

Occupational Safety and Health Administration. 2000. *Ergonomics Standard.* <http://www.osha-slc.gov>, April 22, 2000.

Service Employees International Union. 2000. *Dignity, Rights, and Respect: The SEIU Nursing Home Campaign.* <http://www.seiu.org>, April 22, 2000.

U.S. Congress, General Accounting Office. 1999. *Assisted Living: Quality-of-Care and Consumer Protection Issues in Four States.* GAO-HEHS-99-27. Washington, DC: General Accounting Office.

U.S. Department of Labor. 2000a. *Number of Cases and Incidence Rates of Non-*

fatal Occupation Injuries for Private Industries with 100,000 or More Cases, 1998. <http://www.dol.gov>, April 22, 2000.

————. 2000b. *Fastest Growing Occupations Covered in the 2000–01 Occupational Handbook, 1998–2008.* <http://www.dol.gov>, April 22, 2000.

Yee, D. L. 1994. Will new settings offer better work environments for para-professionals? *Generations* 18 (3): 59–65.

5 African American Use of Residential Care in North Carolina

Elizabeth J. Mutran, Ph.D., S. Sudha, Ph.D., Peter S. Reed, M.P.H., Manoj Menon, M.P.H., and Tejas Desai, M.S.

Little is known regarding the use of long-term-care facilities by African Americans other than a few simple facts. First, it is well documented that African Americans use nursing homes less than whites (Belgrave, Wykle & Choi, 1993; Greene & Ondrich, 1990; Hing, 1987; Kemper & Murtaugh, 1991; Mui & Burnette, 1994; Salive et al., 1993; Smith, 1993; Wallace et al., 1997). Second, this lower use of nursing facilities by minorities is not the result of a lower need for care. Several studies have found that despite greater disability, elderly African Americans were placed in nursing homes at between one-half and three-quarters the rate of elderly whites, and that they underused services that could improve quality of care (Belgrave, Wykle & Choi, 1993; Greene & Ondrich, 1990; Hing, 1987; Smith, 1993). Mui and Burnette (1994) wrote that whereas whites used more in-home and nursing home services, minorities used more informal helpers. Wallace and colleagues reported similar findings in 1997, demonstrating that African American frail adults with three to five dependencies in activities of daily living were more likely to use unpaid home care or no care than were whites with the same dependency level. They also found that only one-third of African Americans with such limitations were in nursing homes, while more than one-half of whites with similar limitations were using such facilities. Unpaid home care was the sole source of assistance for approximately 45 percent of African Americans who needed care, with less than one-third of whites using only unpaid help.

In addition, it is known that a change in usage is occurring. For the past few decades, the African American rate of long-term-care use has been gradually converging with that of whites. Burr (1990) suggests that this may be due to increased African American participation in government programs such as Medicaid and Medicare. According to the National Center for Health Statistics (Brooks, 1996), the concentration of

African Americans in skilled nursing facilities has been steadily increasing, growing 65 percent from 1974 to 1985, whereas white use appears stable. Though white seniors of both sexes have higher rates of institutionalization, evidence suggests that use by African American men and women is increasing relative to their white counterparts (Burr, 1990).

If this trend is witnessed in skilled nursing facilities, what can be said about African American use of residential care? This is a system of care that serves populations unable to live in a completely independent manner, who need help with personal care but are not in need of skilled services. Rates of institutionalized care utilized by the U.S. Census to assess use sometimes blur the distinction between types of homes (Pynoos & Golant, 1996), but residential care facilities are indeed distinct types of living arrangements. The type of housing called "board and care" (also known as adult-care homes, domiciliary care homes, small congregate homes, or shared housing) forms one specific and rapidly growing segment of these alternate facilities. North Carolina has more than the national average number of these facilities and has fewer than the average number of nursing homes, with a distinctive reliance on the former as a substitute for the latter (Bolda, 1991). North Carolina refers to these facilities as adult care. Homes with less than seven residents are designated as *family care homes*, and larger homes are termed *homes for the aged*. They offer congregate meals and generally shared rooms. At the time the data presented in this chapter were collected (1994), neither Medicare nor Medicaid paid for residents of these homes, although some assistance was available from a state fund for the medically needy.

Little is known about racial differences in the use of such homes. One recent study compared small board-and-care homes that provided a familial care setting in Cleveland and Baltimore (Morgan, Eckert & Lyon, 1995). The study found that the facilities differed by the race of the operator. Homes that were owned and operated by African Americans were smaller, had more shared space, charged lower fees, and had lower profits. They also tended to have a slightly more racially diverse clientele, although in general, homes served residents of a particular racial group, typically matching that of the operator. However, the study also found similarities across homes operated by African Americans and whites on key interpersonal and service dimensions. These included the level of service provision, the social or support networks of operators and residents, operator attitudes about the burden of caregiving, motivations of altruism and service provision rather than profit-making, and an emphasis on a family atmosphere. These similarities may be due to the study's focus on the smaller homes. Though the study did assess resident satisfaction, concluding that residents were on the whole satisfied with their living situation and that there was a good fit between needs and service provisions, there was little discussion of racial differences in this dimension.

It is not clear whether such findings are noted in other states. The situation is complicated by the variation from state to state in the definition and regulation of these homes. Thus, generalizing findings from one state to another is problematic. There is little research regarding the existence and quality of racially separate residential care. Nonetheless, there are proposed explanations as to why facilities may be susceptible to providing services exclusively to one racial group. Nursing homes may have higher racial integration as a result of nondiscrimination policies of Medicaid and Medicare certification, but this is not true of residential care facilities. Residential care costs are often not paid by these federal programs, placing ability to pay as a primary contributor to use. The majority of such care is financed through a combination of savings, personal income, and Social Security Disability Income payments (Hawes et al., 1993; Mor, Sherwood & Gutkin, 1986; Namazi et al., 1989). Due to disparities in level of income and resources, this may create a situation in which African Americans cannot afford to be placed in the same facilities as whites. In addition to economic considerations, size may play a role in racial separation of residential care. Most adult-care homes are small, which may enable specialization by race (Dittmar, 1989; Mor, Sherwood & Gutkin, 1986).

The key issues involved in the assessment of the role of race in the field of residential care are (1) attitudes toward residential care, (2) willingness to use residential care, (3) separation by race, (4) access to care, and (5) differences in the quality of residential care. The study discussed here adds to current knowledge of race vis-à-vis residential care by studying a sample of elderly persons living in the community, their caregivers, and a group of elderly persons residing in adult-care homes. The study examined the community dwellers' attitudes toward living in an adult-care home versus being cared for by family. It also observed the organization of care and satisfaction with care among adult-care homes.

The Conceptual Framework: Attitudes toward Rest Home Use

Researchers who have examined differences in use of services by racial groups usually investigate either the economic factors that limit use or speculate on the differences in values or cultures among racial groups regarding family care. Researchers highlighting racial and ethnic differences between the *use* of long-term care and the *need* for care have speculated that attitudes toward care influence the placement of elderly persons (Mui & Burnette, 1994; Mutran & Ferraro, 1988). Cultural explanations are often invoked as the reason for differential use, but this is often assumed rather than demonstrated (Belgrave, Wykle & Choi, 1993). Lee, Peek, and Coward (1998) were able to establish a cultural difference between racial groups, showing that aged African Americans regarded assistance from their children as more normative than did aged white parents. Although Kelley (1994) reported that African American caregivers believed it was their duty and obligation to care for their elders at home and that using formal services could be considered a failure, this was not contrasted to white caregivers' views. There has been an increased call recently for studies of racial variation in attitudes toward long-term care (Tennstedt & Chang, 1998; Wallace et al., 1998).

Most of the studies considering attitudes treat them as if they were static and unvarying over generations. This approach ignores social causation of attitudes and does not allow for social change. Yet if any social change is occurring, it is more likely to be reflected in the views of the younger generation. With seniors often placed in institutions by people other than themselves, it is the view of the younger generation toward residential care that may influence the actual use of such facilities by elders. It may be that racial differences in attitudes toward service use are converging among the younger generation or among the caregivers of elderly persons, a possibility that was investigated in the study presented here. The study used a conceptual model of attitudes toward service use that allowed consideration of the social causation of attitudes, examining how race and socioeconomic status could affect both attitudes toward and use of services (Sudha & Mutran, 1999).

Description of the Adult-Care Home Study

Research Questions

This chapter addresses three areas dealing with adult-care homes, one type of residential care facility. First, it asks whether African American and white elderly persons are equally willing to consider using an adult-care home. Second, it asks whether African American and white adult family members are equally willing to consider placing their elderly relatives in such a facility. Third, it looks at a sample of adult-care homes and describes the diversity or lack of diversity found in the racial composition of the homes. Diversity or the lack thereof may affect the home in which the elderly person is placed. These issues were addressed using data collected between 1994 and 1997 as part of a study on adult-care homes in North Carolina.

Sample: Community Dwellers and Their Caregivers

Counties in North Carolina with a minority population of at least 10 percent, a population size greater than 50,000, and at least five family-care homes and two homes for the aged formed the sampling frame for the study. Twenty-nine of one hundred counties met these eligibility criteria. The counties were divided into four strata (urban high-minority, rural high-minority, urban low-minority, and rural low-minority) based on the size of the total population and the percent of minority population. *Urban* referred to counties with populations greater than 100,000, and *rural* described counties with a lower population. Low-minority counties were those where the minority population was less than 19 percent. From these four strata, a sample of four counties was randomly selected from each urban stratum, as well as a random sample of six counties from each rural stratum, yielding a total of twenty counties.

The study had two parallel components. One addressed family caregiving in the community, and one examined many similar issues for residents of adult-care homes. The community sample was used to answer the first two questions of the study and the residential sample to address the third. To develop the community sample, persons age 65 and over were randomly selected from the twenty sampled counties using the Medicare Beneficiary Utilization tape of the Health Care Financing Administration (HCFA). A total of 4,236 elderly persons were randomly identified from the HCFA tape; however, approximately 21 percent could not be located despite repeated attempts. Of the remaining 3,332 persons, 411 persons (12%) refused to be screened for eligibility. The remainder were screened to be sure they were residing in the community (i.e., not in any adult-care facility) and were frail (i.e., had some difficulty performing one or more activities of daily living or instrumental activities of daily living). A further 2,069 did not meet these two criteria, had moved, or were deceased. This resulted in a pool of 852 persons from which a final sample was drawn. Of these, 683 individuals were randomly selected to meet the target sample size, with oversampling of African Americans; eight persons refused to participate further. The remainder were administered the Short Portable Mental Status Questionnaire; of these, 138 were unable to complete the questionnaire because of mental incompetence or physical frailty. Thus, 537 elderly persons remained who were eligible and willing to be interviewed over the telephone and included in analysis, reflecting a response rate of approximately 79 percent of the target sample. This group included 283 African Americans and 254 whites.

The caregivers of the frail seniors were also interviewed. All caregivers of the original sample of 683 elderly persons were eligible to participate in the study. The caregivers were identified in one of two ways. The elderly person was asked to identify his or her primary caregiver during the screening call; if the call to the home revealed that the elderly person was unable to communicate, the interviewer asked to speak to the caregiver and to identify that person's relationship to the older person. There were 108 frail elders who did not have family caregivers. Thirty-six caregivers refused, 7 caregivers had problems in communicating, and in 12 instances the elderly person refused to give the name of the caregiver. Out of 683 possible caregivers, 361 caregivers were interviewed whose care recipient had also been interviewed. In addition, 146 caregivers of those elders who were unable to or refused to participate were interviewed. This gave a response rate of about 74 percent among eligible caregivers. Analyses were conducted on 492 caregivers (265 African Americans and 227 whites).

Elderly people and caregivers were asked similar questions in separate survey questionnaires, and their answers were analyzed separately. These data were used to answer the questions of whether African American and white elders were equally willing to consider using an adult-care home and whether African American and white adult caregivers were equally willing to consider placing their elder in such a home. It was expected that the caregivers would be more willing to consider this option than elders would be.

Sample: Adult-Care Homes and Their Residents

To study racial issues in these homes, adult-care homes in the twenty selected counties were alphabetized in two separate lists. One list was of the homes with fewer than seven residents (family-care homes); the other was of the larger homes (homes for the aged). The homes were listed alphabetically within the alphabetized counties. Each list of homes was numbered 1 to N, where N = the number of homes within each randomly selected county. The Proc Plan procedure of the statistical package SAS was used to randomly generate N numbers for both types of homes within each county. The first three numbers generated for each type of home were used to select the family-care homes and homes for the aged by matching the corresponding numbers to the alphabetized list. An alternate list was also generated. This list would be used in the event that the first list was not sufficient to achieve the desired sample size of 350 residents in family-care homes and 350 residents in adult-care homes, each having 175 of each racial group. This proved to be the case, as only the desired sample size of whites in homes for the aged was reached at the end of the first list. To achieve the desired sample size of African Americans in homes for the aged, as well as the sample of both races in family-care homes, it was necessary to approach the homes on the second list. Homes were approached in accordance with their order on the list. Only high-minority homes for the aged (defined as having over 60% African American residents) were approached from the alternate list, since the target sample size for whites had already been reached. It was necessary to use only the first three counties on the alternate list to complete the sample for the larger homes. These three counties were urban low-minority counties. Fifty-seven homes for the aged and 135 family-care homes were approached as a result of the sampling procedure, with a total of 40 homes for the aged and 106 family-care homes agreeing to participate. The overall recruitment rate was 76 percent (70% of the homes for the aged and 79% of the family-care homes).

In the family-care homes, all residents age 65 and over were eligible to participate. In each of the homes for the aged, a list of all residents age 65 and over was generated and a random selection was made. To provide a more meaningful sample for the purpose of this study, African Americans were intentionally overrepresented. In addition, the Short Portable Mental Status Questionnaire (Pfeiffer, 1975) was administered to those who were physically able to communicate and willing to participate. Based on a cutoff point of four correct responses to ten questions, 386 respondents met the criterion for mental competence. Three hundred fifty-five completed the questionnaire. Ninety-three percent of the sampled residents in homes for the aged and 96 percent of those in family-care homes agreed to be in the study.

Responsible parties were identified either from the records of the homes or with help from the resident or administrator. The term *responsible parties* was used because for some residents the responsible party was the adult home specialist or a legal guardian. Such responsible parties were limited in their knowledge on some issues concerning the care and placement of the resident. Eighty-seven percent of all responsible parties agreed to be interviewed.

Measuring Attitudes toward Adult-Care Homes

This study used nine items to assess the desire for home care versus acceptance of long-term rest home care (a more colloquial name for adult-care home). Exploratory factor analysis was used to investigate the underlying factor structure of these items, and three dimensions were found. One dimension was a positive attitude toward family care; a second dimension was a negative attitude toward rest home care; a third dimension was the unwillingness or willingness to consider placement in a rest home. A positive attitude toward family care was measured by four similarly worded items administered to both elderly persons and caregivers. The items asked persons to agree or disagree with the following statements: "Homes are for people with no family," "Elderly people are always better off with family or friends than in rest homes," "Adult children should have to care for elderly parents," and "If family loved you, they would never place you in a rest home." A higher score on the construct indicated greater preference for family care.

For the negative attitude toward rest homes, four similarly worded statements for the elderly person and for the caregiver were again used. The items included "I would rather die than go to a rest home" or, if speaking to the caregiver, "I would rather the elderly person die than go to a rest home" (reverse coded for consistent direction with the other items); "Rest homes are pleasant places" (reverse coded); "Homes are where people go to die"; and "People in homes are lonely and depressed" (reverse coded). Higher scores on this construct indicated a more negative perception of rest homes. This factor structure and the item loadings were tested to see whether they were the same for African Americans as for whites. Using confirmatory factor analysis, it was concluded that the items worked equally well with both groups. The fact that the measurement model was statistically equivalent for both racial groups suggests that the process of attitude formation is similar for these two groups and for both caregivers and elders.

The third construct, unwillingness to enter a rest home, was measured by a single item with a three-point response scale among elderly persons and a dichotomous response among caregivers. Seniors were asked if "it would be OK with you to go to a rest home," with responses of *yes, somewhat,* and *no.* Caregivers were asked if "it would be OK with you for the elderly person [in your care] to go to a rest home," with responses of *yes* or *no.* Coding of these responses for analysis led to examining unwillingness to enter a rest home (for elderly persons) or to place an elderly person in one (caregivers).

Data Analysis

The research questions were investigated by conducting separate analyses of attitudes toward rest homes (adult-care homes) among elderly persons living in the community and their caregivers. The analysis specifically focused on racial contrasts in attitudes and determinants of attitudes, using multivariate statistical techniques. Characteristics of the sample of adult-care homes and of the residents of those homes were also described. Information on all homes in the selected counties was used in constructing weights for the sampled homes for the analysis describing the differences in residents in the different types of homes. The weights took into account the probability a given home was selected from all homes in the county and the probability a given person was selected, given the home's selection. In addition, whether African Americans and whites were indeed using different facilities was investigated, and the implications of the findings for the quality of care being received by members of different racial groups was considered.

Willingness to Use Adult-Care Homes:
Elders' and Caregivers' Attitudes

Results

Table 5.1 gives the descriptive characteristics of the frail elders living in the community and their caregivers. African American and white frail elders living in the community were similar in age, gender, self-rating of health, and number of medical conditions. The mean age of the elders was approximately 76 years, and 70–76 percent of the frail elders living in the community were female. In terms of their health, approximately 65 percent rated their health as fair or poor rather than excellent or good, and they experienced an average of four medical conditions.

On many other variables there were significant differences between African American and white elders living in the community as frail individuals. Many of the disadvantages of minority populations were reflected, with African American seniors being less educated and having fewer economic resources. Fewer were married and fewer had children. Perhaps as a consequence of disadvantaged socioeconomic status, African American elders had more difficulty performing the activities of daily living as well as the instrumental activities of daily life, such as shopping or getting out and about. Despite some studies showing that African Americans feel they can expect help from their families (Kelley, 1994), this group of African American elders received less help from their family ties than whites received. Frail African American elders also had less paid help (21% vs. 30% for whites). The church was the one source of support in which African Americans fared better than whites, with 24 percent receiving help from their church, whereas only 16 percent of whites had such help.

In terms of the type of preferred care, these older racial groups did not differ in their willingness to consider using adult-care homes; however, they differed in the reasons why. Older African Americans strongly favored care by their family members, while white elders felt a comparatively greater dislike of adult-care homes.

Turning to a description of African American and white caregivers, reported in the last two columns of table 5.1, African American and white caregivers, like the elders themselves, were alike in age and in their self-rating of health. The caregivers were also equally likely to be free of impairments that limited their activities. Caregivers averaged 49–51 years of age, and approximately 20 percent rated their health as fair or poor. The

Table 5.1. Descriptive Statistics: Means or Proportions Reporting Various Characteristics

	Elderly Persons		Caregivers	
	White (N = 254)	African American (N = 283)	White (N = 137)	African American (N = 181)
Demographics				
Age	75.62	75.76	51.10	49.28
Proportion male	0.30	0.24	0.29*	0.19
Proportion currently married	0.43**	0.31	0.64***	0.39
Proportion with children	0.76***	0.63	0.40	0.48
Proportion with other relatives residing within an hour's drive	0.60**	0.73		
Proportion high school graduates	0.50***	0.28	0.85	0.79
Proportion financially needy	0.03***	0.25	0.18***	0.52
Proportion reporting friend or family member ever stayed in rest home	0.84***	0.53	0.75***	0.51
Health status				
Self-perceived health status (fair/poor)	0.63	0.68	0.17	0.22
ADL/IADL[a] dependency score (elderly persons); activity-limiting conditions (caregivers)	11.69*	13.39	0.27	0.25
Number of self-reported medical conditions	3.98	3.94	—	—
Number of elders' medical conditions reported by caregivers	—	—	4.53*	4.05
Caregiving situation				
Caregiver feels hardship/stress taking care of elder	—	—	2.13**	1.65
Negative effect on caregiver's life	—	—	2.99***	2.06
Someone shares caregiving	—	—	0.39	0.40

(continued)

Table 5.1. (*Continued*)

	Elderly Persons		Caregivers	
	White (N = 254)	African American (N = 283)	White (N = 137)	African American (N = 181)
Proportion with duration of care ≥5 years	—	—	0.55	0.63
Care recipient's ADL score	—	—	4.60**	5.72
Needs help taking care of elderly person	—	—	0.27	0.25
Receives care from				
Friends	0.25	0.25	—	—
Church	0.16*	0.24	—	—
Paid caregiver	0.30*	0.21	—	—
Family	0.75*	0.68	—	—
Attitude				
Dislikes rest homes	10.94***	9.56	9.77*	9.08
Likes family care	10.55***	11.56	9.88***	11.15
Unwilling to use rest home care	1.88	1.95	0.48	0.41

Note: ADL = activity of daily living; IADL = instrumental activity of daily living.
*$p < .05$ across racial groups
**$p < .01$ across racial groups
***$p < .001$ across racial groups

caregivers were also alike in the percent having children, but other measures distinguished African American and white caregivers. Most caregivers were women, but this was especially true among African Americans (81% vs. 71% for whites). A larger percentage of white elders had male caregivers than did African Americans. Among caregivers as a whole, only a little more than half were married, but this was more often the case among whites than among African Americans (39% vs. 64% for whites). Also, African American and white caregivers, like their elders, differed in terms of socioeconomic status. African American caregivers were considerably more likely to be financially needy, resembling North Carolina's percentage of minority elders below poverty levels.

About 75 percent of whites were likely to have had someone close to them use a rest home, whereas only about 50 percent of African Americans had had that experience. Both groups were equally likely to have someone share caregiving tasks with them, and the majority of both groups did not need additional help. White caregivers were assisting elders with multiple health problems, but African American caregivers were assisting elders who were functionally more limited in the activities of daily living and instrumental activities. The caregivers also differed in their perceptions of how caregiving affected their lives. White caregivers, more often than African American caregivers, reported that their lives were negatively affected by caregiving and that they felt more stress. In terms of preference for care, the pattern among caregivers was the same as among the frail elders themselves.

The relationship between race and preference for family care, or race and dislike of adult-care homes, called for further investigation. Given the different socioeconomic backgrounds and resources of the two groups, one must question whether the relationship between race and attitudes toward source of care exists after controlling for these differences. A second possibility is that some variables have a stronger influence on the preferences of one racial group than on the other. In other words, there may be some statistical interaction effects. To answer the first question, the preference for family care was regressed on the other variables listed in table 5.1, and dislike of rest homes was regressed on the same set of variables with the omission of preference for family care. The relationships were modeled so that preference for family care, the most commonly preferred choice of care, was predicted in part by dislike of rest homes. The entire set of variables was then used to predict the willingness to use rest homes. Although the results of the regressions are not presented here (see Sudha and Mutran, 1999, for further details), the findings are discussed below. To answer the second question regarding whether race moderated or altered the effects of some variables on the preference for family care, the dislike of rest homes, or the willingness to use rest homes, two methods of examining statistical interactions were used. These included t-tests for the differences in slopes of separate equations for African Americans and whites and a linear structural equation approach. These methods did not reveal any statistical interactions. The regression slopes were similar for both groups.

Discussion

Frail older African Americans prefer family care more than do whites, and frail older whites dislike rest home care more than do African Americans. Multivariate analysis indicated that the white preference for family care appears indirect, operating through a dislike of more formal residential care. Older African Americans prefer family care but do not exhibit a strong dislike of residential care. Other characteristics that contributed to a feeling that families should be the source of care include older age, being male, being in poor health, and having less than a high school education. Very little besides being white is related to a strong dislike of rest homes. One variable, having help from church members, contributes to more positive feelings toward this type of residential care. There are several possible explanations for this finding. It could be measurement error; for example, social desirability might affect those who were most engaged in religion. Also, religious persons might not be as condemnatory of others. In addition, it might be that church members work to help those who have no family. Overall, the unwillingness of elderly persons to use a rest home was influenced by differences in preference toward family care and negative views of the adult-care homes themselves.

The regression analyses also showed that, like frail older persons, white caregivers disliked adult-care homes more than African American caregivers; however, the preference for family care was only marginally different, with African Americans preferring family help only slightly more. Those who felt stress in caregiving were less favorable toward family care than those who felt less stress. The major association seen in the caregiver data is the strong correlation between dislike of adult-care homes and a preference for family care. In terms of identifying who might dislike adult-care homes, other than on the basis of race, caregivers who were economically needy disliked rest homes, whereas those caring for frail persons with multiple health problems had more favorable views.

Were caregivers in this study, regardless of race, equally willing or unwilling to use residential care? The answer was yes: the unwillingness to use adult-care homes was associated primarily with the degree to which the caregiver felt negative toward such facilities and also with being male, with caring for a senior with multiple health problems, and, to some extent, with being more educated. Racial group membership did not have a significant impact on caregivers' willingness or unwillingness to use residential care.

Adult-Care Homes and Their Residents: Different Rest Home Facilities for Whites and African Americans?

Results

As African Americans increase their use of residential care, it is important to look specifically at the facilities that they use, and ask whether they are the same facilities as those used by whites. It is also important to evaluate the potential impact of separate facilities on the care received by residents. This section describes the findings of the North Carolina (NC) Adult Care Home Study concerning the existence of racially separated homes. It also describes the varying characteristics of the racially distinct residential care facilities. Finally, differences in satisfaction with the care received by residents of African American facilities and those of white facilities are discussed.

A major goal of the NC Adult Care Home Study was to determine whether racial diversity existed within the residential care facilities or whether the facilities were racially separate. This is a different issue than the rate of use, focusing on which homes older persons actually enter once the decision is made. The results confirmed the lack of racial diversity among recipients of residential care: the great majority, 128 of 146 homes surveyed (88%) exhibited a resident population that was either at least two-thirds white or at least two-thirds African American. In the predominantly white facilities, 93 percent of the residents were white. There were 80 such homes in the study, with a total resident population of 1,146 persons; only 80 (7%) were African American. In predominantly African American facilities, 92 percent of the residents were African American. There were 48 such facilities in the study, housing 461 residents with only 35 (8%) whites. Of the 18 homes that were not predominantly white or African American, 50–64 percent of residents were either African American (13 facilities) or white (5 facilities). Such figures clearly show that, at least for this sample, there is a definite division between white and African American residential care facilities.

There were 40 large homes in the study and 106 smaller homes. The larger homes were predominantly white facilities (60%). Only 9 (22%) of the larger homes served mostly African Americans. Eighteen percent served persons of both racial groups. The larger white homes had higher monthly charges, at $1,468 per month, in comparison to the larger African American homes, which charged an average of $1,180 per month. The rate of pay for the more racially integrated homes was at an intermediate level. Of the 106 family-care homes, 53 percent were white and 37 percent African American. The remaining 10 percent were not classified as white or African American homes. The mean monthly rate for a family-care home was $1,065 for a white home and $984 for an African American home.

White and African American homes were distinct in several other ways. African American homes typically housed a higher proportion of males, whether in homes for the aged or in family-care homes. On average, white homes had less than 20 percent male residents. The larger African American homes had 55 percent male residents, and on average the smaller homes had 33 percent male residents. The residents of white and African American homes also differed in their relationship with the next of kin and source of payment. Fifty-seven percent of the white residents had a spouse or a child listed in their records as the next of kin. Only 36 percent of the African Americans had as close a relative listed as the next of kin. This may reflect the facts that African Americans are more likely to care for their relatives at home, and placement is more likely when there is a shortage of close family members. White homes had a larger proportion of residents paying privately (60%). In comparison, only 10 percent of African Americans pay privately. This difference in source of payment also reflects the amount of resources available to the home, since private-pay residents traditionally help subsidize the care of those receiving public funds.

Most health indicators did not significantly differ across homes, although there were a few differences in clientele with limitations in activities of daily living at the time of admission. As shown in table 5.2, a larger percentage of residents in African American homes needed assistance in dressing and personal hygiene. Once an older person and her or his family or responsible party started looking for placement, different issues emerged. African Americans reported encountering more difficulties in finding a home because of the behavioral problems of the elder. As a result, African American homes were significantly more likely to house residents who had these problems. Residents of white homes were more likely to report difficulty in finding a home they liked.

Table 5.2. Percentage of Residents Needing Assistance
with Selected Activities at Time of Admission

	White Homes	African American Homes
Bathing	60.1%	61.5%
Dressing	30.2**	45.5
Toileting	13.8	25.1
Hair grooming	37.1	52.4
Skin care	32.5*	48.5
Shaving	19.7**	44.2
Mouth care	21.3**	43.3
Getting in or out of bed	11.8	23.8
Ambulation	18.6	22.8
Feeding	4.8	11.8

*$p < .05$ across homes
**$p < .01$ across homes

Table 5.3. Mean Satisfaction Rating of Residents in Family-Care Homes
and Homes for the Aged, by Site and Race

	Family-Care Homes		Homes for the Aged	
	White	African American	White	African American
Most people living here get best possible care	3.56	3.49	3.57	2.57***
I am getting all the care I need	3.62	3.60	3.61	2.19***
The staff gives me enough attention	3.53	3.67*	3.48	2.52***
The staff spends as much time as necessary with me	3.42	3.60*	3.28	2.62***
The staff here goes out of their way to be nice	3.56	3.36*	3.43	2.44***

Note: Satisfaction: 1 = not satisfied; 4 = highly satisfied.
*$p < .05$ across homes
***$p < .001$ across homes

Table 5.3 shows that there are significant differences between the level of satisfaction of residents of African American homes and those of white homes. These analyses used statistically constructed weights for the homes and examined separate satisfaction measures among residents of larger versus smaller African American and white homes. The data show a difference between family-care homes and homes for the aged. In small family-care homes, all homes show a fairly high level of resident satisfaction, but on two of the five items, residents of African American homes were significantly more satisfied in their evaluation of the care received. On one of the five indicators, white homes had a more satisfied population. These three items highlighted the commitment of the staff and the attention they give to the residents. In the larger homes for the aged, the differences in satisfaction are more pronounced. Residents of white homes were on average more satisfied with the quality of their care.

Discussion

These data suggest that the factors predicting satisfaction are sensitive to the context in which care is given. African Americans appear more amenable to the intimacy of small, family environments. White residents show comparable levels of satisfaction regardless of type of home. These findings may be explained in part by the characteristics of the homes, which were previously described. Because the family-care homes have fewer residents, perhaps there is more personal attention given to each resident and a better quality of interpersonal communication, negating the racial differences manifested in the larger facilities. It is also possible that the motivations of the caregivers and home owners or operators play a role in the amount and type of care provided to the residents of the smaller homes. In their study of small board-and-care homes (those housing eight or fewer residents, with a coresiding home operator), Morgan, Eckert, and Lyon (1995) found that the operators were motivated by a desire to help others by providing a familial care setting to elderly persons, and not by financial or profit considerations. To the extent that this may be more often the case in a smaller home, perhaps the residents not only receive better care but also perceive the care to be of high quality and thus have a higher level of satisfaction.

It can be stated, then, that once a decision to enter a facility is made, African Americans enter facilities marked by different characteristics than do whites. With this determination made, it becomes important to consider why there are racially separate facilities. One way of viewing this is in terms of the different situations impacting white and African American residents, including various demographic and social characteristics, resources, and care needs. In terms of demographic characteristics predisposing an individual to be placed in a specific facility, the NC Adult Care Home Study found that African American homes have significantly more males than do white homes. This, along with other demographic characteristics, may help to explain the differences in use. Because men in general are more likely to be cared for at home with marital partners as caregivers, the men in these homes are more likely to be those without family.

The data also suggest that costs play a role, with African American facilities serving a poorer population and African American facilities costing less than white facilities. In addition, African American facilities have a significantly higher percentage of residents who rely on state funds to pay for their care. This economic difference may translate to fewer resources for a home, which could affect staffing ratios and other structural differences. These differences may have an impact on the quality of care. Since poverty rates are higher among African Americans, it seems likely that some African Americans may be choosing a facility on the basis of lower cost; even though such facilities may provide high-quality interpersonal interaction, they may not be able to afford the same quality of meals or furnishings as more expensive homes. If it is true that the price of a facility is related to the quality of care provided, the result is that people with fewer means tend to use lower-quality facilities.

In evaluating the level of need of residents, evidence using the individual as the unit of analysis showed that there was no difference between African American and white individuals in their health and physical functioning. However, using the facility as the unit of analysis did show differences between the functioning of residents of predominantly white facilities and those of predominantly African American facilities. For example, African American facilities have residents with significantly lower mental competency scores, which is consistent with the contention that African Americans remain in the community longer. An alternate explanation is that racially different facilities are providing for different needs and thus attract a specific, racially and functionally distinct resident population.

Conclusions

African Americans' preference for family care does not go hand in hand with greater disfavor toward adult-care homes. Instead, the pattern of results suggests that minorities' attitudes toward family care and institutional care are partly determined by socioeconomic background and experiences. The preference for family care does reflect African American kinship bonds (Stoller & Rose, 1994); however, it is also in part a reflection of a perceived lack of acceptable institutional alternatives, not of a cultural predisposition to disdain institutional care. Notably, multivariate regression analyses indicated that although minority elders are more unwilling to consider entering an adult-care home, their caregivers show no racial difference in reluctance to place a senior in such a residential care facility. This shows that attitudes toward extrafamilial care might be converging over generations, but it also highlights the importance of establishing whether residential care facilities for seniors are providing appropriate and high-quality care for members of all racial groups and whether the residents are satisfied with their dwellings.

These findings on adult-care homes make it clear that there is limited diversity within residential care facilities and that this homogeneity may be associated with practical, social, and economic considerations. Correspondingly, there is diversity across facilities. It is important to understand the differences in order to ensure quality of care and remove inequalities that may be based on the race or ethnicity of the older person. Because African Americans and whites are not evenly distributed across facilities, questions concerning equal access and the process by which people choose, or are placed in, a facility remain and are in need of further research. The NC Adult Care Home Study found that different issues faced African Americans and whites once a decision was made to enter a residential care facility. For white older persons and their families, the major problem was to find a place that the elderly person liked. However, for African Americans, the major problem was to find a facility willing to admit the elderly person. This suggests that whites have a greater range of choices and the luxury of looking for a place to please the care recipient, whereas African Americans may struggle to find a place to accept the care recipient. These factors hold implications for the satisfaction of the residents.

Resident satisfaction with a facility is an established measure of the quality of care (Berwick, 1987; Clearly & McNeil, 1988). In the described study, the type of facility related to the satisfaction level of minority residents. Among residents of larger homes, those in predominantly white homes were significantly more satisfied across several dimensions, including overall care, care needed, staff attention, and courtesy. This may be due to the attention paid to finding a facility that the elder might like.

A caveat is also due here. There are several potential explanations for the differences in satisfaction with care. Differences in satisfaction may result from a preference for family care that corresponds with the comparatively higher satisfaction that African Americans feel with family-care homes. However, this explanation should be treated cautiously, for if quality-of-care differences exist, it is the resident of these homes who suffers. The assumption that homes with greater resources might provide a higher level of care than facilities with fewer resources should not be ruled out, and it should be remembered that racial composition is correlated with the cost of the facility. The provision of higher levels of care may not be due to the fact that the residents are white but due to the greater resources that white facilities have; also, African American residents have fewer close familial "responsible parties" to monitor their ongoing welfare. Morgan, Eckert, and Lyon (1995) discuss rest home organization and care in terms of the concept of social marginality, pointing out that small board-and-care homes are situated in the margin between in-home care and full-fledged nursing home care. The operators of the homes are positioned between caring for their own family members and providing impersonal professional assistance to clients. In addition, the residents are those who fall between being able to live on their own and needing skilled nursing assistance. The results of the NC Adult Care Home study suggest an added dimension to the social marginality of the minority residential care residents: African Americans who enter a residential care facility have fewer close family networks. This fact, combined with the greater problems minorities encounter in locating a facility, suggests that minority elders who do enter a residential care facility constitute a specifically vulnerable group. In the smaller homes, this vulnerability may be compensated for by greater interpersonal interaction and more individualized care provided by the operators. However, in larger homes the vulnerable residents may feel their marginality. Among this group, therefore, as stated by Brooks (1996), it may be that long-term care provided to the older people of different races is "separate and unequal."

Acknowledgment

This study was supported by Grant NR 03406 from the National Institute on Nursing Research.

References

Belgrave, L. L., Wykle, M. L., & Choi, J. M. 1993. Health, double jeopardy, and culture: The use of institutionalization by elderly African Americans. *Gerontologist* 33:379–85.

Berwick, D. M. 1987. Toward an applied technology for quality measurement in health care. *Medical Decision Making* 8:253–58.

Bolda, E. J. 1991. North Carolina domiciliary care policy: Background and issues. *Long Term Care Advances* 3:1–12.

Brooks, S. 1996. Separate and unequal. *Contemporary Long Term Care* 19:40–46.

Burr, J. A. 1990. Race/sex comparisons of elderly living arrangements: Factors influencing the institutionalization of the unmarried. *Research on Aging* 12:507–30.

Cleary, P. D., & McNeil, B. J. 1988. Patient satisfaction as an indicator of the quality of care. *Inquiry* 25:25–36.

Dittmar, N. D. 1989. Facility and resident characteristics of board and care homes for the elderly. In M. Moon, G. Gaberlavage, & S. J. Newman (eds.), *Preserving Independence, Supporting Needs: The Role of Board and Care Homes.* Washington, DC: Public Policy Institute, American Association of Retired Persons.

Greene, V. L., & Ondrich, J. I. 1990. Risk factors for nursing home admissions and exits: A discrete-time hazard function approach. *Journal of Gerontology* 45:S250–58.

Hawes, C., Wildfire, J., & Lux, L. 1993. *The Regulation of Board and Care Homes: Results of a Survey in the 50 States and the District of Columbia: National Summary.* Washington, DC: American Association of Retired Persons.

Hing, E. 1987. Use of nursing homes by the elderly: Preliminary data from the 1985 National Nursing Home Survey. National Center for Health Statistics, Advance Data No. 135, May 14. National Center for Health Statistics, Hyattsville, MD.

Kelley, J. D. 1994. African American caregivers: Perceptions of the caregiving situation and factors influencing the delay of the institutionalization of elders with dementia. *ABNF Journal,* July–August, 106–9.

Kemper, P., & Murtaugh, C. M. 1991. Lifetime use of nursing home care. *New England Journal of Medicine* 324:595–629.

Lee, G. R., Peek, C. W., & Coward, R. T. 1998. Race differences in filial responsibility expectations among older parents. *Journal of Marriage and the Family* 60:404–12.

Mor, V., Sherwood, S., & Gutkin, C. 1986. A national study of residential care for the aged. *Gerontologist* 26:405–17.

Morgan, L. A., Eckert, J. K., & Lyon, S. M. (eds.). 1995. *Small Board-and-Care Homes: Residential Care in Transition*. Baltimore: Johns Hopkins University.

Mui, A. C., & Burnette, D. 1994. Long-term care service use by frail elders: Is ethnicity a factor? *Gerontologist* 34:190–98.

Mutran, E. J., & Ferraro, K. F. 1988. Medical need and use of services among older men and women. *Journal of Gerontology: Social Sciences* 43B:S162- 71.

Namazi, K. H., Eckert, J. K., Kahana, E., & Lyon, S. M. 1989. Psychological well-being of elderly board and care home residents. *Gerontologist* 29:511– 16.

Pfeiffer, E. 1975. A short portable mental status questionnaire for the assessment of organic brain deficit in elderly patients. *Journal of the American Geriatrics Society* 23:433–41.

Pynoos, J., & Golant, S. 1996. Housing and living arrangements for the elderly. In R. H. Binstock & L. K. George (eds.), *Handbook of Aging and the Social Sciences*. 4th ed. San Diego: Academic Press.

Salive, M. E., Collins, K. S., Foley, D. J., & George, L. K. 1993. Predictors of nursing home admission in a biracial population. *American Journal of Public Health* 83:1765–67.

Smith, D. B. 1993. The racial integration of health facilities. *Journal of Health Politics, Policy, and Law* 18:851–69.

Stoller, E. P., & Rose, C. G. 1994. The diversity of American families. In E. P. Stoller & R. C. Gibson (eds.), *Worlds of Difference: Inequality in the Aging Experience*. Thousand Oaks, CA: Pine Forge Press.

Sudha, S., & Mutran, E. J. 1999. Ethnicity and eldercare: Comparison of attitudes toward adult care homes and care by families. *Research on Aging* 21:570–94.

Tennstedt, S., & Chang, B. H. 1998. The relative contribution of ethnicity versus socioeconomic status in explaining differences in disability and receipt of informal care. *Journal of Gerontology: Social Sciences* 53B:S61–70.

Wallace, S. P., Levy-Storms, L., Andersen, R. M., & Kington, R. 1997. The impact by race of changing long-term care policy. *Journal of Aging and Social Policy* 9:1–20.

Wallace, S. P., Levy-Storms, L., Kington, R. S., & Andersen, R. M. 1998. The persistence of race and ethnicity in the use of long-term care. *Journal of Gerontology: Social Sciences* 53B:S104–12.

II Diversity in Profile
Assisted Living in Four States

6 An Overview of the Collaborative Studies of Long-Term Care

Sheryl Zimmerman, Ph.D., Philip D. Sloane, M.D., M.P.H., J. Kevin Eckert, Ph.D., Verita Custis Buie, M.S., Joan F. Walsh, Ph.D., Gary Grove Koch, Ph.D., and J. Richard Hebel, Ph.D.

Despite the prevalence and diversity of residential care/assisted living (RC/AL) (see part 1), there are virtually no comparative outcome data in this area, and even less is known regarding the relationship of the structure and process of care to resident quality of life. To begin to address these issues, two grants were funded in 1996 by the National Institute on Aging: "Medical and Functional Outcomes of Residential Care" (Sheryl Zimmerman, principal investigator; J. Kevin Eckert, co–principal investigator), and "Alternatives to Nursing Home Care for Alzheimer's Disease" (Philip D. Sloane, principal investigator). In consideration of their similar goals and design, the efforts of these two grants were integrated and conducted cooperatively under the title "The Collaborative Studies of Long-Term Care" (CS-LTC).

The CS-LTC is the largest, most comprehensive study of RC/AL ever undertaken, and it is the first to examine and compare the relationship of the structure and process of care with outcomes for this population. The primary aim is to determine adverse medical outcomes, change in functional status, and health service utilization over one year and to discover how they relate to resident-level characteristics and the quality (structure and process) of care in RC/AL and nursing homes, for persons residing in RC/AL and similar persons residing in nursing homes. Between October 1997 and November 1998, CS-LTC study staff enrolled 2,839 residents and collected data on-site from 233 facilities; outcome data were collected through November 1999. A wealth of descriptive data were collected during subject enrollment and constitute the basis of part 2 of this book. These data address resident characteristics, the physical environment and process of care, aging in place, care for persons with dementia, economics and financing, and interpersonal connectedness. This chapter presents an overview of the methods of the CS-LTC, to allow the subsequent findings to be put into context.

Sampling Design

State Selection and Regional Determination

As explained in chapter 1, no national standards exist for RC/AL; state regulations differ, and RC/AL exhibits great interstate and intrastate variability. Therefore, as the CS-LTC was designed, the inclusion of multiple states was a paramount consideration. It was also necessary that they be in proximity to each other, to enable on-site data collection. After consultation with national experts, including Robert Mollica, Rosalie Kane, Catherine Hawes, and Keren Brown-Wilson; a review of state regulations; consideration of other research currently being conducted; and evaluation of logistical considerations, four states were identified that reflect the variation of this field: Florida, Maryland, New Jersey, and North Carolina. In the eastern United States, New Jersey has progressed the furthest in defining new-model RC/AL, including a provision for Medicaid funding. It is among the states with the broadest parameters for admission and retention and allows extensive services, thus enabling aging in place. Nationally, Florida contains almost 10 percent of all licensed RC/AL beds, and North Carolina has almost one-half of all RC/AL Medicaid beneficiaries. Maryland is notable in comparison because its regulations were only beginning to be developed at the inception of the CS-LTC; also, it is less penetrated by new-model RC/AL (discussed below).

To increase efficiency in data collection, a purposive sample of counties (i.e., a sampling region) was selected within each state. Data on county characteristics were obtained from the 1994 Area Resource File, the 1996 U.S. Census Website, the 1995 physician listings, and the 1996 hospital listings, as well as from lists of licensed homes in each county, to help assure the selection of a representative sampling region. The following criteria were used to select the region: (1) *the number and proportion of facilities:* each region must contain at least 15 percent of the state's RC/AL facilities of each type; (2) *rural/urban diversity:* each region must include both urban and suburban areas (defined as being in or outside of a Standard Metropolitan Statistical Area); and (3) *state representativeness:* when compared with the entire state, a proposed sampling region must fall within 30 percent of the state mean on each of eight measures listed in table 6.1. These criteria were met in all four states with one exception. North Carolina exhibited a large proportion of primary-care physicians, but on examination this excess was found to be confined to a few counties

Table 6.1. Representativeness of Collaborative Studies of Long-Term Care Sample: Regional and State Distributions of Demographic and Health-Related Variables

Demographic Variable	Region	State	Region/State
Florida			
Per capita income	$19,336	$20,650	94%
Over age 65	19.4%	18.6%	104%
Nonwhite	14.4%	16.9%	85%
Employed	49.8%	48.2%	103%
Below poverty level	12.5%	14.4%	87%
Primary-care M.D.s[a]	10.0	10.9	92%
Hospital beds[a]	25.6	22.7	113%
Nursing home beds[a]	35.8	29.6	121%
Maryland			
Per capita income	$20,743	$23,908	87%
Over age 65	11.8%	11.3%	104%
Nonwhite	34.2%	29.0%	118%
Employed	54.1%	53.4%	101%
Below poverty level	8.8%	9.9%	89%
Primary-care M.D.s[a]	28.5	26.2	109%
Hospital beds[a]	32.3	31.3	103%
Nursing home beds[a]	52.6	54.2	97%
New Jersey			
Per capita income	$27,989	$26,876	104%
Over age 65	14.3%	13.7%	104%
Nonwhite	21.1%	20.7%	102%
Employed	49.9%	50.2%	99%
Below poverty level	7.9%	9.2%	86%
Primary-care M.D.s[a]	18.0	18.1	99%
Hospital beds[a]	29.5	9.4	100%
Nursing home beds[a]	47.0	47.2	100%
North Carolina			
Per capita income	$21,494	$18,670	115%
Over age 65	11.9%	12.1%	95%
Nonwhite	21.7%	24.4%	89%
Employed	53.6%	50.2%	107%
Below poverty level	10.7%	13.0%	82%
Primary-care M.D.s[a]	27.2	14.4	189%
Hospital beds[a]	41.6	32.1	129%
Nursing home beds[a]	46.6	41.7	112%

[a]Number per thousand persons over age 65 years.

and was considered to not reflect a true lack of variation. In Florida, Maryland, and North Carolina, the sampling region consisted of two noncontiguous blocks of counties, to capture the geographic diversity within these states.

Facility Strata

The CS-LTC aimed to present a comprehensive picture of RC/AL; other studies in this subject area have been limited by an exclusive focus on smaller homes (e.g., see Morgan, Eckert & Lyon, 1995) or on other select types of facilities, such as apartment-style assisted living. To achieve broad representation, the CS-LTC defined RC/AL as facilities or discrete portions of facilities, licensed by the state at a non-nursing-home level of care, that provided room, board, twenty-four-hour oversight, and assistance with activities of daily living. Three types of RC/AL homes were then identified, all of which were studied: facilities with fewer than sixteen beds, larger homes of the traditional board-and-care type, and new-model facilities with sixteen or more beds. To arrive at an operational definition of this new model of care, 66 facilities were identified in New Jersey and Maryland, half of which were known to be new-model, based on licensure status or expert knowledge of the investigators. A telephone survey of these facilities was conducted, and the data were analyzed to determine which combination of questions yielded the highest sensitivity and specificity in identifying new-model RC/AL. Based on the results, inclusion criteria were specified: the facilities must have sixteen or more beds; must have been built after January 1, 1987; and must meet at least one of the following additional criteria: (1) at least two different private pay monthly rates, depending on resident need, (2) 20 percent or more of its resident population requiring assistance in transfer, (3) 25 percent or more of its resident population incontinent daily, or (4) either an RN or an LPN on duty at all times. It is important to recognize that the definition of *new-model* is a research construction only, permitting clarity and uniformity in data collection and interpretation; it does not necessarily represent a pure or distinct model of RC/AL.

New-model facilities constitute one stratum used in the sampling scheme. Smaller facilities (fewer than sixteen beds) were selected as a stratum because the structure and process of care in these facilities have been reported to be distinctly different from those in large facilities (e.g., smaller RC/AL facilities tend to be managed by individuals as opposed to corporations, have a higher level of operator involvement, and are more homelike) (Morgan, Eckert & Lyon, 1995). A third stratum of RC/AL ("traditional") incorporates all other facilities, those with sixteen or more beds that do not operationally subscribe to the new model, as described herein. Nursing homes served as a fourth stratum.

Facility and Resident Selection

The sampling frame consisted of all RC/AL facilities and nursing homes within each selected region. To maximize efficiency and assure an elderly sample, several additional selection criteria were applied to the facilities under study. The following types of facilities were excluded: those that primarily served persons with mental illness or developmental disability, small RC/AL facilities that housed fewer than four persons age 65 and older, large RC/AL facilities that housed fewer than ten residents age 65 and older, and nursing homes with fewer than forty residents. Exclusions based on size resulted in minimal loss to the sampling pool. Nursing homes were further stratified to reflect variation in size: nursing homes within each state were ordered by size, and homes were divided into three fractiles. Facilities were randomly selected from a stratified list of all licensed nursing homes and RC/AL facilities, provided by state departments and agencies. Within each state, nursing homes were randomly selected such that three were from the largest one-third of homes, three from the middle third, and four from the smallest one-third of homes. In reference to RC/AL facilities, because the CS-LTC aimed to equally include residents from each type of facility, more small facilities were required than others, because they house fewer residents. A total of 233 facilities were recruited from October 1997 to November 1998 (113 small, and 40 from each of the other three types).[1]

Among eligible facilities, the overall recruitment rate was 59 percent. To compare enrolled facilities with refusals, 49 nonparticipating facilities were contacted and administered forty-two questions related to facility and resident characteristics; forty-four administrators (90%) responded. Nonparticipating RC/AL facilities differed from participating facilities in three areas: they had more owners working more hours in the facility; they had more rate levels; and they housed a slightly less impaired resident population (e.g., 4.6% vs. 9.9% were chairfast, and 1.2% vs. 4.2% were unable to transfer). There were no differences in reference to proprietary status; affiliation with other long-term-care facilities; facility age, size, or occupancy rate; and resident age, ethnicity, or race. Nonparticipating nursing homes had a higher occupancy rate than participating nursing homes and less resident impairment (e.g., 53.6% vs. 65.8% were incontinent, and 4.4% vs. 24.0% were unable to transfer). There were no differences in reference to the other variables listed above.

Within each state, subjects over the age of 65 were sampled to obtain equal numbers across the strata. In nursing homes, additional eligibility criteria were applied, to selectively recruit two subgroups of subjects who were hypothesized to have relevance for RC/AL: (1) residents with dementia who required no more than supervision to transfer, ambulate, and/or eat; and (2) residents who required physical assistance to transfer, ambulate, and/or eat (but did not require physical assistance for all three activities), regardless of dementia status. The first group was thought to be similar to many current RC/AL residents. The latter group was anticipated to have fewer counterparts among current RC/AL residents, but to be rapidly growing. In facilities with fewer than sixteen beds, all eligible persons were approached to participate. In larger facilities, the target number of residents was 19 (RC/AL) or 20 (large nursing homes); in some cases these numbers were increased slightly (to 24 or 26 for new-model and traditional facilities, respectively, and 28 for nursing homes), to compensate for facilities with too few eligible residents. Residents who met the eligibility criteria were randomly selected for inclusion. Consent was obtained from residents or a significant other if the resident was unable to provide his or her own consent. A total of 2,839 residents were enrolled in the CS-LTC; 2,078 (73%) were residents of RC/AL facilities. Overall, only 8 percent of eligible residents and/or their family members refused to participate, ranging from 5 percent in smaller facilities to 11 percent in new-model facilities. Table 6.2 gives the numbers of facilities and residents in the CS-LTC sample.

The goal was to recruit a similar number of facilities across states (32 "small" and 10 of each other type, per state) and to enroll a similar number of residents across facility types and states (25% of residents from each facility type and from each state), but the numbers of facilities and subjects who actually participated deviated slightly from these quotas. Maryland provided the most "small" facilities (33 facilities, 29% of the sample), and New Jersey provided the fewest (21 facilities, 19% of the sample). In terms of resident recruitment, Maryland provided the most subjects (804

Table 6.2. Number of Facilities and Subjects Enrolled in the Collaborative Studies of Long-Term Care, per Facility Type, by State

Facility Type	Facilities	Residents	Facilities	Residents
	Florida		*Maryland*	
<16 beds	29	172	33	212
≥16 beds, traditional	10	150	10	180
≥16 beds, new-model	10	179	10	202
Nursing homes	10	169	10	210
Total	59	670	63	804
	New Jersey		*North Carolina*	
<16 beds	21	146	30	135
≥16 beds, traditional	10	163	10	155
≥16 beds, new-model	10	202	10	182
Nursing homes	10	208	10	174
Total	51	719	60	646

residents, 28% of the sample), and North Carolina provided the fewest (646 residents, 23% of the sample).

Data Collection and Instruments

Facility and resident baseline evaluations were conducted on-site. The measures used in the CS-LTC were selected, modified, or designed to assess the structure and process of RC/AL and the status of residents at the time of study recruitment and through one year of follow-up, by means of interviews and structured observation. Table 6.3 presents an overview of the key quantitative baseline measures and data sources, which are discussed below. Data from those that are used in the chapters in part 2 are described in more detail in the various chapters. In addition to the quantitative measures that are described, the CS-LTC included a qualitative component: the fourteen evaluators who traveled across all four states and spent multiple hours in each facility were asked to maintain field journals, and they participated in group and individual interviews with the principal investigators. Some of the data from their interviews and journals are presented in chapter 13.

Table 6.3. Key Measures, by Data Source, for the Collaborative Studies of Long-Term Care

Facility-level measures

Observation:	Therapeutic Environment Screening Survey for Residential Care
	Resident and Staff Observation Checklist: Quality of Life Indicators
	Philadelphia Geriatric Center Affect Rating Scale
Report:[a]	Policy and Program Information Form

Resident-level measures

Performance:	Mini-Mental State Examination
	Gait, Balance, Strength
Report:	Charlson Comorbidity Index[b]
	MDS Cognition Scale[c]
	MDS-ADL Self-Performance Index[c]
	Instrumental Activities of Daily Living[c]
	Cornell Scale for Depression in Dementia[c]
	Cohen-Mansfield Agitation Inventory[c]
	Multidimensional Observation Scale for Elderly Subjects (social withdrawal)[c]

[a]Administrator or other administrative staff person provided information regarding the facility.
[b]Resident or primary-care provider (if the resident was unable) provided information regarding the resident's medical condition and history.
[c]Primary-care provider provided information regarding resident's functional status.

Facility-Level Measures

Data related to environmental characteristics derived from expert observation using the Therapeutic Environment Screening Survey for Residential Care (TESS-RC). This measure is a refinement of the TESS-NH, which evolved from the TESS 2+ and the TESS (Sloane & Matthew, 1990; Sloane, Mitchell, Long & Lynn, 1995; Sloane et al., 2000). The TESS-RC is completed through a structured observation of the facility and collects data on indicators believed to reflect each of the goals of quality care: safety and security, resident orientation, stimulation without stress, privacy or personal control, facilitation of social interaction, continuity with the past, and cleanliness and maintenance. Chapter 8 uses this measure to describe the facilities participating in the CS-LTC.

The process of care was measured with self-report and observational measures. The Resident and Staff Observation Checklist: Quality of Life

Indicators (RSOC-QOLI) is an unobtrusive observer-rated checklist of the social environment. Residents, staff, and visitors were observed for 15–30 seconds to determine resident activity, behavior, alertness, location, grouping, mobility, and restraints; quality of interaction and appearance also were noted. The RSOC-QOLI was developed from the RSOC (Matthew & Sloane, 1991); interrater reliability for RSOC items evaluated on two hundred observations found agreement on individual items (for categorical variables) ranging from 95 percent to 100 percent and correlations (for continuous scales) ranging from 0.81 to 1.0. The RSOC-QOLI has been further adapted to incorporate the six-item Philadelphia Geriatric Center Affect Rating Scale (Lawton, Van Haitsma & Klapper, 1996), a validated observation tool that evaluates facial expression, body movement, and other nonverbal cues to assess positive as well as negative affect.

The process of care was also assessed with a modification of the Policy and Program Information Form (POLIF), one of five instruments constituting the Multiphasic Environmental Assessment Procedure (Moos & Lemke, 1996). It includes scales that assess philosophical policies such as the extent to which facilities impose limitations on resident behavior (i.e., functional impairment or problem behavior) and the degree of freedom or control, choice, and privacy afforded to residents. Studies using the POLIF have found that it discriminates between different long-term-care settings as well as the types of residents who reside therein (Perkins, King & Hollyman, 1989; Philip et al., 1989; Benjamin & Spector, 1992). Chapter 9 draws heavily on these data.

Additional data regarding the structure and process of care were collected regarding the physical plant (e.g., size, age, location, availability of social and assistive resources), medical care availability (e.g., access to physicians, RNs, LPNs, and specialists; the capability to take X-rays or draw blood on-site; having a defibrillator or staff who are trained in cardiopulmonary resuscitation), the proximity of health care facilities (e.g., hospitals) and linkages with home health providers and mental health centers, administration (e.g., staff-resident ratios and turnover; salaries), programming (e.g., availability of social or activity therapy, family involvement, preventive and other medical and rehabilitative services), expenditures and revenues (payer mix; revenues, rates, maintenance and other costs), staff experience, medication storage and supervision, and integration of community services. These measures were developed after careful review of surveys used in other RC/AL studies, as well as the investigators' own work in long-term care. Data from these instruments are used in many of the following chapters.

Resident-Level Measures

A great deal of data have been collected directly from the resident or the care provider for each of the 2,839 subjects enrolled in the CS-LTC, including information regarding the resident's age, gender, race, ethnicity, marital status, education, finances, and history (e.g., length of stay in the facility; residence before admission). Information regarding medical conditions from which to calculate a Charlson Comorbidity Index score (Charlson et al., 1987) also was obtained. The Charlson index is a validated method of classifying comorbidity that predicts short- and long-term mortality and replaces direct measures of illness severity that require prospective data collection. This index assigns weights for each comorbid condition, approximately equal to the one-year relative risk of death for that condition. Additional related data were collected on vision, hearing, medications, restraint use, and advance directives.

Cognitive status was directly evaluated with the Mini-Mental State Examination (MMSE) (Folstein, Folstein & McHugh, 1975), a thirty-point continuous scale derived from brief interviews. The MMSE is particularly well suited for persons living in RC/AL, many of whom have early and midstage dementia, because ceiling and floor effects are least problematic in these persons. The MMSE has a test-retest reliability of .80 to .95, an internal consistency of .54 (low education) to .96 (medical patients), and well-established validity (Tombaugh & McIntyre, 1992). Cognition was also assessed from data provided by caregivers, using the MDS Cognition Scale (MDS-COGS) (Hartmaier et al., 1994), developed from the Minimum Data Set (Morris et al., 1990). The MDS-COGS is a valid measure that assesses the presence and severity of cognitive impairment, with sensitivity, specificity, and chance-corrected agreement (kappa) above .80. Data on cognitive status and other resident-level measures are presented in chapters 7 and 11.

Activities of daily living were assessed through observed physical performance and care-provider reports. A ten-minute battery of performance tests assessed gait, balance, and lower extremity strength and endurance (including walking eight feet and rising from and returning to the seated position five times). These performance measures have been administered to more than five thousand community-dwelling persons participating in the EPESE (Established Populations for Epidemiologic Studies of the Elderly). They evidence a wide distribution of performance and distinguish a gradient of risk for mortality and nursing home admission even among those at the high end of the functional spectrum (Guralnik et al., 1994; Fried et al., 1996). The level of independence in performing physical tasks of daily living was also rated with the MDS-ADL Self-Performance Index (MDS-ADL), a ten-item categorical scale of dependency in activities of daily living (ADLs) (Morris et al., 1995). The MDS-ADL assigns subjects a score based on dependency over the previous seven days in bed mobility, eating, locomotion, transfer, toileting, dressing, and personal hygiene; scores range from 1 (total dependence in the late-loss ADLs of bed mobility and eating) to 10 (independence in all). Interrater reliabilities for individual MDS-ADL items exceed .90. Instrumental activities of daily living were assessed with items developed from work in RC/AL and specifically reflect those type of activities in which this population might engage, such as cleaning their room and maneuvering outside of the facility.

Depression was assessed by care-provider report on the Cornell Scale (Alexopoulos et al., 1988), an observer-rated scale of depressive symptomatology designed to rate depression in persons with dementia. This scale is the only depression scale validated for long-term-care populations with dementia; its interrater reliability (kappa = .67) and internal consistency (alpha = .84) are good. Behavior was assessed by the care provider using the short (14-item) version of the Cohen-Mansfield Agitation Inventory (CMAI) (Cohen-Mansfield, 1986), a scale that identifies the frequency of reported agitated behaviors over the previous two weeks. The CMAI has excellent concurrent validity and internal consistency. Two items related to resisting care, abstracted from the MDS, also were assessed. Questions regarding social functioning in the preceding seven days were adapted from work in RC/AL populations and include items such as going to the barber or beauty shop, attending senior adult day care, and working on a hobby. Social withdrawal was assessed with a seven-item scale of the Multidimensional Observation Scale for Elderly Subjects (Helmes, Csapo & Short, 1987), which measures contact with and interest in people, events, and activities. Additional items relate to hallucinations and delusions.

Special Considerations

Dementia-Specific Care Areas

Because special care units for persons with dementia are emerging in RC/AL and because the structure and process of care in these units are likely to differ from other areas, the CS-LTC was designed to obtain information about special care. However, not all facilities are consistent in their definition and use of the term *special care;* to clarify matters, the CS-LTC used the term *dementia-specific care area,* defining it as a portion of the facility (or the entire facility) that is designated as an Alzheimer disease or dementia unit and in which 75 percent or more of the residents have a diagnosis of Alzheimer disease or a related disorder. Data were collected separately for these areas and are reported in chapter 11. Facility-level scores for RC/AL facilities that had both dementia-specific and non-dementia-specific care areas were derived as weighted averages according to the number of beds in each area for continuous data or by choosing the value for the larger area, for categorical data.

Analytic Issues

All chapters in part 2 present data by facility type (stratum). The CS-LTC aimed to examine a broad spectrum of RC/AL facilities and residents. To achieve maximum diversity, it developed a stratified sample and collected data from a similar number of facility types and residents per state; data collection was not designed to be representative of each state or of all four states overall. Therefore, the study presents a picture of facilities and residents within three RC/AL strata (i.e., fewer than 16 beds, larger traditional facilities, and larger new-model facilities). To efficiently focus on RC/AL that served elderly clients, exclusion criteria were instituted (i.e., facilities that serve primarily persons with diagnoses of mental illness or developmental disability, small RC/AL that house fewer than 4 persons age 65 and older, large RC/AL that house fewer than 10 residents age 65 and older, and nursing homes with fewer than 40 residents). Therefore, generalizability is limited to facilities that met the eligibility criteria, and the data cannot be merely aggregated across facility types.

Resident-level data collected in facilities with fewer than sixteen beds may be considered to be more representative than those obtained in other facilities, because residents were sampled at equal rates in all small facilities but at differing rates (selection probabilities) within larger facilities;

in small facilities all residents were solicited, but a maximum number of subjects was established in larger facilities. Cautions related to eligibility also apply: subjects include only residents 65 years of age and older, and additional selection criteria were applied in nursing homes.

All data presented in part 2 are to be interpreted with these caveats. A second analytic issue that is common to all chapters relates to the handling of missing data when deriving an aggregated scale or index. If less than 25 percent of the data for that measure was missing, a proportionate score was calculated; if 25 percent or more of the data was missing, the summary measure was considered missing. Additional analytic strategies are presented throughout part 2 as they relate to the topic under discussion.

An Overview of the Collaborative Studies of Long-Term Care Sample

Demographic Characteristics of the Facilities

Select characteristics of facilities participating in the CS-LTC are presented in table 6.4. (Additional information is presented in chapters 8–13, and resident-level data are presented in chapter 7.) Between 15 and 21 percent of each facility type were located in rural communities. Proprietary facilities constitute 58–91 percent of the sample, the least being in nursing homes and the most in smaller RC/AL. Dementia-specific care areas are more prevalent in sampled nursing homes (30%) and new-model facilities (25%) and less prevalent in other RC/AL settings (8%). Facilities with fewer than sixteen beds were much newer than traditional facilities (mean age 13 and 23 years, respectively), and both were older than new-model facilities (mean age 5 years).

Weighted Characteristics of Facilities and Residents

Although data for different facility types cannot be aggregated because of the sampling design, weights can be applied to each facility and each resident to generate stratum-specific state averages and averages across all four states. Tables 6.5 through 6.9 present such weighted data.[2] Based on these estimates, Florida has the most facilities and beds of all types but not the most beds per one thousand population age 65 and older across all facility types. When calculated in reference to the density of the elderly population, North Carolina has the most new-model beds, and Maryland has the most nursing home beds; however, Maryland also has the fewest

Table 6.4. Facility Characteristics of the Collaborative Studies of Long-Term Care Sample

	Residential Care/Assisted Living			Nursing Home
	<16 Beds	Traditional	New-Model	
Number of facilities	113	40	40	40
Number of rural facilities (%)	24 (21%)	7 (18%)	6 (15%)	6 (15%)
Number of facilities for-profit (%)	103 (91%)	26 (65%)	29 (73%)	23 (58%)
Number of facilities with DSCAs (%)[a]	9 (8%)	3 (8%)	10 (25%)	12 (30%)
Number of beds	1,009	1,832	2,604	4,657
Mean facility bed size (SD)	8.9 (3.6)	45.8 (37.5)	65.1 (41.6)	116.4 (50.7)
Mean facility age in years (SD)[b]	12.7 (13.4)	23.0 (16.4)	5.3 (3.0)	24.1 (15.1)
Number of employees[c]	564	829	1307	—

[a]DSCAs = dementia-specific care areas.

[b]One traditional facility had been in operation for 148 years and was excluded from the calculation. The facility in operation for the next longest time had been open for 80 years.

[c]Staffing estimates are based on 159 RC/AL facilities (82%); these data were not obtained for nursing homes.

Table 6.5. Aggregated Four-State Estimates of Facility and Resident Characteristics, Based on the Collaborative Studies of Long-Term Care Sample

	Residential Care/Assisted Living				Nursing Home
	<16 Beds	Traditional	New-Model	All RC/AL	
Facility					
Number of facilities	1,216	877	407	2,500	1,551
Number of rural facilities (%)	248 (20%)	122 (14%)	59 (14%)	429 (17%)	237 (15%)
Number of facilities for-profit (%)	1,171 (96%)	596 (68%)	331 (81%)	2,098 (84%)	909 (59%)
Number of facilities with DSCAs (%)	23 (2%)	104 (12%)	103 (25%)	230 (9%)	531 (34%)
Number of beds	10,301	44,420	25,547	80,268	175,990
Number of beds/1,000 pop. 65+	2	9	5	16	34
Mean facility bed size (SD)	8.9 (3.6)	45.8 (37.5)	65.1 (41.6)	31.0 (0.6[d])	116.4 (50.7)
Mean facility age in years (SD)	12.7 (13.4)	23.0 (16.4)	5.3 (3.0)	15.1 (0.3[d])	24.1 (15.1)
Number of employees[a]	5,325	19,983	12,910	38,218	—

(continued)

Table 6.5. (Continued)

| Resident[b] | Residential Care/Assisted Living | | | | Nursing Home |
	<16 Beds	Traditional	New-Model	All RC/AL	
Number age 65+	7,727	32,556	19,323	59,594	—
Mean resident age (SD)	83.1 (8.2)	84.6 (7.9)	84.5 (7.0)	84.2 (0.6[d])	—
Number male (%)	1,750 (23%)	7,163 (22%)	5,264 (27%)	14,177 (24%)	—
Number nonwhite (%)	730 (9%)	1,275 (4%)	519 (3%)	2,524 (4%)	—
Number with dementia[c] (%)	3,114 (40%)	6,851 (21%)	6,615 (34%)	16,580 (28%)	—
Number mobility dependent[c] (%)	2,341 (30%)	4,638 (14%)	4,309 (22%)	11,288 (19%)	—
Number impaired in 2+ ADLs[c] (%)	4,308 (56%)	11,039 (34%)	8,952 (46%)	14,298 (24%)	—
Number incontinent of urine[c] (%)	2,326 (30%)	4,755 (15%)	5,520 (29%)	12,601 (21%)	—

Notes: The states are Florida, Maryland, New Jersey, and North Carolina. Estimates are based on facilities that met eligibility criteria.

[a]Staffing estimates are based on 159 RC/AL facilities (82%); these data were not obtained for nursing homes.

[b]Resident estimates are of persons age 65+. Resident-level weighted data are not provided for nursing homes because of nonrandom resident sampling.

[c]Cognitive impairment was determined by an MMSE score ≤16; if missing, by an MDS-COGS score ≤16; if missing, by an MDS-COGS score ≥4; if missing ($N = 24$), by a reported diagnosis of dementia. Mobility dependence means requiring assistance in transfer or locomotion (does not include fully independent in wheelchair). Impaired in 2+ ADLs includes transfer, locomotion, eating, toileting, dressing, and bathing. Incontinent of urine means experiencing urinary incontinence on a majority of days.

[d]Standard error.

Table 6.6. Estimates of Florida Facility and Resident Characteristics, Based on the Collaborative Studies of Long-Term Care Sample

		Residential Care/Assisted Living		All	Nursing Home
	<16 Beds	Traditional	New-Model	RC/AL	
Facility					
Number of facilities	737	382	168	1,287	662
Number of rural facilities (%)	49 (7%)	0 (0%)	17 (10%)	66 (5%)	66 (10%)
Number of facilities for-profit (%)	737 (100%)	229 (60%)	168 (100%)	1,134 (88%)	397 (60%)
Number of facilities with DSCAs (%)	0 (0%)	76 (20%)	50 (30%)	126 (10%)	331 (50%)
Number of beds	6,530	28,956	14,314	49,800	73,416
Number of beds/1,000 pop. 65+	2	11	5	18	28
Mean facility bed size (SD)	8.9 (3.0)	75.8 (55.5)	85.2 (63.8)	38.7 (1.1[d])	110.9 (58.6)
Mean facility age in years (SD)	8.9 (4.3)	13.9 (6.0)	6.6 (2.8)	10.1 (0.1[d])	29.1 (12.0)
Number of employees[a]	2,389	10,238	5,057	17,684	—

(continued)

Table 6.6. (Continued)

| | Residential Care/Assisted Living | | | | Nursing Home |
	<16 Beds	Traditional	New-Model	All RC/AL	
Resident[b]					
Number age 65+	4,953	21,965	10,212	37,130	—
Mean resident age (SD)	84.2 (8.3)	84.5 (8.7)	83.3 (7.9)	84.2 (1.0[d])	—
Number male (%)	1,078 (22%)	4,650 (21%)	3,527 (35%)	9,255 (25%)	—
Number nonwhite (%)	168 (3%)	449 (2%)	68 (1%)	685 (2%)	—
Number with dementia[c] (%)	1,887 (38%)	4,409 (20%)	3,490 (34%)	9,786 (26%)	—
Number mobility dependent[c] (%)	1,486 (30%)	2,581 (12%)	1,991 (19%)	6,058 (16%)	—
Number impaired in 2+ ADLs[c] (%)	2,766 (56%)	6,926 (32%)	4,267 (42%)	13,959 (38%)	—
Number incontinent of urine[c] (%)	1,417 (29%)	3,278 (15%)	2,812 (28%)	7,507 (20%)	—

Notes: Estimates are based on facilities that met eligibility criteria.

[a]Staffing estimates were not obtained for nursing homes.

[b]Resident estimates are of persons age 65+. Resident-level weighted data are not provided for nursing homes because of nonrandom resident sampling.

[c]Cognitive impairment was determined by an MMSE score ≤16; if missing, by an MDS-COGS score ≥4; if missing, by a reported diagnosis of dementia. Mobility dependence means requiring assistance in transfer or locomotion (does not include fully independent in wheelchair). Impaired in 2+ ADLs includes transfer, locomotion, eating, toileting, dressing, and bathing. Incontinent of urine means experiencing urinary incontinence on a majority of days.

[d]Standard error.

Table 6.7. Estimates of Maryland Facility and Resident Characteristics, Based on the Collaborative Studies of Long-Term Care Sample

	Residential Care/Assisted Living				Nursing Home
	<16 Beds	Traditional	New-Model	All RC/AL	
Facility					
Number of facilities	137	36	27	200	212
Number of rural facilities (%)	4 (3%)	11 (31%)	5 (19%)	20 (10%)	0 (0%)
Number of facilities for-profit (%)	133 (97%)	18 (50%)	14 (52%)	165 (83%)	106 (50%)
Number of facilities with DSCAs (%)	12 (9%)	0 (0%)	5 (19%)	17 (9%)	64 (30%)
Number of beds	1,216	1,634	1,858	4,708	29,320
Number of beds/1,000 pop. 65+	2	3	3	8	51
Mean facility bed size (SD)	8.9 (3.3)	45.4 (31.3)	68.8 (32.0)	23.6 (1.3[d])	138.3 (66.6)
Mean facility age in years (SD)	7.1 (3.7)	28.3 (22.8)	6.0 (2.7)	10.8 (0.7[d])	23.6 (21.6)
Number of employees[a]	378	536	1,058	1,972	—

(continued)

Table 6.7. *(Continued)*

	Residential Care/Assisted Living				Nursing Home
	<16 Beds	Traditional	New-Model	All RC/AL	
Resident[b]					
Number age 65+	939	1,401	1,496	3,836	—
Mean resident age (SD)	83.5 (7.9)	85.3 (7.2)	85.7 (6.3)	85.0 (0.5[d])	—
Number male (%)	222 (24%)	282 (20%)	345 (23%)	849 (22%)	—
Number nonwhite (%)	106 (11%)	116 (8%)	114 (8%)	336 (9%)	—
Number with dementia[c] (%)	435 (46%)	398 (28%)	539 (36%)	1,372 (36%)	—
Number mobility dependent[c] (%)	350 (37%)	176 (13%)	405 (27%)	931 (24%)	—
Number impaired in 2+ ADLs[c] (%)	585 (62%)	485 (35%)	777 (52%)	1,847 (48%)	—
Number incontinent of urine[c] (%)	372 (40%)	228 (16%)	488 (33%)	1,088 (28%)	—

Notes: Estimates are based on facilities that met eligibility criteria.

[a]Staffing estimates were not obtained for nursing homes.

[b]Resident estimates are of persons age 65+. Resident-level weighted data are not provided for nursing homes because of nonrandom resident sampling.

[c]Cognitive impairment was determined by an MMSE score ≤16; if missing, by an MDS-COGS score ≥4; if missing, by a reported diagnosis of dementia. Mobility dependence means requiring assistance in transfer or locomotion (does not include fully independent in wheelchair). Impaired in 2+ ADLs includes transfer, locomotion, eating, toileting, dressing, and bathing. Incontinent of urine means experiencing urinary incontinence on a majority of days.

[d]Standard error.

Table 6.8. Estimates of New Jersey Facility and Resident Characteristics, Based on the Collaborative Studies of Long-Term Care Sample

	Residential Care/Assisted Living				Nursing Home
	<16 Beds	Traditional	New-Model	All RC/AL	
Facility					
Number of facilities	40	182	54	276	333
Number of rural facilities (%)	4 (10%)	0 (0%)	5 (9%)	9 (3%)	33 (10%)
Number of facilities for-profit (%)	29 (73%)	127 (70%)	38 (70%)	194 (70%)	200 (60%)
Number of facilities with DSCAs (%)	11 (28%)	0 (0%)	16 (30%)	27 (10%)	33 (10%)
Number of beds	481	6,406	3,861	10,748	36,996
Number of beds/1,000 pop. 65+	0.4	6	4	10	34
Mean facility bed size (SD)	12.0 (4.3)	35.2 (18.5)	71.5 (29.6)	38.9 (1.2[d])	111.1 (35.6)
Mean facility age in years (SD)	26.9 (24.2)	33.7 (15.6)	3.5 (3.5)	26.8 (0.9[d])	27.8 (11.3)
Number of employees[a]	308	4,204	1,510	6,022	—

(continued)

Table 6.8. (*Continued*)

| | Residential Care/Assisted Living | | | Nursing Home |
	<16 Beds	Traditional	New-Model	All RC/AL	
Resident[b]					
Number age 65+	305	3,933	3,159	7,397	—
Mean resident age (SD)	81.9 (7.6)	83.9 (7.8)	84.1 (7.1)	83.9 (0.7[d])	—
Number male (%)	76 (25%)	987 (25%)	687 (22%)	1,750 (24%)	—
Number nonwhite (%)	15 (5%)	106 (3%)	67 (2%)	188 (3%)	—
Number with dementia[c] (%)	107 (35%)	460 (12%)	794 (25%)	1,361 (18%)	—
Number mobility dependent[c] (%)	61 (20%)	291 (7%)	615 (19%)	967 (13%)	—
Number impaired in 2+ ADLs[c] (%)	114 (37%)	600 (15%)	1,391 (44%)	2,105 (28%)	—
Number incontinent of urine[c] (%)	82 (27%)	272 (7%)	657 (21%)	1,011 (14%)	—

Notes: Estimates are based on facilities that met eligibility criteria.

[a] Staffing estimates were not obtained for nursing homes.

[b] Resident estimates are of persons age 65+. Resident-level weighted data are not provided for nursing homes because of nonrandom resident sampling.

[c] Cognitive impairment was determined by an MMSE score ≤16; if missing, by an MDS-COGS score ≥4; if missing, by a reported diagnosis of dementia. Mobility dependence means requiring assistance in transfer or locomotion (does not include fully independent in wheelchair). Impaired in 2+ ADLs includes transfer, locomotion, eating, toileting, dressing, and bathing. Incontinent of urine means experiencing urinary incontinence on a majority of days.

[d] Standard error.

Table 6.9. Estimates of North Carolina Facility and Resident Characteristics, Based on the Collaborative Studies of Long-Term Care Sample

	Residential Care/Assisted Living				Nursing Home
	<16 Beds	Traditional	New-Model	All RC/AL	
Facility					
Number of facilities	302	277	158	737	344
Number of rural facilities (%)	191 (63%)	111 (40%)	32 (20%)	334 (45%)	138 (40%)
Number of facilities for-profit (%)	272 (90%)	222 (80%)	111 (70%)	605 (82%)	206 (60%)
Number of facilities with DSCAs (%)	0 (0%)	28 (10%)	32 (20%)	60 (8%)	103 (30%)
Number of beds	2,074	7,424	5,514	15,012	36,258
Number of beds/1,000 pop. 65+	2	8	6	16	40
Mean facility bed size (SD)	6.9 (2.3)	26.8 (6.4)	34.9 (23.8)	20.4 (0.4[d])	105.4 (32.2)
Mean facility age in years (SD)	12.5 (7.8)	17.2 (12.1)	5.2 (2.0)	12.7 (0.3[d])	16.0 (11.4)
Number of employees[a]	2,250	5,005	5,285	12,540	—

(continued)

Table 6.9. (Continued)

| | Residential Care/Assisted Living | | | Nursing Home |
	<16 Beds	Traditional	New-Model	All RC/AL	
Resident[b]					
Number age 65+	1,529	5,257	4,456	11,231	—
Mean resident age (SD)	82.1 (8.8)	84.5 (8.0)	84.7 (6.4)	84.3 (0.6[d])	—
Number male (%)	374 (24%)	1244 (24%)	706 (16%)	2,324 (21%)	—
Number nonwhite (%)	441 (29%)	604 (11%)	270 (6%)	1,315 (12%)	—
Number with dementia[c] (%)	686 (45%)	1,584 (30%)	1,791 (40%)	4,061 (36%)	—
Number mobility dependent[c] (%)	445 (29%)	1,590 (30%)	1,299 (29%)	3,334 (30%)	—
Number impaired in 2+ ADLs[c] (%)	843 (55%)	3,028 (58%)	2,516 (56%)	6,387 (57%)	—
Number incontinent of urine[c] (%)	456 (30%)	977 (19%)	1,562 (35%)	2,995 (27%)	—

Notes: Estimates are based on facilities that met eligibility criteria.

[a]Staffing estimates were not obtained for nursing homes.

[b]Resident estimates are of persons age 65+. Resident-level weighted data are not provided for nursing homes because of nonrandom resident sampling.

[c]Cognitive impairment was determined by an MMSE score ≤16; if missing, by an MDS-COGS score ≥4; if missing, by a reported diagnosis of dementia. Mobility dependence means requiring assistance in transfer or locomotion (does not include fully independent in wheelchair). Impaired in 2+ ADLs includes transfer, locomotion, eating, toileting, dressing, and bathing. Incontinent of urine means experiencing urinary incontinence on a majority of days.

[d]Standard error.

traditional and new-model beds. New Jersey warrants mention by having the least facilities with fewer than sixteen beds and the second-least new-model and nursing home beds, relative to the size of the elderly population. State variation is evident based on geography, as well: 3–5 percent of all RC/AL facilities are in rural areas in New Jersey and Florida, compared to 45 percent in North Carolina. Finally, RC/AL employs more than thirty-eight thousand workers across the four states (including full- and part-time staff members), almost one-half of whom work in Florida.

In reference to long-term-care residents over the age of 65 across all four states, 76 percent are female, 4 percent are nonwhite, and their mean age is 84.2 years (SE = 0.6). Twenty-eight percent are cognitively impaired, the highest rates consistently exhibited in facilities with fewer than sixteen beds. The four-state rates of dependence range from 19 percent (mobility) to 21 percent (incontinence) to 24 percent (two or more ADL dependencies). Maryland and North Carolina have the highest acuity levels in these areas (24%, 28%, 48% in Maryland, and 30%, 27%, 57% in North Carolina, respectively), and New Jersey has the lowest levels (13%, 14%, 28%).

Conclusion

As indicated in tables 6.5–6.9, the four strata and four states in the CS-LTC appear to have captured much of the diversity of the RC/AL industry. Variation across strata and states is considerable, in both facility and resident characteristics. These findings are gratifying and suggest that the selection decisions outlined in this chapter achieved their goal of representing a wide range of RC/AL facilities. Thus, although the results of the CS-LTC analyses cannot be generalized beyond the study sample, it is not unreasonable to expect the results from this sample to reflect in large measure the RC/AL industry as it exists in much of the United States.

Notes

1. The numbers of facilities and residents to be enrolled were determined based on power requirements for the longitudinal analyses.

2. Facility-level weights were derived for each facility type by (1) telephone screening to determine the number of eligible facilities in each selected region, (2) multiplying the proportion of eligible facilities in the region by the number of facilities in the state to derive the number of eligible facilities in the state,

and (3) dividing the number of eligible facilities in the state by the number of participating facilities, to obtain the number of eligible facilities in the state that each participating facility represented as a weight. Resident-level weights within each facility were derived by multiplying the facility-level weight by a second-level weight for the number of eligible residents in the facility represented by those in the study. Second-level weights were calculated for each facility by (1) determining the number of eligible residents (over age 64) in the facility and (2) dividing the number of eligible residents by the number of participating residents.

References

Alexopoulos, G. S., Abrams, R. C., Young, R. C., & Shamoian, C. A. 1988. Cornell scale for depression in dementia. *Biological Psychiatry* 23:271- 84.

Benjamin, L. C., & Spector, J. 1992. Geriatric care on a ward without nurses. *International Journal of Geriatric Psychiatry* 7:743–50.

Charlson, M. E., Pompei, P., Ales, K. L., & MacKenzie, C. R. 1987. A new method of classifying prognostic comorbidity in longitudinal studies: Prognostic development and validation. *Journal of Chronic Diseases* 40:373–83.

Cohen-Mansfield, J. 1986. Agitated behaviors in the elderly. II. Preliminary results in the cognitively deteriorated. *Journal of the American Geriatrics Society* 34:722–27.

Folstein, M. F., Folstein, S. E., & McHugh, P. R. 1975. Mini-mental State: A practical method for grading the cognitive state of patients for the clinician. *Journal of Psychiatric Research* 12:189–98.

Fried, L. P., Bandeen-Roche, K., Williamson, J. D., Prasada-Rao, P., Chee, E., Tepper, S., & Rubin, G. S. 1996. Functional decline in older adults: Expanding methods of ascertainment. *Journal of Gerontology: Biological and Medical Sciences* 51:M206–14.

Guralnik, J. M., Simonsick, E. M., Ferrucci, L., Glynn, R. J., Berkman, L. F., Blazer, D. G., Scherr, P. A., & Wallace, R. B. 1994. A short physical performance battery assessing lower extremity function: Association with self-reported disability and prediction of mortality and nursing home admission. *Journal of Gerontology: Medical Science* 49:M85–94.

Hartmaier, S., Sloane, P. D., Guess, H., & Koch, G. 1994. The MDS Cognition Scale: A valid instrument for identifying and staging nursing home residents with dementia using the Minimum Data Set. *Journal of the American Geriatrics Society* 42:1173–79.

Helmes, E., Csapo, K. G., & Short, J. A. 1987. Standardization and validation of the Multidimensional Observation Scale for Elderly Subjects (MOSES). *Journal of Gerontology* 42(4):395–405.

Lawton, M. P., Van Haitsma, K., & Klapper, J. 1996. Observed affect in nursing home residents with Alzheimer's disease. *Journal of Gerontology: Psychological Science and Social Sciences* 51B:3–14.

Mathew, L. J., & Sloane, P. D. 1991. Care on dementia units in five states. In P. D. Sloane & L. J. Mathew (eds.), *Dementia Units in Long-Term Care.* Baltimore: Johns Hopkins University Press.

Moos, R. H., & Lemke, S. 1996. *Evaluating Residential Facilities: The Multiphasic Environmental Assessment Procedure.* Thousand Oaks, CA: Sage.

Morgan, L. A., Eckert, J. K., & Lyon, S. M. (eds.). 1995. *Small Board-and-Care Homes: Residential Care in Transition.* Baltimore: Johns Hopkins University Press.

Morris, J. N., Fries, B. E., & Morris, S. 1999. Scaling ADLs within the MDS. *Journal of Gerontology: Medical Science* 54:M546–53.

Morris, J. N., Hawes, C., Fries, B. E., Phillips, C. D., Mor, V., Katz, S., Murphy, K., Drugovich, M. L., & Friedlob, A. S. 1990. Designing the national resident assessment instrument for nursing homes. *Gerontologist* 30 (3): 293–307.

Perkins, R. E., King, S. A., & Hollyman, J. A. 1989. Resettlement of old long-stay psychiatric patients: The use of the private sector. *British Journal of Psychiatry* 155:233–38.

Philip, I., Mutch, W. J., Devaney, J., & Ogston, S. 1989. Can quality of life of old people in institutional care be measured? *Journal of Clinical and Experimental Gerontology* 11:11–19.

Sloane, P. D., Long, K. M., Mitchell, C. M., Zimmerman, S. I., & Weisman, G. 2000. Therapeutic Environment Screening Survey for Nursing Homes (TESS-NH). <http://www.unc.edu/depts/tessnh/>, December 22, 2000.

Sloane, P. D., & Mathew, L. J. 1990. The Therapeutic Environment Screening Scale. *American Journal of Alzheimer's Care* 5(6):22–26.

Sloane, P. D., Mitchell, C. M., Long, K., & Lynn, M. 1995. *TESS 2+ Instrument B: Unit Observation Checklist—Physical Environment: A Report on the Psychometric Properties of Individual Items, and Initial Recommendation on Scaling.* Chapel Hill: University of North Carolina.

Tombaugh, T. N., & McIntyre, N. J. 1992. The Mini-Mental State Examination: A comprehensive review. *Journal of the American Geriatrics Society* 40:922–35.

7 Resident Characteristics

Leslie A. Morgan, Ph.D., Ann L. Gruber-Baldini, Ph.D., and Jay Magaziner, Ph.D., M.S.Hyg.

Residents are a focal point in the study of residential care/assisted living (RC/AL), since their needs should drive the creation of the facilities and services. As new forms of RC/AL emerge, it is critical to understand the characteristics of residents in order to plan for an aging population. Questions such as what types of elderly individuals select (or have selected for them) which types of housing and care can illuminate the dynamics in this emergent field. Profiling residents' characteristics and needs also clarifies the niche that RC/AL fills in the health care system and better enables those designing both policies and regulations and those running facilities to respond to preferences and care needs of the growing elderly population.

RC/AL is changing, with concomitant changes in the characteristics of residents. Specifically, the rising standards for entry into nursing homes, along with the aging in place of residents in lower-skilled steps along the continuum of care, have meant that more impaired residents now reside in RC/AL settings than was the case even ten years ago (Dittmar et al., 1983; Hawes et al., 1995; Newcomer, Breuer & Zhang, 1993). Research has shown considerable diversity in the functional status of residents in RC/AL facilities in Florida, with nursing home residents clearly demonstrating more severe functional decrements (Polivka, Dunlop & Brooks, 1997). Such dynamics suggest that it is important to revisit regularly the changing profile of residents in RC/AL.

This chapter has three purposes. The first purpose is to provide descriptive data on the sample of residents participating in the Collaborative Studies of Long-Term Care, directing attention to the three types of RC/AL settings from which the data were obtained. We anticipated variations in residents across facility types, since a complex and relatively poorly understood system of evaluation and referral has created streams of residents moving into and among various types of care (see McAuley &

Usita, 1998; Speare, Avery & Lawton, 1991). In addition, changes in the types of facilities that are operating and in bed availability at any given time and in any given locality influence the alternatives for placement when a person needs personal care or support in activities of daily living but does not require nursing care. Within this first purpose, we describe four major domains of resident characteristics. The first descriptive domain is the sample's sociodemographic characteristics, including age, race, marital status, educational attainment, and prior residency. In a second set of variables, we describe physical health characteristics, including both health conditions and functional measures. Third, since it is an important issue in RC/AL, we describe cognitive and mental-health indicators. Fourth, we include data on the social networks and activities of residents in RC/AL.

A second purpose of this chapter is to examine the profiles of this sample in comparison with two sets of information: existing studies of residents in other RC/AL settings and data on other, related populations, such as nursing home residents and home care recipients. To the extent possible, we use comparable, national or state-level data on these various populations to put our sample's characteristics into a larger context. Used for comparison are the National Home and Hospice Care Study (NHHCS) (Haupt, 1998) and the 1996 Nursing Home Component of the Medical Expenditure Panel Survey (MEPS) (Krauss & Altman, 1998).

A third purpose of the chapter is to selectively examine the relative roles of facility type, state location of a facility, and facility size in shaping the sampled residents' characteristics. The four states from which the data were obtained (Florida, Maryland, New Jersey, and North Carolina) vary in their regulatory and policy histories with regard to RC/AL and in current support for non-nursing-home alternatives for care. The states also vary in their willingness to support aging in place (see chapter 10). For these reasons, we anticipated that residents in facilities of various types and across states may show important variation in their characteristics. Also, since size is thought to be of importance in RC/AL (Morgan, Eckert & Lyon, 1995; Sherman & Newman, 1988), its inclusion to clarify differences in resident characteristics is essential.

Methods

The data presented in this chapter were collected for the Collaborative Studies of Long-Term Care (CS-LTC), a four-state study of 193 RC/AL facilities and their residents. The methods are presented in chapter 6. Briefly, facilities were stratified into three types (strata): those with fewer than sixteen beds, larger facilities that are newer and purpose-built (new-model), and larger facilities that are more traditional. A cross-sectional sample of residents was selected in each facility, including all residents age 65 and older in small facilities and a random sample of up to twenty elderly residents in all other facilities. Data were collected directly from residents and care providers for these 2,078 RC/AL residents.

Information on demographics, medical conditions, use of medical care services, and impairments in vision or hearing were reported by the resident or by the care provider if the resident was unable to respond or chose not to respond; care-provider proxies completed the forms in 61 percent of cases. Items on physical activities of daily living, modified from the Minimum Data Set (MDS) (Morris et al., 1990), were rated by staff caregivers. Although instrumental activities of daily living (IADLs) were also rated by staff, 40 percent or more of residents had not performed most of these activities in the prior week, so we do not report them here. Care providers also responded to questions with regard to incontinence and use of any of seven categories of mobility devices or support (resident used a cane or walker, or pushed a wheelchair; wore a brace or prosthesis; wheeled self or used an electric cart or a scooter; was wheeled by another person; was lifted manually or mechanically; used a transfer aid; used a trapeze). Behavioral problems were evaluated by staff with the National Institute on Aging—Special Care Unit Common Core version of the Cohen-Mansfield Agitation Inventory (CMAI) (Cohen-Mansfield & Billig, 1986), a fourteen-item scale identifying the frequency of agitated behaviors in the prior two weeks. Items related to depression and mood were drawn from staff reports using the Cornell Scale for Depression in Dementia (Alexopoulos et al., 1988). Cognitive functioning was evaluated by use of the MDS Cognition Scale (MDS-COGS) (Hartmaier et al., 1994), with data obtained from care providers, and the Mini-Mental Status Examination (MMSE) (Folstein, Folstein & McHugh, 1975), with data obtained from direct evaluation of residents. Care providers also provided information on availability of social support from kin and others, as well as contact frequency. The measure of participation in social activities in the facility was derived from Dittmar and co-workers 1983. Social interaction was evaluated through a reverse scoring of the eight-item withdrawn behavior scale of the Multidimensional Observation Scale for Elderly Subjects (MOSES) (Helmes, Csapo & Short, 1987).

Most analyses are descriptive, providing data on a wide range of resident characteristics by the three strata of RC/AL used in the study. We have also selectively included regression analyses to examine some of the interrelationships of the variables being measured and specifically to examine the role of size and state in addition to stratum in understanding the profile of resident characteristics. Either logistic or linear least squares regression techniques were employed as appropriate, using two models. The simple regressions included only stratum comparisons, utilizing traditional homes as the comparison category to establish whether stratum differences were statistically significant in light of the respondent clustering created by the sampling design. The more complete models included state (using New Jersey as the basis of comparison), stratum, and size (number of beds) to determine whether stratum variations held up when state and size (or other selected control variables) were introduced.

Given the stratified design by which the facilities were sampled, the descriptive results reported here are best interpreted as a profile of our sample, not as representing the population of RC/AL residents in general nor of those in the four states studied in particular. (The weighted estimates presented in chapter 6 can be used for this purpose.) However, resident selection was representative, and the data provide a wealth of information about cross-sectional characteristics and needs of residents from all types of RC/AL settings. Finally, it is important to note that the percentages presented in the following tables represent percentages of our sample in a stratum of facilities, not percentages of a resident population in that type of RC/AL setting.

Resident Profile

Demographic Characteristics

Data describing the demographic characteristics of the CS-LTC sample, divided into the three RC/AL strata, are presented in table 7.1. Comparisons with existing studies of RC/AL residents reveal consistencies in terms of the demographic profile.

Table 7.1. Collaborative Studies of Long-Term Care Residential Care/Assisted Living Resident Sample Sociodemographic Profile, by Facility Type (%)

	<16 Beds (N = 665)	Traditional (N = 648)	New-Model (N = 765)
Age: above 85	46.2%	57.4%	52.5%
Female	76.0	76.8	74.9
Race or ethnicity			
White	85.1	92.4	94.9
African American	10.1	5.6	4.2
Other	4.7	2.0	0.9
Marital status			
Widowed	67.4	67.3	73.3
Married	10.0	9.6	13.8
Other	21.0	22.4	11.7
Education			
Less than 12 years	38.1	30.8	27.4
12 years	31.6	29.7	32.8
13+ years	30.3	39.5	39.8
Prior housing arrangement			
Community	64.8	64.5	65.3
Supportive housing or health care	35.2	35.5	34.7
Current tenure in facility			
Less than 1 year	37.3	37.7	42.7
1–3 years	24.5	21.0	29.2
3+ years	38.2	41.3	28.1

Age. Prior research in RC/AL facilities finds most residents to be elderly but that some facilities house mixed-age populations, including younger, physically or mentally disabled adults (Hawes et al., 1995; Lair & Lefkowitz, 1990, Newcomer, Breuer & Zhang, 1993). For example, 29 percent of residents over age 65 in small Maryland homes were 85 or older (Morgan, Eckert & Lyon, 1995); Hawes and colleagues reported that 64 percent of all residents were over age 75, with one-third over 85 (Hawes et al., 1995). Earlier studies by Dittmar, Mor, and colleagues found fewer (38%–42%) over age 75 (Dittmar et al., 1983; Mor, Sherwood & Gutkin, 1986). Some types of facilities have an age criterion for admission, but many others admit only on the basis of need for functional or medical support, resulting in a more age-mixed population.

Data for the CS-LTC sample confirm the "graying" of RC/AL populations, since a majority of sample members in two of the strata (52.5% for new-model and 57.4% for traditional facilities) are over age 85. Only in the smaller facilities (fewer than 16 beds) was the proportion of the sample over age 85 slightly below half (46.2%). (Note that the CS-LTC data are also affected by the fact that only residents over age 65 were sampled. Not only do these facilities serve the "older population," but like other RC/AL settings, they are primarily serving the "old-old."

Gender. Residents in most RC/AL facilities (with the exception of Veterans Administration facilities) are predominantly female. This is not a surprising finding, given the longer life expectancy of women, which advances the risks of both widowhood and functional impairment requiring supportive care (Dittmar et al., 1983; Hawes et al., 1995; Mor, Sherwood & Gutkin, 1986). Over two-thirds of board-and-care home residents in Maryland were female (Morgan, Eckert & Lyon, 1995). Sex ratios are more balanced among younger residents, who more commonly are admitted to RC/AL because of mental or physical disabilities (Lair & Lefkowitz, 1990). As expected, three-quarters or more of CS-LTC sample members are women, with little variation across strata (table 7.1).

Race or Ethnicity. Most studies estimating state or national populations in RC/AL show that the African American population is underrepresented (Hawes et al., 1995; Lair & Lefkowitz, 1990; Newcomer, Breuer & Zhang, 1993). Hawes and colleagues (1995) reported 91 percent of residents in their ten-state study to be white. Whether because of economic factors, discrimination, or cultural preferences, RC/AL providers serve fewer African Americans and other minorities than would be expected, even given their differential mortality (for an exception, see Fonda et al., 1996). Data from Hawes and associates (1995) found that smaller homes included more minority elders. Morgan, Eckert, and Lyon (1995) reported that 69 percent of residents in the small homes they studied were white, even in a region with a large African American population. Residents in board-and-care homes, some of which are less expensive, also house fewer poor and minority residents than expected (Dittmar et al., 1983; Hawes et al., 1995; Morgan, Eckert & Lyon, 1995).

The racial-ethnic breakdown for the CS-LTC sample confirms the finding of Hawes and colleagues. Smaller homes served more African Americans and residents of other races than either the traditional or the new-model homes. The new-model homes showed the least racial diversity, with nearly 95 percent of CS-LTC residents in the white, non-Hispanic category, although the percentage for the traditional facilities was quite similar (92%).

Marital Status. Studies in RC/AL settings tend to be consistent in showing a majority of residents as unmarried, although the percentages and marital history vary (Dittmar et al., 1983; Hawes et al., 1995; Lair & Lefkowitz, 1990). The majority of residents in facilities serving the elderly are widowed, with smaller percentages divorced or never married. Some individuals who are in RC/AL settings with chronic mental health problems may never have married because of those problems (Bartels, Mueser & Miles, 1997). Hawes and associates (1995) reported only 13 percent of their sample to be currently married and another 19 percent as never married.

Residents in the CS-LTC sample mirror these trends, with majorities widowed (from 67.4% in the homes of fewer than sixteen beds to a high of 73.3% in new-model facilities). Other marital statuses of residents vary somewhat by stratum, with relatively few residents in the new-model facilities (11.7%) falling into the "other" category (never married, divorced, or separated). Since marital status and economic security are correlated in the older population, this item is one of several that is suggestive of relative economic advantage among those in new-model facilities, especially in comparison to the facilities with fewer than sixteen beds.

Education. Educational attainment is seldom reported in studies of older persons utilizing long-term care. Profiles of the educational attainment of aged populations show high percentages who have a high school education or less, with relatively small numbers having completed college work or degrees (Kominski & Adams, 1994). The sample in the CS-LTC shows educational attainment above average for older adults, with some variation across strata. Though the proportion of sample members in each stratum completing high school was very close, variations occurred for those with less than high school education, with a higher percentage (38.1%) of residents in homes of fewer than sixteen beds and a lower percentage (27.4%) of those sampled from new-model facilities falling into this category. Both traditional and new-model homes had about four of ten residents who had completed some education beyond high school, again suggesting socioeconomic differences in the sample.

Prior Housing and Current Tenure in RC/AL. Another issue seldom described in studies of RC/AL is the prior housing arrangement from which the resident entered. Morgan, Eckert, and Lyon (1995) found that prior residence varied by state, with more Ohio residents having arrived from community settings (62%) than was the case for residents in Maryland (26%). Mor, Sherwood, and Gutkin (1986) reported that only 19 percent of their sample had prior experience in RC/AL. Data for the residents in the CS-LTC sample are remarkably consistent across strata. Thirty-five percent of the residents came to their current housing or care environment from some other supportive housing or health care setting, including hospitals, nursing homes, and other similar facilities. The remaining majority of residents moved into their current RC/AL setting from housing in the community, including their own homes or apartments, the homes of relatives or friends; or senior apartments or retirement communities without health care or supervision. For a majority of CS-LTC residents studied, then, their current RC/AL setting was their first step from unsupported community living. Logistic regressions showed significant differences by state, with residents from North Carolina and Florida significantly less likely to have entered from the community than their peers sampled in other states.

A related and important concept is the length of current tenure in the RC/AL setting for residents at the time they were enrolled in the study. Two earlier studies of board-and-care homes (Dittmar et al., 1983; Morgan, Eckert & Lyon, 1995) each found an average of 3.5 years, but tenure varies by the housing type, state, and regulations regarding aging in place. Over 60 percent of residents in Cleveland-area board-and-care homes had tenures of under a year, compared to about 30 percent in the Baltimore area (Morgan, Eckert & Lyon, 1995). Hawes and colleagues (1995) reported in their ten-state study that residents studied had been in the RC/AL setting somewhat less time on average (mean = 2.8 years).

One reason to expect stratum variation in the CS-LTC is the shorter amount of time in operation (by definition) for the new-model facilities. As expected, tenures beyond three years were less common among residents in the new-model facilities, but distributions were very similar for homes of fewer than sixteen beds and those in the traditional stratum. Significant minorities of residents in these latter two strata (38.2%–41.3%) had been in residence for three years or more at the time of enrollment, compared to only 28.1 percent in new-model facilities. When current tenure was used in its continuous form in regression, the shorter tenure for residents for the new-model homes was statistically significant. When state and size were added to the regression, residents both from facilities located in Florida and from new-model facilities had significantly shorter current tenures in RC/AL. When controls for length of time in operation were added, however, the coefficient for new-model facilities became nonsignificant. The presence of many new-model facilities in Florida and state policies with regard to aging in place may partially account for this difference.

In sum, the data on the demographic characteristics of the CS-LTC suggest that the profile of residents is in most ways quite similar to those found in prior studies of assisted living or board-and-care facilities. There are some distinctions by stratum suggesting the likely socioeconomic advantage of those in new-model facilities, which are often more expensive and private-pay.

Physical Functioning

A key concern among policymakers and practitioners has to do with the degree to which RC/AL has a niche in terms of providing supportive care to those with significant physical impairments who do not require the highly medicalized and expensive services of a nursing home. Table 7.2 presents data on selected aspects of functional health and impairments among the residents sampled for the CS-LTC.

Activities of Daily Living. Prior studies in RC/AL facilities show impairments in physical functioning for many, but not all, residents. Since some facilities house mixed populations including the chronically mentally ill, a subset of residents function with few or no limitations as measured by indexes such as the activities of daily living (Lair & Lefkowitz, 1990). Most residents in a California study showed at least some limitation in functioning in physical or instrumental tasks of daily living (Newcomer, Breuer & Zhang, 1993). Residents in both states studied by Morgan, Eckert, and Lyon (1995) demonstrated significant impairments in bathing, dressing, and grooming, with 20–60 percent of residents over 65 having dependencies in these areas. There is also a correlation in most data between resident age and the degree of impairment (Lair & Lefkowitz, 1990), and in California there is greater physical impairment among residents of smaller homes (Newcomer, Breuer & Zhang, 1993). Nearly half of the residents in a ten-state study of board and care received assistance in one or more activities, but few (7%) had help with four or more (Hawes et al., 1995). In that study, 45 percent of residents had help

Table 7.2. Collaborative Studies of Long-Term Care Residential Care/Assisted Living Resident Sample Sociodemographic Profile, by Facility Type

	<16 Beds (N = 665)	Traditional (N = 648)	New-Model (N = 765)
Activity: limited assistance to total dependence, in %			
Bed mobility	15.1%	5.3%	9.8%
Transfer	22.6	8.3	18.3
Locomotion on unit	19.8	8.5	13.8
Dressing	42.9	22.8	34.4
Eating	12.1	5.0	7.4
Toilet use	32.9	16.0	25.1
Personal hygiene	45.3	21.8	33.2
Bathing	62.5	52.3	59.2
Mean number of dependencies	2.48	1.40	1.97
3 or more of 6 core dependencies[a]	37.1%	14.9%	25.4%
Mobility: uses mobility device	51.9%	62.9%	62.0%

[a]Six core dependencies exclude bed mobility and personal hygiene.

with bathing, 20 percent with dressing, and 9 percent with mobility. Hawes and colleagues concluded that board-and-care-home residents are significantly less impaired on average than the residents studied concurrently in nursing homes, reflecting their expected niche in the continuum of care.

Table 7.2 lists the percentage of the resident sample in each stratum who have some dependency in each of eight activities of daily living (ADLs). The findings suggest the usual variation among activities, with the greatest percentage of residents across strata having dependencies in bathing (52.3%–62.5%), personal hygiene (21.8%–45.3%), and dressing (22.8%–42.9%). Fewer residents in the sample faced problems with eating, bed mobility, and locomotion. Surprisingly, between 33 and 43.7 percent of residents across the three strata were reported to have dependencies in none of the eight ADL items.

There are significant variations by stratum in the level of impairment of the residents in the sample. The stratum of smaller homes (fewer than 16 beds), where all older residents were included in the sample, showed the highest percentages, with dependencies on each of the ADL items and the highest average number of dependencies overall (mean = 2.48). Logistic regression by stratum on those with three or more dependencies in ADL items (out of a possible 8) found that residents in the traditional facilities are significantly less impaired (mean = 1.4) relative to either new-model or smaller facilities. New-model residents fell in the middle on many individual ADL items and in their mean score for impairments (mean = 1.97). A fuller logistic regression including stratum, state, and number of beds found that being a resident in North Carolina was also associated with more ADL impairments and that stratum differences remained significant.

Table 7.2 also includes data on residents having limitations in three or more of the six most commonly employed ADL items (omitting bed mobility and personal hygiene). Using this standard shows again that residents in traditional-stratum facilities are least functionally impaired of our three strata (14.9%), with more residents in new-model (25.4%) and smaller homes (31.7%) meeting this criterion of impairment. This criterion enables a more direct comparison with the nursing home resident data presented later.

Medical Conditions. In examining the literature on the most common medical conditions experienced by residents in RC/AL, degenerative joint disease, circulatory and heart problems, and hypertension were the most commonly reported among board-and-care home residents by Dittmar and associates (1983). Common health problems in the Hawes and associates study (1995) included arthritis or rheumatism (42%), high blood pressure (28%), diabetes (11%), and asthma or other lung problems (11%).

Incontinence is also a common condition for residents in board-and-care homes (Hawes et al., 1995), with increasing probability of incontinence with age (Lair & Lefkowitz, 1990). Hawes and associates (1995), for example, found that 23 percent of the residents in board-and-care homes in ten states experienced urinary incontinence. Incontinence is slightly more common for women than for men in some studies (Lair & Lefkowitz, 1990).

Many of these same medical conditions appear in the sample of CS-LTC residents (data are excluded from table 7.2). The most frequently reported conditions were a complex of arthritis, rheumatism, degenerative joint diseases, and similar ailments (ranging from 44.7% in small facilities to 52.1% in new-model homes); high blood pressure (ranging from

42.2%–49.5% across strata); and vision problems, including glaucoma, cataracts, and macular degeneration (ranging from 34.7% in homes of fewer than sixteen beds to 46.4% in traditional facilities). Other medical conditions reported in 25–40 percent of residents across strata included coronary problems (angina, arrhythmia, etc.), fractures, mental or psychiatric illnesses, and dizziness or balance problems. In these conditions there were only minor variations across strata.

Urinary incontinence is common in the CS-LTC sample and varies significantly by stratum. Whereas only 14.4 percent of the sampled residents from the traditional facilities were reported to be frequently or completely incontinent, the percentages were over twice as high in both the facilities with fewer than sixteen beds and the new-model facilities (33% and 30.6%, respectively). A fuller logistic regression, including state, stratum, and bed size, showed that residents in Maryland were significantly more likely to be reported as incontinent, that stratum variations remained in force, and that there was a slight decline in incontinence associated with larger facility size.

Impairments in sight or hearing can seriously limit the ability of an older person to continue living independently. It is therefore noteworthy that significant minorities (27.3%–32.2%) of the CS-LTC sample from each stratum report these types of impairment. Differences across strata are minor.

Use of Medical Services. Another way of examining the severity of physical health problems is through the frequency with which residents in RC/AL use medical services such as hospitals, emergency rooms, rehabilitation facilities, or nursing homes. Prior research in RC/AL settings has indicated that, because of multiple impairments, 89 percent of residents in board and care reported visiting a physician within the prior twelve months, 32 percent had an overnight hospital stay, and 28 percent were treated in the emergency room (Hawes et al., 1995). Similar findings were reported for residents in California assisted living facilities (Newcomer, Breuer & Zhang, 1993).

Data on the CS-LTC sample show significant use of these more intensive medical settings. In a six-month period, one resident in every five or six required admission to the hospital (16.7% in new-model facilities versus 19.3% and 19.8% for traditional facilities and those with fewer than sixteen beds). Fewer residents (5.8%–6.2%) needed a stay in a nursing home or rehabilitation center during a comparable time frame. Moderate percentages (14.3% in traditional facilities, 15.9% in small, and 17.1% in new-model homes) had required a visit to the emergency room in the previous six months.

Use of Mobility Devices. The use of mobility devices in RC/AL settings is high in prior studies, with almost one-fourth of board-and-care-home residents using a walker (23%), 19 percent using canes, and 15 percent using wheelchairs (Hawes et al., 1995). In the CS-LTC sample, over half (51.9%–62.9% across strata) of residents were reported to use one or more devices to assist with mobility, with the percentages lowest in the homes of fewer than sixteen beds. Logistic regression results showed that the lower use of mobility devices in smaller homes was statistically significant; in the fuller regression model, small facilities were still significantly less likely to use devices, as were residents in North Carolina and in Maryland compared to other states.

Cognitive Functioning and Mental Health

Chronic mental disorders, including Alzheimer disease and other dementias, chronic mental illness, and developmental disabilities, appear widely in the RC/AL population (Bartels, Mueser & Miles, 1997; Dittmar et al., 1983; Hawes et al., 1995; Mor, Sherwood & Gutkin, 1986; Morgan, Eckert & Lyon, 1995; Rovner & Katz, 1993). Data on the CS-LTC sample related to these topics are presented in table 7.3 and described below.

Cognitive Impairment. Estimates of the prevalence of cognitive impairment in RC/AL populations vary widely, depending on the criteria used. In a nationally representative sample of residents in personal care homes, about one-third of those over 80 were characterized as having dementia of some type (Lair & Lefkowitz, 1990). Cognitive impairment not related to mental illness was reported to involve about one in four residents of the board-and-care homes studied by Hawes and colleagues (1995), with 40 percent of residents overall having some level of cognitive impairment. Residents in California licensed facilities have both cognitive impairment and behavioral problems, with the rates inversely related to the size of the facility (Newcomer, Breuer & Zhang, 1993). A study of small board-and-care homes by Morgan, Eckert, and Lyon (1995) found that nearly one-third of their resident sample evidenced significant cognitive impairment, based on the MMSE. Similar percentages of cognitive impairment among elderly persons in assisted living are reported in the United Kingdom (Jagger & Lindesay, 1997).

Table 7.3. Collaborative Studies of Long-Term Care Residential Care/Assisted Living Resident Sample Cognitive Functioning, Behavioral Problems, and Depression Indicators, by Facility Type (%)

	<16 Beds (N = 665)	Traditional (N = 648)	New-Model (N = 765)
Cognitive status[a]			
Intact	36.9%	55.1%	48.0%
Mild–moderately impaired	31.7	29.5	25.3
Severely impaired	31.4	15.4	26.7
Behavioral problems[b]			
Cursing, verbal aggression	21.6	16.4	16.5
Complaining	16.2	10.9	14.5
Pacing, aimless wandering	15.4	11.4	17.8
Constant requests for attention	19.7	11.8	15.2
Repetitive sentences	16.8	12.0	14.4
General restlessness, repetitious mannerisms	14.9	10.0	12.7
1+ CMAI behaviors	48.9	36.4	39.0
Resists taking medications	9.8	6.1	9.0
Resists assistance with ADLs	15.9	9.1	15.6
Hallucinations or delusions	18.3	11.0	10.7
Depression[c]			
Anxious, worrying	35.1	37.7	35.9
Easily annoyed, irritable	31.5	24.2	27.5
Sad expression, tearful	25.2	23.9	25.5
Slow movements, speech, reactions	23.1	18.4	20.3

Note: ADLs = activities of daily living.
[a]Based on MDS-COGS score, with 0–1 indicating intact, 2–4 indicating mild–moderately impaired, and 5 or greater indicating severely impaired.
[b]The first six items are the most commonly reported items from the Cohen-Mansfield Agitation Index (CMAI) (Cohen-Mansfield & Billig, 1986).
[c]Most commonly reported items from the Cornell Scale for Depression in Dementia (Alexopoulous et al., 1988).

Data presented in table 7.3, using items identical to those in the Minimum Data Set, suggest that there are substantial numbers in the CS-LTC sample with moderate to significant cognitive impairment and that there is notable variation across strata. In the traditional facilities, for example, slightly over half (55.1%) of the sampled residents achieved a score reflecting intact cognition, whereas substantially fewer (36.9% and 48.0%) in facilities with fewer than sixteen beds and in the new-model facilities were cognitively intact. Small facilities contained the highest percentages of residents with severe impairment (31.4%), compared to a low of 15.4 percent in traditional homes. At both extremes, the new-model homes held an intermediate position.

Mental Health and Behavioral Problems. Behavioral problems, including violence, wandering, and other disruptions such as yelling, may be related either to dementia or to chronic mental illness. Homes are frequently not well oriented to caring for mentally ill individuals, who do not fit into the expected demographics or usual service needs of an elderly clientele (Gottesman et al., 1991; Rovner & Katz, 1993).

Studies of board-and-care homes showed about one-third of residents experiencing non-dementia-related mental or emotional problems (Dittmar et al., 1983; Hawes et al., 1995; Lair & Lefkowitz, 1990; Spore et al., 1996). In most cases, these are chronically mentally ill individuals, some of whom are also elderly. One analysis reported that 28 percent of residents had previously spent some time in a mental hospital (Mor, Sherwood & Gutkin, 1986). Two studies (Dittmar et al., 1983; Hawes et al., 1995) identified psychiatric conditions in approximately one-third of residents in board-and-care homes. One study described 31 percent of residents overall as being upset or yelling, 11 percent as wandering, and 11 percent as physically hurting others (Lair & Lefkowitz, 1990). In a study of California assisted living residents, 70 percent of those living in small to midsized facilities evidenced one or more behavioral problems (Newcomer, Breuer & Zhang, 1993).

Table 7.3 presents two sets of data on behavioral problems. First is a set of items from the Cohen-Mansfield Agitation Inventory (CMAI) (Cohen-Mansfield & Billig, 1986). Substantial minorities of the sample were reported to evidence problems with several of the fourteen items. Among the most commonly reported behavioral problems were cursing and verbal aggression, complaining, pacing or wandering aimlessly, constant requests for attention, repetitive statements, and restlessness or repetitious mannerisms. Overall percentages were highest in the homes of fewer than sixteen beds (48.9% compared to 36.4% for traditional and 39.0% for new-model facilities).

The other behavioral data relate to three specific behaviors causing problems with care: resistance to medications and to care and the presence of hallucinations or delusions. Fewer than one in ten residents in the CS-LTC sample resisted taking medications. The traditional homes reported somewhat fewer residents with this problem than the other two strata. Somewhat more common is resistance to ADL assistance, reported for about one in six residents in homes of fewer than sixteen beds and in new-model facilities. Similarly, this behavioral issue was less commonly reported for the residents in the traditional stratum homes. Hallucinations or delusions were reported in 18.3 percent of residents of small facilities and fewer of the residents in new-model and traditional homes (10.7% and 11.0%, respectively).

Depression. Depression is commonly reported in care settings for the elderly. Some level of depression was found for a majority of an assisted living sample in California (Newcomer, Breuer & Zhang, 1993). Depression is connected to poor health and functioning as well as mortality in RC/AL settings, but the direction of potential causal relationships is not entirely clear (Parmelee, Katz & Lawton, 1992b; Rovner & Katz, 1993). A comparison of nursing home and congregate apartment dwellers found lower rates of depression for those in apartments at both initial evaluation and a one-year follow-up evaluation (Parmelee, Katz & Lawton, 1992b). A second comparison of nursing homes and congregate housing (Grayson, Lubin & Van Whitlock, 1995) found higher rates of depressive affect among residents in assisted living compared to nursing homes, contrary to Parmelee and associates' findings (1992a).

Table 7.3 includes several items from the Cornell index used to evaluate depression in dementia patients. The items listed were those most commonly reported for residents in the CS-LTC sample. Over a third of the sampled residents in each stratum were reported to be anxious and worrying (35.1%–37.7%); smaller but substantial minorities were reported to be easily annoyed or irritable (24.2%–31.5%), to be sad or tearful (23.9%–25.5%), or to have slow movement, speech, or reactions (18.4%–23.1%). Variations among strata are modest, and many of these conditions could be indicative of medical, psychiatric, or cognitive problems as well as depression.

Social Functioning and Support

Isolation is possible in RC/AL facilities, especially among residents lacking spouses, children, or other geographically proximate kin (Morgan, Eckert & Lyon, 1995) and those who may have moved into the RC/AL

Table 7.4. Collaborative Studies of Long-Term Care Residential Care/Assisted Living Resident Sample Kin Network and Social Functioning Indicators, by Facility Type (%)

	<16 Beds (N = 665)	Traditional (N = 648)	New-Model (N = 765)
Availability of kin			
Proximate spouse	9.2%	8.5%	11.8%
Proximate other relative or friend	86.9	83.3	88.9
Contact with kin in prior two weeks			
Visited 1+ days	78.6	69.4	83.3
Spoke on phone 1+ days	52.6	57.1	58.9
Has a confidant	69.3	69.7	78.2
Contact with confidant in prior two weeks			
Visited 1+ days	62.1	60.8	70.5
Spoke on phone 1+ days	38.9	41.2	46.8
Participation in social or recreational activities in prior week			
0–5 activities	51.1	43.3	37.5
6–10 activities	41.9	45.7	50.1
11–17 activities	11.7	18.1	20.0
Social Interaction Scale[a]			
0–8	14.5	8.8	10.8
9–16	27.6	28.8	27.1
17–24	57.9	62.4	62.1

[a]Based on the Multidimensional Observation Scale for Elderly Subjects (MOSES), with higher scores indicating more engagement (Helmes, Csapo & Short, 1987).

environment from mental health institutions, thereby lacking a community network. Because of their health limitations, residents often remain in the facility (Hawes et al., 1995), requiring that visits be initiated by friends or family. Concerns regarding the adequacy of informal supports available to those living in RC/AL or other long-term-care settings are often paired with consideration of the degree to which social interaction needs are met by programs and friendships within the setting. Table 7.4 presents data relevant to these considerations for the CS-LTC sample of residents.

The Availability of Informal Supports: Family and Friends. In their study of board-and-care-home residents, Hawes and colleagues (1995) reported that almost 20 percent had no visitors in the prior 30 days and another 24 percent had only one or two visits. Tilson (1990) found that fewer than half of residents had visitors at least once a month. About half of the residents in facilities of various sizes in California had had visits from friends or family within 14 days, with slightly more contact among residents in larger homes (Newcomer, Breuer & Zhang, 1993). Morgan, Eckert, and Lyon (1995) found that half to two-thirds of residents in small homes had children but that siblings, spouses, grandchildren, and other kin were included among visitors as well. About one in four residents in a California-based study had no relatives within a one-hour drive of the facility in which they lived (Newcomer, Breuer & Zhang, 1993).

Data from the CS-LTC sample suggest that the availability of kin and confidants is substantial among residents sampled across all RC/AL strata. Although relatively few residents reported a proximate spouse (8.5%–11.8%), an expected result given that few are married, substantial percentages report a proximate relative or friend other than spouse (83.3%–88.9%), with only minor variation across strata. Seven or eight of every ten sampled residents across strata were reported by care providers as having a confidant or someone to whom they felt close, including family or friends. Percentages of the sample having a confidant were substantially lower for those lacking a spouse or relative within a one-hour drive (ranging from 45.9% to 54.4%).

Visiting was common across strata by both kin and confidants. Visiting by kin within the past two weeks ranged from a low of 69.4 percent in traditional facilities to a high of 83.3 percent in new-model facilities, with results from a simple logistic regression demonstrating that stratum differences were significant when comparing traditional to the other two strata. Somewhat lower percentages (60.8%–70.5%) were reported for visiting by confidants. Speaking to members of these same groups on the telephone during the prior two weeks was less common than visiting (52.6% in homes with fewer than 16 beds to 58.9% in new-model homes for kin; 38.9% in the smaller homes to 46.8% in new-model facilities for conversations with confidants). Having a confidant and having visitors or telephone calls is slightly more common in the new-model homes, a fact that may be explained in part by the higher percentage of that group who are currently married. Examination of these patterns among those lacking a spouse (or having a distant spouse) showed no differences; residents who had neither spouse nor kin within a one-hour drive were less likely to have visits or phone conversations. Kin visits for this group dropped to 45.3 percent in homes with fewer than sixteen beds and 51.6 percent in new-model facilities, and confidant phone contacts were half to two-thirds the levels reported in table 7.4 for the full sample (data not shown).

Activities and Interaction within the Home. The role of formal, planned activities in the new field of RC/AL is likely to be the subject of ongoing debate and discussion in terms of outcomes and costs. In their study of board-and-care homes, Hawes and her colleagues (1995) reported limited interaction among residents, but half of the residents spent most or all of their time involved in formal activities in the home. Newcomer, Breuer, and Zhang (1993) found that about one-quarter of residents in the homes they studied had participated in no structured activities in the prior two weeks; relatively few individuals were very active (participating in five or more activities).

The CS-LTC study included a list of seventeen formal social and recreational activities that might take up the time and attention of their residents, including activities outside the home (e.g., shopping or browsing in stores, going to the movies, going out to eat, going to the barber or beauty shop, or attending adult day care), formal facility activities (e.g., attending arts and crafts classes, playing cards and table games), and individual activities (e.g., writing letters, listening to the radio, reading newspapers or books). Participation in certain activities is likely to be constrained for some individuals by illness or cognitive impairment. In addition, formal activity availability may be limited by the facility itself because of its size, budgetary constraints, or policies and procedures.

Data for the CS-LTC sample, presented in table 7.4, show that there is substantial variation by stratum in the degree to which residents had engaged in social and recreational activities during the prior seven days, according to care-provider reports. In facilities with fewer than sixteen beds, over half of the residents were reported to undertake five or fewer of the activities listed, compared to the traditional homes (43.3%) and the new-model homes (37.5%), a difference found to be statistically significant in a simple regression. There was a corresponding difference at the upper range of activities, with slightly fewer sampled residents in the smallest facilities participating in at least eleven of the listed activities compared to those in the other two strata. A fuller regression analysis, however, showed that including bed size or comorbidity/ADL impairment of residents, both correlated with the smallest stratum, removed the significant effect for lower participation in smaller homes.

The final data presented in table 7.4 reflect the social functioning interaction scale, which is a reverse-coded version of the eight-item MOSES withdrawal scale; higher scores indicate more engagement. Care providers indicated how frequently a resident undertook social activities such as initiating contact, taking interest in activities, responding to social contacts, and volunteering to help other residents. Scores for the CS-LTC sample suggest that majorities of residents across all three strata are socially engaged, with relatively few residents scoring in the lowest category across strata (from 8.8% in traditional homes to 14.5% in those with fewer than 16 beds). Majorities of residents were evaluated in the top third of this scale across all strata, regardless of physical and cognitive impairments. Differences across strata were small, suggesting that the size or type of facility was not related to the degree to which such interactions were reported.

Summary: Who Resides in RC/AL?

It is unclear how residents with various types of impairment are sorted into the various forms of assistive environments and what the consequences are of aging in place (when it is permitted or encouraged to occur) once they have moved to RC/AL. The increase of special-care units or facilities specializing in dementia care suggests that there may be a current tendency for environments to specialize in serving select groups. In their study of board-and-care homes in ten states, however, Hawes and her colleagues (1995) found complex resident mixes in most homes, with cognitive impairment, mental illness or mental retardation/developmental disabilities, and physical impairments present in a majority of the facilities studied.

In this section we identify four subgroups of residents within the CS-LTC sample that are distinct in their needs and in the basis for placement in RC/AL. The first is those who are suffering significant cognitive impairment but whose physical health is relatively good. Several studies have demonstrated that often those with dementia experience relatively few physical comorbidities in early and middle stages (Albert et al., 1996). This means that their care needs are quite distinct from the second group, who are largely cognitively functional but experience functional limitations resulting from physical health conditions. A third group is composed of individuals who are afflicted with significant levels of both cognitive and physical impairment. A fourth group consists of any remaining individuals who are experiencing limited impairment on either the cognitive or the physical dimension.

To define these subtypes we used the following criteria: the cognitively impaired were those with scores under 17 on the MMSE or greater than 3 on the MDS-COGS; the physically impaired were those with dependencies in three or more of the six core ADL items typically used for nursing home studies. (This definition represents the nursing home standard mentioned earlier.) The dually impaired met both criteria, and the less impaired group met neither criterion.

Table 7.5 presents data for this distribution of the resident sample, by stratum. Across the three strata, it is clear that relatively few individuals (6%–11%) were placed in RC/AL solely because of severe limitations in health indicated by ADL impairments. (The standard we have applied with the ADLs is fairly high, however, since it reflects the level of functioning reported for 83 percent of nursing home residents nationally.) Most residents show cognitive limitations or a combination of both physical and cognitive limitations. Examining cognitive impairments, 14–20 percent of residents are experiencing significant cognitive impairment without significant physical limitations; RC/AL facilities are serving a substantial component of individuals with primarily cognitive problems. For those we have labeled dually impaired, experiencing significant levels of both cognitive and physical limitations, percentages of residents are moderate (9%–21%) and vary by stratum. Twenty-one percent of residents in smaller homes, 21 percent of new-model residents, and only 12 percent of residents in traditional homes met both criteria. Those who met neither criterion constituted a significant proportion of the residents in each stratum: nearly three-quarters in traditional homes (71%) and about half in new-model facilities (56%) and in the smaller homes (48%).

These data indicate that incapacities related to everyday functioning, such as the mobility limitations and problems with bathing, dressing, and personal care outlined earlier, have brought many of the residents into RC/AL settings, rather than the extremity of their physical impairments per se. These limitations are likely to be related to cognitive problems more than simply physical limitations. Clearly, this resident population is different from a nursing home population in being less impaired overall;

Table 7.5. Collaborative Studies of Long-Term Care Residential Care/Assisted Living Resident Sample Cognitive and Physical Functioning, by Facility Type (%)

	<16 Beds (N = 638)	Traditional (N = 618)	New-Model (N = 747)
Cognitively impaired[a]	20%	14%	18%
Physically impaired[b]	11	6	9
Dually impaired	21	9	16
Less impaired[c]	48	71	56

[a]Cognitively impaired residents were those scoring less than 17 on the Mini-Mental State Examination (Folstein, Folstein & McHugh, 1975). If data were missing, MDS-COGS score (Hartmaier et al., 1994) of greater than 3 was used. In a few cases (N = 17) diagnosis was used.
[b]Physically impaired included residents with dependencies in 3 or more activities (transfer, locomotion, dressing, eating, toileting, bathing).
[c]These residents met neither of the above criteria.

however, they do have notable levels of cognitive or dual impairment (23%–41% in these combined categories across strata).

Comparisons with Other Long-Term-Care Settings

A consistent question with regard to nonmedical forms of care, such as RC/AL, is whether or not they serve a distinctive niche apart from the more intense medical care provided in nursing homes, hospices, and so forth. In this section we draw comparisons where possible with other long-term-care settings to try to discern the degree to which RC/AL is currently serving a distinct and coherent population of residents.

Demographics

In terms of demographics, there are selective age differences between the sample for the CS-LTC and other long-term-care populations. The sample from the National Home and Hospice Care Survey (NHHCS) includes significant percentages (27.6% overall) of their sample under the age of 65; but among those 65 and over, fewer than half are over the age of 80 (46.8% among home health care users and 40.9% in hospice care) (Haupt, 1998). Recent data on the nursing home population suggest that, although some residents are under age 65 (8.8%), nearly half are over 85 (49.3%) (Krauss & Altman, 1998). Thus, the residents sampled in the CS-

LTC study are older than those utilizing home and hospice care and similar to the resident age distribution reported for nursing homes.

In terms of gender, nursing homes have resident populations that are over two-thirds female (71.6%), according to national data (Krauss & Altman, 1998). Haupt (1998) reports that the majority of individuals using hospice care are male (50.3%), in contrast to most other care settings, including home health care recipients (63.5% female). Again, the sample of CS-LTC residents shows similarity both to nursing homes and other users of LTC by consisting predominantly of women.

Data on the nursing home population suggest that the great majority of users (88.7%) are white, with African Americans underrepresented (8.9%) (Krauss & Altman, 1998). African Americans are better represented in the population using hospice services but are again underrepresented as users of home health care services, according to NHHCS data (Haupt, 1998). African American seniors do not substitute home health care for care in skilled nursing facilities; instead, they experience differences in need, preference, or access that require additional research to clarify (Cagney & Agree, 1999). Except for facilities in the stratum below sixteen beds in the CS-LTC, African Americans are less represented in this sample than even in nursing homes.

According to recent estimates, 29 percent of the population receiving home care in the United States are currently married, and hospice recipients are substantially more likely to be married (43.7%) (Haupt, 1998). Among nursing home residents (Krauss & Altman, 1998), a clear majority are widowed (59.8%), with only a small percentage (16.6%) currently married. In the case of marital status, the CS-LTC sample mirrors these trends, with more residents who are unmarried, mostly as a result of widowhood, and a small percentage currently married.

Health

Recent data on nursing homes report that 83.3 percent of residents were receiving assistance with or facing total dependency in three or more of the six core ADLs described earlier (Krauss & Altman, 1998). Assistance was most common for bathing (96.5%), followed by dressing (88.2%) and toileting (79.7%), with dependencies increasing with age and somewhat higher among female residents (Krauss & Altman, 1998). In comparison to nursing home populations, then, those in the CS-LTC sample show significant percentages in each stratum reporting ADL limitations, but the overall percentages reporting the most common functional impairments are substantially lower than in nursing home populations, as befits the less medicalized care they receive.

Several of the medical conditions confirmed to be common in the CS-LTC sample also appear frequently among the nursing home population (45.5% heart disease, 36.6% hypertension, 24.3% arthritis, 21.2% stroke) (Krauss & Altman, 1998). The NHHCS data suggest a different profile, especially for those utilizing hospice services. By far the most common diagnosis among hospice patients is cancer, followed by diseases of the circulatory system. In contrast, those using home health care services have diseases of the circulatory system, diabetes, musculoskeletal problems, and other, ill-defined conditions (Haupt, 1998), presenting a profile more similar to those in RC/AL despite their somewhat younger ages. Krauss and Altman (1998) report that 11.3% of nursing home residents experience bladder incontinence, but an additional 37.6% have combined bowel and bladder incontinence. Thus, the CS-LTC sample evidences a profile of health conditions that, though showing some variation across strata, largely parallels prior research in other LTC populations.

Cognitive and Mental Functioning

Some research suggests that newly admitted nursing home residents may have much higher rates of dementia than has been reported (Rovner & Katz, 1993), but results vary significantly depending on the methodology and types of information included in a diagnosis (Magaziner et al., 2000). Data from the MEPS on the nursing home population (Krauss & Altman, 1998) show 47.7 percent with dementia but suggest that over two-thirds of residents present some memory problems or problems in orientation, with rates rising among the oldest group (85 and older). An expert panel reviewed multiple sources of information and found that 48.2–53.3 percent of newly admitted residents in Maryland displayed dementia, with variations by facility size and urban location (Magaziner et al., 2000). In general, it appears that the cognitive impairment levels are slightly greater in nursing homes than in RC/AL.

More than two-thirds (68.4%) of nursing home residents in one study had one or more psychiatric symptoms (Lair & Lefkowitz, 1990), with more women than men involved. For nursing home residents, behavioral problems such as socially inappropriate behavior (14.5%), resistance to care (12.5%), verbally abusive behavior (11.8%), and wandering (9.4%)

are reported for notable segments of resident samples. Recent data on the nursing home population characterize one resident in five as having depression (Krauss & Altman, 1998). Frequently, residents in nursing homes are prescribed psychoactive medications, in large measure to address behavioral symptoms (Rovner & Katz, 1993). Many of these behavioral problems also occur in RC/AL, with some of them related to dementia.

Summary

In most ways, the residents sampled for the CS-LTC mirror the findings of other studies on the residents of RC/AL settings. Demographically, they match most of the parameters reported in the literature, suggesting that the CS-LTC sample provides an adequate representation of RC/AL residents. Data presented with regard to demographics suggest that the residents who are housed in the new-model facilities are more socially and economically advantaged, with more education, and that more are married or widowed. This may suggest that these homes are attracting a different clientele, who are more able to afford supportive housing with care as an alternative to reliance on informal supports from family or friends. This contrast is greatest with the homes that have fewer than sixteen beds, where prior research has suggested that a significant percentage of residents have faced lives of disadvantage (Morgan, Eckert & Lyon, 1995).

As with other studies, the residents in the sample for the CS-LTC experience multiple health conditions or cognitive problems that result in a reduction in their ability to live independently and provide self-care. Prior studies of RC/AL do show, as expected, lower levels of physical impairment than residents of nursing homes when measures such as ADLs are utilized. Substantial numbers of the CS-LTC sample experience sensory impairments, mobility limitations, and the occasional need for a hospital stay or emergency room care.

As with other studies of RC/AL settings, the older adults sampled for the CS-LTC experience age-related problems of cognition, long-term problems from mental illness, and symptoms of depression. These conditions certainly contribute to needs for care, and the complexity of the symptoms and problems reported reflect the challenges faced by RC/AL settings that serve general populations with widely ranging needs for care.

Most residents in the CS-LTC sample report proximate kin, having a confidant, and visiting or speaking on the phone with these individuals at least once in the prior two weeks. Since this is not a very high level of contact and some do not even meet this standard, there are likely to be residents receiving insufficient social support from their personal networks. Within the facilities, however, most of the sampled residents evidenced engagement with those around them and some degree of participation in organized social activities. Social activity participation was, however, lower in the homes of fewer than sixteen beds, perhaps because fewer options were offered.

Among the homes, there were some important stratum variations in the resident sample. First, small homes, in addition to reflecting socioeconomic differences, have more younger and more African American residents, more ADL impairments, and more cognitive impairment and behavioral problems. On some grounds, then, it appears that some of the smallest homes have very challenging residents. It remains unclear whether a process of selection might have placed these residents in the smaller homes or whether differences also arise from different policies related to aging in place. In contrast, the traditional-stratum homes seem to have the "healthiest" residents of all three strata. New-model homes are serving an intermediately impaired group in the CS-LTC sample.

Based on the results of this descriptive profile, then, the CS-LTC sample appears to mirror samples from other recent studies of RC/AL and portray some diversity by stratum and by state in the characteristics of residents. The data also indicate that homes in the CS-LTC study serve relatively few individuals experiencing purely physical problems; more often they have residents who are cognitively impaired, often in combination with physical health problems. They also confirm trends toward RC/AL facilities' providing services to fewer young, mentally ill, or poor individuals as the residents become increasingly older adults. These data also confirm Hawes's conclusion that RC/AL currently reflects a distinct niche in the long-term-care continuum by providing care and housing to individuals who are significantly less physically or cognitively impaired than the population in nursing homes.

References

Albert, S. M., Del Castillo-Castaneda, C., Sano, M., Jacobs, D. M., Marder, K., Bell, K., Bylsma, F., Lafleche, G., Brandt, J., Albert, M., & Stern, Y. 1996. Quality of life in patients with Alzheimer's disease as reported by patient proxies. *Journal of the American Geriatrics Society* 44 (11): 1342–47.

Alexopoulos, G. S., Abrams, R. C., Young, R. C., & Shamoian, C. A. 1988. Cornell scale for depression in dementia. *Biological Psychiatry* 23:271–84.

Bartels, S. J., Mueser, K. T., & Miles, K. M. 1997. A comparative study of elderly patients with schizophrenia and bipolar disorder in nursing homes and the community. *Schizophrenia Research* 27 (2–3): 181–90.

Cagney, K. A., & Agree, E. M. 1999. Racial differences in skilled nursing care and home health use: The mediating effects of family structure and social class. *Journal of Gerontology: Social Sciences* 54B (4): S223–36.

Cohen-Mansfield, J., & Billig, N. 1986. Agitated behaviors in the elderly: I. A conceptual review. *Journal of the American Geriatrics Society* 34 (10): 711–21.

Dittmar, N. D., Smith, G. P., Bell, J. C., Jones, C. B. C., & Manzanares, D. L. 1983. *Evaluation of the Board and Care Homes: Summary of Survey Procedures and Findings.* Report to Assistant Secretary for Planning and Evaluation, U.S. Department of Health and Human Services NTIS no. PB83-235747. Denver: Denver Research Institute, University of Denver.

Folstein, M. F., Folstein, S. E., & McHugh, P. R. 1975. Mini-Mental State: A practical method for grading the cognitive state of patients for the clinician. *Journal of Psychiatric Research* 12:189–98.

Fonda, S. J., Maddox, G. L., Clipp, E., & Reardon, J. 1996. Design for a longitudinal study of the impact of an enhanced environment on the functioning of frail adults. *Journal of Applied Gerontology* 15 (4): 397–413.

Gottesman, L. E., Peskin, E., Kennedy, K., & Mossey, J. 1991. Implications of a mental health intervention for elderly mentally ill residents of residential care facilities. *International Journal of Aging and Human Development* 32 (3): 229–45.

Grayson, P., Lubin, B., & Van Whitlock, R. 1995. Comparison of depression in the community-dwelling and assisted-living elderly. *Journal of Clinical Psychology* 51 (1): 18–21.

Hartmaier, S., Sloane, P. D., Guess, H., & Koch, G. 1994. The MDS Cognition Scale: A valid instrument for identifying and staging nursing home residents with dementia using the Minimum Data Set. *Journal of the American Geriatrics Society* 42:1173–79.

Haupt, B. J. 1998. *An Overview of Home Health and Hospice Care Patients: 1996 National Home and Hospice Care Survey.* Advance Data, no. 297. Washington, DC: Centers for Disease Control and Prevention, National Center for Health Statistics.

Hawes, C., Lux, L., Wildfire, J., Green, R., Mor, V., Greene, A., Wilcox, V., Phillips, C. D., Spore, D., & Iannacchione, V. 1995. *A Description of Board and Care Facilities, Operators, and Residents.* Report to the Office of the Assistant Secretary for Planning and Evaluation. Research Triangle Park, NC:

U.S. Department of Health and Human Services, Research Triangle Institute, and Brown University.

Helmes, E., Csapo, K. G., & Short, J. A. 1987. Standardization and validation of the Multidimensional Observation Scale for Elderly Subjects (MOSES). *Journal of Gerontology* 42 (4): 395–405.

Jagger, C., & Lindesay, J. 1997. Residential care for elderly people: The prevalence of cognitive impairment and behavioural problems. *Age and Ageing* 26 (6): 475–80.

Kominski, R., & Adams, A. 1994. *Educational Attainment in the United States: March 1993.* Current Population Reports, P 20-476. Washington, DC: Government Printing Office.

Krauss, N. A., & Altman, B. M. 1998. *Characteristics of Nursing Home Residents, 1996.* MEPS Research Findings no. 5. AHCPR pub. no. 99-0006. Rockville, MD: Agency for Health Care Policy and Research, U.S. Department of Health and Human Services.

Lair, T. J., & Lefkowitz, D. C. 1990. *Mental Health and Functional Status of Residents in Nursing and Personal Care Homes.* DHHS pub. no. PHS-90-3470. Rockville, MD: Public Health Service, National Medical Expenditure Survey Research Findings, Agency for Health Care Policy and Research.

Magaziner, J., German, P., Zimmerman, S. I., Hebel, J. R., Burton, L., Gruber-Baldini, A. L., May, C., & Kittner, S. 2000. The prevalence of dementia in a statewide sample of new nursing home admissions age 65 and older: Diagnosis by expert panel. *Gerontologist* 40 (6): 663–72.

McAuley, W. J., & Usita, P. M. 1998. A conceptual model for the mobility patterns of nursing home admissions. *Gerontologist* 38 (6): 726–34.

Mor, V., Sherwood, S., & Gutkin, C. E. 1986. A national study of residential care for the aged. *Gerontologist* 26 (4): 405–17.

Morgan, L. A., Eckert, J. K., & Lyon, S. M. (eds.). 1995. *Small Board-and-Care Homes: Residential Care in Transition.* Baltimore: Johns Hopkins University Press.

Morris, J. N., Hawes, C., Fries, B. E., Phillips, C. D., Mor, V., Katz, S., Murphy, K., Drugovich, M. L., & Friedlob, A. S. 1990. Designing the national resident assessment instrument for nursing homes. *Gerontologist* 30 (3): 293–307.

Newcomer, R., Breuer, W., & Zhang, Z. 1993. *Residents and the Appropriateness of Placement in Residential Care for the Elderly: A 1995 Survey of California RCFE Operators and Residents.* San Francisco: Institute for Health and Aging, University of California.

Parmelee, P. A., Katz, I. R., & Lawton, M. P. 1992a. Depression and mortality among institutionalized aged. *Journal of Gerontology* 47 (1): P3–P10.

————. 1992b. Incidence of depression in long-term care settings. *Journal of Gerontology: Medical Sciences* 47 (6): M189–96.

Polivka, L., Dunlop, B. & Brooks, M. 1997. *Project Two: The Florida Long-Term Care Elder Population Profiles Survey.* Tampa: Florida Policy Exchange Center on Aging, University of South Florida.

Rovner, B. W., & Katz, I. R. 1993. Psychiatric disorders in the nursing home: A selective review of studies related to clinical care. *International Journal of Geriatric Psychiatry* 8:75–87.

Sherman, S. R., & Newman, E. S. 1988. *Foster Families for Adults: A Community Alternative in Long-Term Care.* New York: Columbia University Press.

Speare, A., Jr., Avery, R., & Lawton, L. 1991. Disability, residential mobility, and changes in living arrangements. *Journal of Gerontology: Social Sciences* 46 (3): S133–42.

Spore, D., Mor, V., Larrat, E. P., Hiris, J., & Hawes, C. 1996. Regulatory environment and psychotropic use in board-and-care facilities: Results of a 10-state study. *Journal of Gerontology A: Biological Science Medical Science* 51 (3): M131–41.

Tilson, D. 1990. *Aging in Place: Supporting the Frail Elderly in Residential Environments.* Evanston, IL: Scott Foresman.

8 The Physical Environment

Philip D. Sloane, M.D., M.P.H., Sheryl Zimmerman, Ph.D., and Joan F. Walsh, Ph.D.

There is little doubt that the physical environment affects the comfort and well-being of residents, staff, and visitors in residential care/assisted living (RC/AL) facilities. The environment's contribution to quality of life is pervasive and extensive. It provides the all-important first impression by which visitors and potential residents often judge a facility. It can aid or hinder staff as they carry out everyday duties such as bed changing, toileting, bathing, and monitoring residents who wander. It can help make family visits pleasant or difficult, depending on its ability to provide privacy and enable activities that residents can share with their loved ones. It can give residents opportunities to feel that they are in a good place; it can provide them with meaningful experiences; it can provide them with comfort, safety, and a sense of home—or it can do none of these things.

Virtually all residents of long-term-care facilities have physical, mental, or cognitive disabilities, and a major function of the physical environment is to help them live as effectively and independently as possible. Residents with dementia are especially challenging, for many of them need to be led to activities, directed to the toilet, and prevented from having experiences that will frighten or confuse them. Given the variety of health problems and disabilities in the population they serve (see chapter 7 for a discussion of resident needs), RC/AL facilities must have environments that are flexible and serve multiple purposes.

The overall goal of physical environments for older persons should be the enhancement of the quality of life. To achieve this goal, environments must address a variety of dimensions, each of which is believed to contribute to quality of life. We approach the physical environment of RC/AL settings by considering seven key dimensions, using a modification of the model proposed by Lawton and associates (1997):

- Safety and security
- Resident orientation

- Stimulation without stress
- Privacy and personal control
- Facilitation of social interaction
- Continuity with the residents' past
- Cleanliness and maintenance

We discuss these seven key dimensions primarily as they apply to RC/AL facilities. Data are provided from the Collaborative Studies of Long-Term Care (CS-LTC), a research study funded by the National Institutes of Health and jointly conducted by scientists from the University of North Carolina at Chapel Hill, the University of Maryland at Baltimore, and the University of Maryland at Baltimore County. The CS-LTC studied a stratified random sample of 193 RC/AL facilities and 40 nursing homes in Florida, Maryland, New Jersey, and North Carolina, each of which received a data-collection site visit by one or more of the study's data-collection teams. Within the study's sample of RC/AL facilities, three strata were studied: facilities with fewer than sixteen beds; facilities with sixteen or more beds constructed since 1987 and containing one or more features associated with new, purpose-built models (termed *new-model facilities*); and other facilities with sixteen or more beds (termed *traditional facilities*). Details of the CS-LTC methods are provided in chapter 6.

This chapter discusses the rationale for each environmental dimension and some strategies that can be used to maximize the goals for each dimension. Data from the CS-LTC on measurable aspects of those goals are presented, by stratum. Also, illustrative data from the CS-LTC are presented as they describe components of "Eden Alternative," a subject of considerable attention in the long-term-care industry. The chapter concludes with a summary of the findings of the CS-LTC and their implications for practice and future research.

Systematic Observation of the Physical Structure of Residential Care/Assisted Living Settings: The Therapeutic Environment Screening Survey for Residential Care

The majority of the data presented in this chapter were gathered by direct observation using the Therapeutic Environment Screening Survey for Residential Care (TESS-RC). The TESS-RC is an instrument designed to be completed in a 30- to 45-minute systematic walk through an RC/AL facility. It systematically gathers information on an entire facility or on a unit within a facility. In the CS-LTC, TESS-RC observations were conducted by trained research staff, most of whom had extensive field experience in long-term care. All data collectors underwent training and periodic reliability evaluations to assure standardization of data collection.

The TESS-RC consists mostly of items from the TESS-NH, which itself is a valid, reliable refinement of the of the TESS 2+ and the original TESS (Sloane et al., 1995, 2000; Sloane & Mathew, 1990). In the development of the TESS-RC, a few items were added that are modifications of those in the Board and Care Walk-Through Observation instrument developed by Research Triangle Institute, the Physical and Architectural Features Checklist developed by Rudolf H. Moos (1992), and a form used by Dr. Rosalie Kane and colleagues at the University of Minnesota in a national survey of assisted living settings. These additional items were added to the TESS-NH to capture elements that are emphasized in the literature on assisted living and for which no available measures could be identified. Examples of the new items include measures of personal control, such as the presence of personal heating and cooling controls in resident rooms, and observations of the presence of plants in resident rooms. Another difference between the TESS-RC and previous versions of the TESS is that the TESS-RC provides counts of individual bedrooms and bathrooms belonging to residents who have enrolled in the study, whereas earlier versions of the TESS involved overall ratings of these rooms. This method of data collection resulted in more precise estimates of environmental characteristics and little opportunity for bias, since resident enrollment in the CS-LTC was random and 92 percent of the residents approached to participate did so (on their own or by proxy consent from family).

Additional data on facility structure were gathered by questionnaires administered to facility administrators participating in the CS-LTC. Data from these sources included information on the facility occupancy, the distribution of beds in rooms, information on the presence of animals and children in the facility, and estimates of resident participation in gardening. Items from these sources and from the TESS-RC were selected that represent measures of the seven primary environmental goals that are the focus of this chapter. Analyses consist of frequencies, means, and other descriptive statistics.

Key Environmental Dimensions

Safety and Security

A primary dimension of physical environments for the frail elderly is the promotion of safety and security (Lawton et al., 1997; Mattiasson & Andersson, 1997). Protection from fire, prevention of injury, and provision of assistance in case of need are among the goals of safety-oriented environmental design. Safety is one of the key issues addressed by legislation relating to RC/AL care buildings. Features such as smoke alarms, multiple exits, and handrail placement are generally mandated by law. Legal building requirements vary by state and the type of certification, and their implementation varies across facilities.

Fire safety is commonly addressed by building codes. This is no surprise, since accounts of rest home patients with cognitive impairment or limited mobility perishing in fires are among the early stimuli for increased regulation of the RC/AL industry. Among the measures to reduce the risk of injury due to fire are the provision of multiple exits in facilities and units, the use of fire-retardant materials, and the installation of sprinkler systems (Brawley, 1998; Regnier, Hamilton & Yatabe, 1995).

Most resident injuries occur as a result of falls, and a number of environmental characteristics can affect the risk of falls. A smooth, even, non-slippery floor surface decreases the chance of falls, since elderly people frequently have impaired vision or walk with a shuffling gait, which can cause them to trip on a slippery or uneven floor (Steinfeld, 1987). Handrails along corridors are necessary for some impaired individuals and can prevent falls for others (AIA, 1985). Bathtubs and showers should have seats available and grab bars present.

Call buttons in rooms allow residents to summon assistance. However, residents with moderate or severe dementia often do not understand what call buttons are and therefore fail to use them even in emergencies; therefore, other design features are needed to enhance staff awareness of the needs of demented residents. Examples include close proximity of resident rooms to staff work areas and motion sensors in resident bedrooms. Bathroom doors should open outward so that if someone is lying on the floor, the door can still be opened (Steinfeld, 1987).

Frail elderly people often have difficulty rising from a seated position. To reduce this problem, chairs should have armrests that extend to the end of the chair, high seats, a supportive back, and space under the seat for the feet during rising. Chairs should also be stable enough to serve as a hand-rail (Brawley, 1998).

Table 8.1 displays TESS-RC data from the CS-LTC on selected safety features, by facility type. These results indicate that nursing homes consistently achieve the highest ratings when compared with the three RC/AL strata. This points out one of the dilemmas in the provision and evaluation of quality in long-term care, which is that nursing home regulations, which were spurred by concerns about safety, have achieved their aim, yet other elements of quality (e.g., autonomy or stimulation) have been lost. A challenge for the RC/AL industry and its regulators will be to strike the proper balance between safety and some of the other goals of environmental design and care provision.

Resident Orientation

When older individuals move into a RC/AL setting, they require time to develop a mental map of the facility. Because of memory and visual-spatial problems, persons with dementia often experience great difficulty in navigating facilities and may never develop a mental map; therefore, they need visual cues to orient them on a continuing basis. Mentally impaired residents and visitors benefit from features that aid orientation as well. Thus, orientation to location and place is an important element of a long-term-care environment (Lawton et al., 1997; Norris-Baker et al., 1999).

A variety of design strategies may aid orientation. Small facility or unit size and adequate lighting are two features that generally appear to be more orienting (Netten, 1989). A building design that includes short hallways or none at all is also believed to aid orientation, because that provides greater visual access to activity areas and individual bedrooms than is possible with long corridors.

Since many halls have identical doors, a number of strategies have been developed to identify personal rooms. These include labeling with the resident's name, displaying personal objects at the entrance, placing one or more pictures of the individual near the doorway, color coding, and direct visual access by keeping the door open. Unfortunately, none of these orientation cues work for everyone. Some residents object to cuing; for example, personal pictures are often disliked by residents, who consider them to be in poor taste or to be an invasion of privacy (Brennan, Moos & Lemke, 1988).

Table 8.1. Selected Safety Features in Facilities in the Collaborative Studies of Long-Term Care, by Facility Type (%)

	Residential Care/Assisted Living			Nursing Home
	<16 Beds (N = 113)	Traditional (N = 40)	New-Model (N = 40)	(N = 40)
Percent of Facilities with Feature				
Handrails in hallways				
Extensive	14.0%	50.0%	62.5%	94.9%
Some present	17.8	21.1	20.0	5.1
Little or none present	68.2	29.0	17.5	0
Slippery and/or uneven floor surfaces in shared social spaces				
None	47.2	55.6	71.1	79.5
Little	43.4	38.9	29.0	20.5
Considerable	9.4	5.6	0	0
Mean Percent of Rooms with Feature				
Handrails in bathrooms				
Extensive	34.9	40.9	37.6	64.4
Some present	38.3	37.9	51.7	31.6
Little or none present	26.8	21.2	10.8	4.0
Resident rooms with slippery and/or uneven floors				
Not at all	78.4	74.0	87.1	92.6
A little	19.6	23.9	12.4	7.1
Considerable	2.0	2.1	0.4	0.3
Resident bathrooms with slippery and/or uneven floors				
Not at all	53.2	60.6	49.7	75.9
A little	45.2	34.2	48.7	24.1
Considerable	1.6	5.3	1.5	0
Exits with a lock, alarm, or continuous direct staff monitoring	37.6	45.3	59.0	68.4
Resident rooms with call buttons	23.0	64.4	72.5	98.8
Resident bathrooms with call buttons	11.9	59.3	84.5	95.1

Locating the bathroom is important, especially for residents with continence problems. Having the toilet visible from the resident's bed eliminates the need for any mental processing other than recognizing a toilet. A picture, graphic, or sign visible from the resident's bed or hallway can serve to orient some residents to the bathroom, as well.

Table 8.2 displays TESS-RC data on the provision of orientation cues in the CS-LTC homes, by stratum. It demonstrates that small homes clearly are much more capable than the other home types of avoiding long, disorienting corridors. Small homes also tend to rely on direct visual cues, such as open doors, to orient residents. Other cues, such as room numbers, personal objects, and photographs of the residents, tend to be utilized more extensively by larger homes, with larger RC/AL homes relying more on personal cues (pictures and mementos) and nursing homes (and larger RC/AL facilities) tending to use room numbers. Overall, the

Table 8.2. Selected Orientation Cues in Facilities in the Collaborative Studies of Long-Term Care, by Facility Type (%)

	Residential Care/Assisted Living			Nursing Home
	<16 Beds	Traditional	New-Model	
Percent of Facilities with Feature				
Configuration of rooms				
No hallways; bedrooms open into living (common) area	6.2%	2.5%	2.5%	0%
Short hallways (≤50 ft.)	85.8	22.5	12.5	2.5
Long hallways (>50 ft.)	8.0	75.0	85.0	97.5
Mean Percent of Rooms with Feature				
Cues to location of resident bedroom				
Door left open	74.5	51.6	33.2	82.9
Name of resident	8.8	8.8	15.4	9.9
Current picture of resident	2.0	4.7	11.4	10.6
Old picture of resident	0.4	2.2	9.6	1.9
Personal object(s)	12.9	28.5	37.6	11.5
Room number (≥2 in. high)	16.2	45.2	53.3	52.2
Identifying colors	0.9	0	0.2	0
Cues to location of bathroom(s)				
Toilet visible from bed	18.5	15.2	2.2	0
Sign or icon visible from bed	3.1	2.4	0.9	2.9

use of cues other than open doors and room numbers is relatively low in all facility types.

Stimulation without Stress

Creating a positive sensory environment for older persons requires both limitation of "bad" stimuli and provision of "good" stimuli. The first step is prevention of potential distractions and hazards, such as glare, uneven lighting, unpleasant odors, and noise. Merely preventing negative stimuli is not enough, however, since that would render the environment sterile and uninteresting. In addition to minimizing noxious, distracting stimuli, the long-term-care environment should offer opportunities for positive stimulation through the provision of tactile, visual, and other opportunities for residents (Lawton et al., 1997).

Normal aging is associated with numerous sensory changes, particularly in the visual and auditory systems, which can adversely affect environmental perception and the performance of daily tasks. A physical environment for the elderly should take these into account. In the eye, a variety of changes decrease illumination of the retina and impair performance in low light (Kline & Scialfa, 1996). Insufficient light can make walking less safe and reading more difficult and generally discourage activity (Brawley, 1998; Hiatt, 1979). Lighting levels that are satisfactory for young adults are inadequate for seniors; because of physiological changes in the eye, the Illuminating Engineering Society of North America recommends that people over 60 be provided with at least twice the light as 20-year-olds (AIA, 1985). Susceptibility to glare increases with age, however, so efforts to provide adequate illumination must be accompanied by glare minimization (Brawley, 1998). A number of features can achieve glare reduction, including overhangs, recessed windows, light shelves in windows, tinted glass, window shades, carpeting, glare-reducing floor and furniture treatments, indirect light fixtures, frosted bulbs, and the absence of windows at the end of hallways (AIA, 1985; Brawley, 1998; Regnier & Pynoos, 1987). Aging also brings a slowing of the speed of adaptation of the eye to different light levels, causing difficulty entering and leaving dark and light areas and trouble seeing shadowed areas in brightly lit rooms (Kline & Scialfa, 1996). For this reason, visibility and safety are increased when lighting is relatively even, without shadows or sudden changes in light level (Brawley, 1998; AIA, 1985).

Most older persons have presbycusis, an age-associated hearing loss that differentially impairs recognition of high-frequency sounds. This hearing loss makes many older persons highly sensitive to distraction from adventitious noises such as the conversation of others, the whirring of vacuum cleaners, and even background music (Elm, Warren & Madill, 1998). Thus, to facilitate conversation and task performance, ambient noise should be minimized in environments for older persons (Kline & Scialfa, 1996). High noise levels also contribute to stress, which can adversely affect mood and health (Welch & Welch, 1970). Particularly bothersome are sudden "pulse" noises, such as intercoms, alarm bells, and shouting, which are associated with startle responses and should be eliminated if possible (Kryter, 1985).

The sense of smell appears to undergo less decline with aging than the other senses (Barber, 1997). As a result, older persons may be especially sensitive to odors. Long-term-care settings should therefore seek to minimize noxious odors, such as the stench of feces and stale urine and the chemical smell of strong cleaning solutions. Positive stimulation with pleasant aromas should be present whenever possible, because such aromas can enhance mood, orientation, and function. One example is having pleasant kitchen odors waft into the living area before a meal.

The concept of stimulation without stress describes the desired balance between minimization of negative stimuli and provision of positive ones (Mace, 1991). In such an environment, noxious stimuli such as glare, uneven lighting, background noise, pulse noises, and unpleasant odors are eliminated. In their place are facilitative stimuli such as adequate, even, glare-free lighting, pleasant odors, and the opportunity to engage in activities that stimulate the senses. Thus, a long-term-care facility should contain objects that residents can touch, pick up, and work with (tactile stimuli) and things that residents find engaging and emotionally positive to look at (visual stimuli).

Table 8.3 presents TESS-RC data related to the degree and quality of stimulation in the CS-LTC homes, by facility type. It demonstrates that new-model homes scored most favorably in all aspects of lighting, including intensity, evenness, and absence of glare in public areas and in resident rooms. The new-model homes also provided more tactile and visual stimulation in comparison with the other facility types. Distracting noises were most prevalent in nursing homes and least frequent in small RC/AL facilities, with the exception of television and radio, which were present to a similar extent (60%–79% of homes) in all four strata. Body excretion

Table 8.3. Selected Indicators of the Degree and Quality of Stimulation in Facilities in the Collaborative Studies of Long-Term Care, by Facility Type (%)

	Residential Care/Assisted Living			Nursing Home
	<16 Beds	Traditional	New-Model	
Percent of Facilities with Feature				
Lighting intensity in hallways				
Ample	42.5%	57.5%	80.0%	75.0%
Good	46.9	30.0	20.0	22.5
Barely adequate or inadequate	10.6	12.5	0	2.5
Lighting intensity in activity areas				
Ample	56.3	57.5	85.0	76.9
Good	33.9	30.0	12.5	20.5
Barely adequate or inadequate	9.8	12.5	2.5	2.6
Glare in hallways				
Little or none	88.4	79.4	85.0	53.9
In a few areas	9.8	18.0	12.5	41.0
In many areas	1.8	2.6	2.5	5.1
Glare in activity areas				
Little or none	82.0	76.9	90.0	46.2
In a few areas	17.1	18.0	10.0	48.7
In many areas	0.9	5.1	0	5.1
Lighting evenness in hallways				
Even throughout	29.5	53.9	64.1	57.5
Mostly even	57.1	23.1	35.9	37.5
Uneven, with many shadows	13.4	23.1	0	5.0
Lighting evenness in activity areas				
Even throughout	39.3	50.0	64.1	45.0
Mostly even	43.8	27.5	33.3	50.0
Uneven, with many shadows	17.0	22.5	2.6	5.0
Distraction due to noise from				
Resident screaming or calling	8.0	15.0	20.0	55.0
Staff talking loudly	5.4	15.0	22.5	17.5
TV or radio	78.6	60.0	77.5	65.0
Loudspeaker or intercom	6.3	20.0	25.0	55.0
Alarm or call bells	8.9	15.0	22.5	65.0
Other noises (e.g., machines)	27.9	25.0	30.0	40.0

(*continued*)

Table 8.3. (*Continued*)

	Residential Care/Assisted Living			Nursing Home
	≤16 Beds	Traditional	New-Model	
Bodily excretion odors in public areas				
Barely or not at all	89.6	80.0	83.3	58.3
In some areas	8.5	14.3	16.7	33.3
Throughout much of area	1.9	5.7	0	8.3
Tactile stimulation available				
Extensively	31.3	22.5	55.0	25.0
Quite a bit	19.6	17.5	15.0	22.5
Somewhat	33.0	55.0	22.5	47.5
None	16.1	5.0	7.5	5.0
Visual stimulation available				
Extensively	44.3	32.5	72.5	32.5
Quite a bit	21.2	27.5	17.5	37.5
Somewhat	30.1	37.5	10.0	30.0
None	4.4	2.5	0	0
Neighborhood attractiveness				
Very attractive	25.0	27.5	42.5	12.5
Attractive	57.1	52.5	42.5	60.0
Unattractive	8.0	17.5	2.5	12.5
Very unattractive	9.8	2.5	12.5	15.0
Mean Percent of Rooms with Feature				
Lighting intensity in resident rooms				
Ample	55.5	56.4	73.4	52.0
Good	33.8	30.3	23.6	43.3
Barely adequate or inadequate	10.7	13.3	3.1	4.6
Glare in resident rooms				
Little or none	91.1	87.2	94.6	63.7
In a few areas	8.5	12.4	5.4	34.2
In many areas`	0.4	0.4	0	2.1
Lighting evenness in resident rooms				
Even throughout	47.9	55.3	69.0	45.4
Mostly even	40.9	29.6	24.8	41.6
Uneven, with many shadows	11.1	15.1	6.2	13.0

odors were least prevalent in small homes, of intermediate prevalence in both of the larger RC/AL home types, and most noticeable in nursing homes.

Privacy and Personal Control

Individuals in American society value privacy and personal control as important standards of living. Until recently, however, long-term-care facilities have placed little emphasis on these objectives. Privacy features, such as a private room and bathroom, are valued because control of lights, room temperature, door locks, television use, and other room features must be shared by residents in a multiple-occupant room (Wilson, 1996). Greater privacy has costs, however: increased building size (in square feet), more bathrooms, and greater travel distances for staff. It also makes surveillance and assistance by staff more difficult. A decline in physical competence does not, however, decrease the desire for privacy. To increase opportunities for privacy in semiprivate rooms, each resident should ideally have his or her own window, storage space, television, and telephone, with a solid barrier between the two resident spaces. Rooms housing more than two people provide little privacy.

Part of what makes a room truly private is the ability to control who exits and enters. Being able to lock the door is a simple, and the most common, method of providing this control. A lock on the door is a physical symbol of a commitment to privacy, independence, and autonomy (Regnier, Hamilton & Yatabe, 1995). A lock is of less importance to privacy than the number of people housed in a room, however.

Another aspect of privacy is the ability to carry out certain personal activities, such as bathing, urination, defecation, and cleaning of the teeth, without the intrusion of others. Although physical and cognitive disabilities often make staff assistance with these tasks necessary, access to the bathroom is an important measure of privacy. One's own toilet with bath or shower provides the most privacy; a bathroom down the hall shared by many residents provides the least.

Personal control is facilitated by privacy; however, a number of other environmental features can also enhance control over one's personal environment. The presence of a telephone or telephone connection in a room allows the resident to communicate with the outside world without using a public phone. Individual control of heating and air conditioning is important for resident comfort, as older people often have narrower comfort zones of temperature than the young (Kalymun, 1990). Windows that open to the outdoors allow additional temperature control, as well as permitting the resident access to fresh air whenever desired.

Table 8.4 displays TESS-RC data on indicators of privacy and personal control in CS-LTC facilities. It demonstrates a clear distinction between the three RC/AL strata, all of which house the majority of their residents in private rooms, and nursing homes, where private rooms are rare. The proportion of new-model homes' residents who have private rooms is similar to the proportion in traditional RC/AL facilities, suggesting that private rooms are a longstanding feature of the RC/AL industry rather than a new phenomenon. Private baths, however, tend to be most common in new-model facilities and more common in traditional homes than in small RC/AL and nursing homes.

In the area of autonomy and personal control, new-model homes consistently demonstrated a higher prevalence of the features observed. Thus, individualized heating and air conditioning controls, kitchen appliances, telephone connections, and door locks were all observed more commonly in new-model facilities than in the other three strata. Nursing homes tended to have the fewest locks on resident doors, but they did provide individual thermostats more often than small and traditional RC/AL homes did.

Facilitation of Social Interaction

People are social animals. Developing friendships, working and socializing with others, and spending meaningful time with loved ones are important elements of a satisfying life for most people. In this respect, long-term-care institutions have the potential to be superior living situations when compared with the homes of many older persons, especially those who live alone, reside in unsafe neighborhoods, or are separated from family. However, developing and maintaining friendships, though important to long-term-care residents, can also be difficult in these settings (Mattiasson & Andersson, 1997; Reed, Payton & Bond, 1998). The physical environment can help facilitate meaningful social interaction through the provision of a variety of public and private spaces for couples and groups (Lawton et al., 1997). Multiple-occupancy bedrooms are not a good way to facilitate social interaction; the negative consequences of im-

Table 8.4. Selected Indicators of Privacy and Personal Control in Facilities in the Collaborative Studies of Long-Term Care, by Facility Type (Mean %)

	Residential Care/Assisted Living			Nursing Home
	<16 Beds	Traditional	New-Model	
Resident rooms that are private	60.2%	62.1%	72.5%	18.3%
Residents who are in private rooms	54.3	65.4	63.6	18.1
Semiprivate rooms with provision for privacy other than a curtain	0.4	0	1.6	0
Residents living in rooms with three or more residents	1.8	2.7	0.5	4.7
Resident rooms with				
Individualized heating controls	13.1	60.7	81.9	75.3
Individualized air conditioning controls	15.4	54.8	81.9	76.2
Own kitchen or kitchenette	0.9	4.3	36.9	0
Telephone or telephone connection	39.3	72.1	93.4	71.1
One or more windows that open	95.9	97.5	99.8	99.1
Ability to lock door from inside	41.9	48.5	77.9	14.8
Ability to lock door from outside	25.8	48.2	74.9	13.5
Residents with				
Private bath	8.4	39.1	63.4	11.0
Private toilet only	7.5	11.1	5.4	13.6
Semiprivate bath	7.0	4.7	10.6	18.8
Semiprivate toilet only	1.9	3.4	1.8	25.0
Shared bath	16.4	11.3	16.5	7.7
Shared toilet	1.1	8.2	1.4	18.4
No direct toilet or bath access	59.6	22.3	0.9	5.6
Toilet shared by two or more residents	44.1	25.2	23.7	32.7

pingement on privacy and personal space by roommates generally exceeds their value as companions. Instead, a facility's public spaces and living areas should be designed to foster social interaction.

There is no consensus in the literature that the presence of more social spaces is better. Some design experts advocate a focal point in a facility where residents can gather and interact (Regnier, Hamilton & Yatabe, 1995). Others note that having multiple social spaces allows for a greater variety of functions, activities, and interactions. For example, a library can serve as a site for discussions, a chapel as the hub for religious activities and family meetings, and a living area with a kitchen as a focus for crafts and group activities (Kalymun, 1990). Having a focal point and having many social spaces are not mutually exclusive goals; with care, both can coexist in a facility. Innovative design features that promote social interaction include clustered entry doors to private apartments, groupings of rooms into small subunits, and clustered furniture arrangements conducive to conversation (Regnier, Hamilton & Yatabe, 1995).

Four items in the TESS-RC can be considered primarily to be indicators of facilitation of social interaction. These, and the results by stratum, are presented in table 8.5. The mean of 2.2 residents per common or activity area in small RC/AL homes suggests the greatest ease of having intimate conversation in these facilities; traditional and new-model homes are intermediate (5.9–6.0 residents per public room), and nursing homes provide little opportunity for small social gatherings (14.9 residents per public room). All four home types tended to have an approximately even split between dining-oriented public rooms and those furnished for nondining activities.

Table 8.5. Selected Environmental Characteristics That Facilitate Social Interaction in Facilities in the Collaborative Studies of Long-Term Care, by Facility Type

	Residential Care/Assisted Living			Nursing Home
	<16 Beds	Traditional	New-Model	
Mean number of residents in facility per common or activity area	2.2	5.9	6.0	14.9
Mean percent of social spaces with dining tables, per facility	47.3%	38.6%	41.8%	55.3%
Percent of Facilities with Feature				
Kitchen appliances in public area(s) for resident and family use				
Full kitchen	21.4%	18.0%	30.0%	0%
Selected appliances	8.0	12.8	15.0	0
None present	70.5	69.2	55.0	100
Absence of routine television use in the main activity area	43.4	50.0	55.0	65.0

Two other indicators of the facilitation of social interaction noted in the TESS-RC are the presence of kitchen appliances in public areas, which can facilitate a variety of food-related activities, and the absence of routine television use in the main public area. In the CS-LTC, no nursing homes had public kitchens, whereas a significant minority of RC/AL homes in all three strata did. Kitchens were most prominent in new-model facilities. Routine television was, however, more common in all RC/AL facility types than in nursing homes. It was particularly prevalent in the small homes.

Continuity with the Residents' Past

People enter long-term-care facilities with a long personal history of exposure to and adoption of social patterns, technologies, and cultural symbols (Norris-Baker et al., 1999). Ideally, people should be able to remain in contact with such familiar, personally meaningful settings and activities while residing in a RC/AL facility (Reed, Payton & Bond, 1998). The physical environment can foster this continuity by including elements that facilitate these linkages to the residents' past (Lawton et al., 1997).

"Homelikeness" is one element of continuity with the past. A homelike environment may ease the transition into the RC/AL setting, improve mood and decrease depression, and reduce agitation (Rowles, 1979; Cohen-Mansfield & Werner, 1998). To a large extent, homelikeness is equated with noninstitutional elements: small instead of large public areas, furniture made of fiber and wood instead of plastic and metal, the lack of public address systems, and the presence of personal possessions in resident rooms (Kalymun, 1990; Regnier, Hamilton & Yatabe, 1995). There is no universally applicable definition for *homelike*, however, since *home* means different things to different people. So, to some extent homelikeness should involve a fit between the resident and the facility.

The presence of personal pictures and mementos, noninstitutional furniture, and homelike decor are the observed environmental indicators of continuity of the past in the TESS-RC. Table 8.6 reports the results for these variables among the facilities in the CS-LTC. It indicates that all three strata of RC/AL scored higher than nursing homes on all three of these indicators of continuity, with the disparity being especially great in the provision of homelike and noninstitutional public areas. Within the RC/AL homes, the small homes tended to provide a more noninstitutional, homelike setting than the others, and the new-model homes ap-

Table 8.6. Selected Structural Indicators of Continuity with the Past in Facilities in the Collaborative Studies of Long-Term Care, by Facility Type (%)

	Residential Care/Assisted Living			Nursing Home
	<16 Beds	*Traditional*	*New-Model*	
Percent of Facilities with Feature				
Degree of homelikeness in public areas[a]				
Very homelike	80.5%	30.0%	57.5%	17.5%
Moderately homelike	15.9	40.0	27.5	12.5
Somewhat homelike	2.7	27.5	15.0	32.5
Not homelike	0.9	2.5	0	37.5
Percent of Rooms with Feature				
Three or more personal pictures or mementos in bedrooms	80.2	81.1	90.6	77.6
Noninstitutional furniture in bedrooms	91.2	76.8	87.6	35.5

[a]Elements considered "homelike" included patterned or visually textured fabric and wood on furniture; use of multiple furniture styles in the same room; furniture arrangement in small clusters (with chairs at right angles to each other); paper or border prints on walls; nonvinyl, nonterrazzo floor treatments; and lamps or incandescent lighting fixtures.

peared to more consistently provide for personal pictures and mementos to be part of room decor.

Cleanliness and Maintenance

Long-term-care facilities should be clean and well-maintained. Cleanliness is both aesthetic and health-promoting, for people feel and function better in a clean environment. For example, clutter in hallways can constitute a safety hazard, impairing residents' use of handrails and potentially promoting falls. A certain amount of clutter, however, can be homelike, for people normally place objects on dressers, tables, and chairs as a matter of convenience. Thus, cleanliness should not be equated with a sterile absence of personal objects or tactile stimuli; instead, it should be judged by the amount of dirt and trash present in the environment and the absence of potentially hazardous clutter.

Maintenance is required by virtually everything that staff and residents use. Items that are in poor repair are often not functional and may constitute hazards. Examples of maintenance needs in a facility include loose handrails, broken doorknobs, broken chairs, exposed wires or extension cords, and wheelchairs with missing parts. A well-maintained area has no visible repair needs. An area in need of some repairs will need only minor corrections, such as a little painting, the repair of a broken handle, or the repair of curtains. An area in need of extensive repairs has multiple broken fixtures, which may create a hazardous environment for the residents.

Table 8.7 displays the TESS-RC ratings of cleanliness and maintenance in the facilities in the CS-LTC. New-model RC/AL facilities were consistently rated highest in all categories of cleanliness and maintenance. Among the other types of homes, nursing homes tended to score the best in maintenance. Cleanliness scores showed no consistent pattern. Results were consistent for both social spaces and resident rooms.

Scales in the Collaborative Studies of Long-Term Care Environmental Data

As evidenced in the preceding tables, many discrete TESS-RC items reflect similar dimensions of the physical environment. The ability to create scales from these items was assessed. Specifically, nine groups of TESS-RC items thought to represent discrete dimensions of the physical environment were aggregated into additive measures and evaluated according to standard scale-development parameters, using Cronbach's alpha and factor analysis (DeVillis, 1991). To permit items to contribute equally, those that were not dichotomous were converted to variables with ranges from 0 to 1 and the mean was computed.

Three of the nine item combinations were validated as potential scales (i.e., as items whose values are caused by an underlying construct). These three scales reflect the dimensions of safety, lighting, and cleanliness-maintenance. They are summarized below:

Safety. Nine items are included: exits controlled for unauthorized resident exit; floor surface (slippery/uneven) in shared social spaces, hallways, resident rooms and bathrooms; handrails in halls and bathrooms; and call buttons in rooms and bathrooms. Cronbach's alpha is .77.

Lighting. Nine items included: light intensity in halls, activity areas,

Table 8.7. Selected Indicators of Cleanliness and Maintenance in Facilities in the Collaborative Studies of Long-Term Care, by Facility Type (%)

	Residential Care/Assisted Living			Nursing Home
	<16 Beds	Traditional	New-Model	
Percent of Facilities with Feature				
Cleanliness of social spaces				
Very clean	79.3%	74.4%	90.0%	73.0%
Moderately clean	18.0	25.6	10.0	27.0
Poor level of cleanliness	2.7	0	0	0
Cleanliness of hallways				
Very clean	78.2	74.4	95.0	73.7
Moderately clean	20.9	25.6	5.0	26.3
Poor level of cleanliness	0.9	0	0	0
Maintenance of social spaces				
Well maintained	79.1	77.5	97.4	84.6
In need of some repairs	20.0	22.5	2.6	15.4
In need of extensive repairs	0.9	0	0	0
Maintenance of hallways				
Well maintained	82.6	75.0	100	90.0
In need of some repairs	15.6	25.0	0	10.0
In need of extensive repairs	1.8	0	0	0
Mean Percent of Rooms with Feature				
Cleanliness of resident rooms				
Very clean	79.9	72.9	89.9	85.2
Moderately clean	18.5	22.8	9.8	14.7
Poor level of cleanliness	1.6	4.4	0.2	0.3
Cleanliness of resident bathrooms				
Very clean	73.0	66.0	86.1	74.1
Moderately clean	23.4	26.9	13.7	22.1
Poor level of cleanliness	3.6	7.1	0.1	3.8
Maintenance of resident rooms				
Well maintained	81.6	75.4	97.0	87.7
In need of some repairs	17.3	23.8	2.9	12.3
In need of extensive repairs	1.0	0.8	0.1	0
Maintenance of resident bathrooms				
Well maintained	65.6	69.3	93.0	77.4
In need of some repairs	30.1	28.1	6.5	22.4
In need of extensive repairs	4.4	2.6	0.5	0.1

Table 8.8. TESS-RC Mean (SD) Scale Scores in Facilities in the Collaborative Studies of Long-Term Care, by Facility Type

	Residential Care/Assisted Living			Nursing Home
	<16 Beds	Traditional	New-Model	
Safety	0.51 (0.16)	0.68 (0.22)	0.77 (0.14)	0.90 (0.07)
Lighting	0.75 (0.19)	0.76 (0.21)	0.89 (0.10)	0.77 (0.18)
Cleanliness–maintenance	0.88 (0.17)	0.86 (0.18)	0.97 (0.06)	0.90 (0.11)

Note: Each scale represents a mean of multiple items, and ranges from 0 (worst) to 1 (best).

and resident rooms; glare in halls, activity areas, and resident rooms; and light evenness in halls, activity areas, and resident rooms. Cronbach's alpha is .84.

Cleanliness and maintenance. Eight items are included: maintenance of shared social spaces, halls, resident rooms, and bathrooms; and cleanliness of shared social spaces, halls, resident rooms, and bathrooms. Cronbach's alpha is .91.

Mean scores on the three TESS-RC scales for the facilities in the CS-LTC are provided in table 8.8. They indicate that the scales appear to perform well and to have the ability to identify differences by stratum. Safety, for example, is scored highest in nursing homes, lowest in small homes, and intermediate in the two types of larger RC/AL homes. Lighting scores are highest in the new-model facilities and similar across the other three strata. Cleanliness-maintenance scores do not vary substantially by facility type; however, there is a tendency for new-model homes to receive higher scores, for nursing homes to be intermediate, and for the traditional and small RC/AL homes to be lowest.

Physical Environmental Features of Edenization

In recent years, a variety of innovative approaches to the physical setting of long-term-care facilities have been developed. One approach, which has been subject to considerable publicity, is the "Eden Alternative." Full-fledged "Edenization" includes more than the physical environment; it also includes staff autonomy and control, the use of teams, and the assignment of primary staff responsibility for residents, among other elements (Thomas, 1994). However, the physical environmental components of Edenization represent the most significant innovation of the approach.

Edenized facilities attempt to surround their residents with living things. Plants are placed in resident rooms and public areas. Cats and dogs roam freely, expanding the benefits of pet therapy to an entire facility. Birds are present in cages in many resident rooms and public areas. Children, often by agreement with nearby day care centers, are regular visitors to the facility and interact actively with the residents. In addition, residents are encouraged to go outdoors, both for sunlight and for the mood-enhancing benefits of the outdoors (Thomas, 1994).

In the CS-LTC, on-site observers noted the presence or absence of plants in common areas and resident rooms, the ease of access to the outdoors, the attractiveness of the outdoor area, and the availability of gardening activities. In addition, based on information provided by facility administrators, statistics were compiled on the number of cats, dogs, birdcages, and fish tanks per one thousand residents and on the degree of involvement of the residents in activities involving children and gardening. These data are presented in table 8.9.

There is considerable variation within and across strata in the degree to which physical aspects of Edenization were present in CS-LTC facilities. Plants were relatively rare in all types of facilities; a minority of facilities and resident rooms in all strata had extensive plants. Direct resident access to the outdoors was common, particularly in traditional and new-model RC/AL facilities. Gardening activities were relatively rare, and few residents were reported to participate regularly. The same was true for all types of pets. The typical facility had no pets. Cats and dogs were the most common facility pets; they were most frequently found in small facilities, and to a lesser extent in new-model facilities.

Conclusion: Functionality, Esthetics, and Quality in Environmental Design in Residential Care/ Assisted Living Facilities

Physical design requires accommodation to the needs of a variety of residents, attention to staff needs and function, concern for visitors and family, adherence to regulations, and observance of budgetary constraints. While addressing these multiple and sometimes conflicting issues, facil-

Table 8.9. Selected Physical Environmental Features of Edenization in Facilities in the Collaborative Studies of Long-Term Care, by Facility Type

	Residential Care/Assisted Living			Nursing Home
	<16 Beds	Traditional	New-Model	
Percent of Facilities with Feature				
Presence of plants in common areas				
Extensive	11.9%	21.6%	25.6%	22.5%
Somewhat	41.3	40.5	38.5	40.0
None	46.8	37.8	35.9	37.5
Level of access to outdoors from facility				
Adjacent area, residents free				
to go out on own	75.2	90.0	90.0	70.0
Adjacent area, staff must				
accompany residents	22.1	5.0	2.5	17.5
Outdoor area some distance from				
resident living space	1.8	0	7.5	5.0
No outdoor access	0.9	5.0	0	7.5
Attractiveness of outdoor area				
Very	42.5	44.7	75.0	40.0
Somewhat	49.6	34.2	25.0	37.5
Not at all	7.1	15.8	0	15.0
No outdoor area	0.9	5.3	0	7.5
Gardening activities available				
At least weekly	20.9	21.6	15.4	15.4
Occasionally (< monthly)	44.5	62.1	56.5	58.9
Mean Percent of Rooms with Feature				
Presence of plants in resident rooms				
Extensive	2.5%	12.3%	16.0%	6.4%
Somewhat	11.0	18.4	22.4	13.9
None	81.1	65.3	61.4	79.8
Estimated Mean[a]				
Cats per 1,000 residents	68	9	25	9
Dogs per 1,000 residents	65	7	18	5
Birdcages per 1,000 residents	16	14	19	3
Fish tanks per 1,000 residents	16	12	14	6
Percent of residents engaged				
in activities involving children				
at least once a week	18.1	11.2	5.5	4.2
Percent of residents gardening				
at least once a week	7.5	2.3	2.4	1.1

[a]Estimates of numbers and rates provided by facility administrators; means computed based on facility occupancy.

ity design is expected to be both functional and aesthetic. Needless to say, these demands represent a significant challenge. Furthermore, though much has been written about "quality" facility design, little empirical outcome-based data exist to validate that these tenets are associated with favorable outcomes.

These issues underscore the fact that the TESS-RC measures have significant limitations. The measures are based on the opinions and advice of experts, but many items have not been tested in empirical studies to determine whether they affect resident outcomes. An outcome-based instrument would identify which environmental factors effect favorable resident outcomes, an issue that future analyses of the CS-LTC data and other studies of RC/AL will surely address. Also, the current items do not necessarily represent qualities that are desirable to all residents and staff. Finally, they fail to measure some important concepts, most notably the ability of the environment to support resident functional abilities and the "fit" between the environment and individual resident needs or desires.

Despite these caveats, the data presented in this chapter represent a rich descriptive profile of long-term-care facilities in the four CS-LTC states. They indicate that there is tremendous variation both within and across facility types as represented by the study strata. The degree of variation suggests that the TESS-RC methodology may provide useful information. Thus, it is quite possible that a structured walk through a facility or unit, perhaps using a select number of TESS-RC items, could potentially be useful to families or others who want to objectively evaluate aspects of the environment that are important to consumers.

In the meantime, the TESS-RC items and domains provide a useful method of conceptualizing and describing the physical environment of long-term-care facilities and of comparing groups of facilities with one another. Through such awareness of the various domains of the physical environment, designers, planners, administrators, and owners can approach facility design with greater attention to the goals and functional needs of facility users, ideally achieving improved quality of life within long-term-care facilities.

References

American Institute of Architects. 1985. *Design for Aging: An Architect's Guide.* Washington, DC: AIA Press.

Barber, C. E. 1997. Olfactory activity as a function of age and gender: A comparison of African and American samples. *International Journal of Aging and Human Development* 44 (4): 317–34.

Brawley, E. C. 1998. Environment: A silent partner in caregiving. In M. Kaplan & S. B. Hoffman (eds), *Behaviors in Dementia*. East Peoria, IL: Health Professions Press.

Brennan, P., Moos, R., & Lemke, S. 1988. Preferences of older adults and experts for physical and architectural features of group living facilities. *Gerontologist* 28:1, 84–90.

Cohen-Mansfield, J., & Werner, P. 1998. The effects of an enhanced environment on nursing home residents who pace. *Gerontologist* 38:2, 199–208.

DeVellis, R. F. 1991. *Scale Development*. Newbury Park, CA: Sage.

Elm, D., Warren, S., & Madill, H. 1998. The effects of auditory stimuli on functional performance among cognitively impaired elderly. *Canadian Journal of Occupational Therapy* 65:30–36.

Hiatt, L. 1979. The importance of the physical environment. *Nursing Homes*, September–October, 2–10.

Kalymun, M. 1990. Toward a definition of assisted living. In L. A. Pastalan (ed.), *Optimizing Housing for the Elderly*. New York: Haworth Press.

Kline, D. W., & Scialfa, C. T. 1996. Visual and auditory aging. In J. E. Birren & K. W. Schaie (eds.), *Handbook of the Psychology of Aging*, 4th ed. San Diego: Academic Press.

Kryter, K. D. 1985. *The Effects of Noise on Man*. Orlando: Academic Press.

Lawton, M. P., Weisman, G. D., Sloane, P., & Calkins, M. 1997. Assessing environments for older people with chronic illness. In J. A. Teresi, M. P. Lawton, D. Holmes, & M. Ory (eds.), *Measurement in Elderly Chronic Care Populations*. New York: Springer.

Mace, N. 1991. *Dementia Care: Patient, Family, and Community*. Baltimore: Johns Hopkins University Press.

Mattiasson, A. C., & Andersson, L. 1997. Quality of nursing home care assessed by competent nursing home patients. *Journal of Advanced Nursing* 26:1117–24.

Moos, R. 1992. *The Board and Care Walk-Through Observation*. Palo Alto: Stanford University Center for Health Care Evaluation.

Netten, A. 1989. The effect of design of residential homes in creating dependency among confused elderly residents: A study of elderly demented residents and their ability to find their way around homes for the elderly. *International Journal of Geriatric Society* 4:143–53.

Norris-Baker, C., Weisman, G., Lawton, M. P., Sloane, P., & Kaup, M. 1999. Assessing special care units for dementia: The Professional Environmental Assessment Protocol. In E. Steinfeld & G. S. Danford (eds.), *Enabling En-*

vironments: Measuring the Impact of Environment on Disability and Rehabilitation. New York: Kluwer Academic/Plenum Publishers.

Reed, J., Payton, V. R., & Bond, S. 1998. The importance of place for older people moving into care homes. *Social Science and Nursing* 46:859–67.

Regnier, V., Hamilton, J., & Yatabe, S. 1995. *Assisted Living for the Aged and Frail: Innovations in Design, Management, and Financing.* New York: Columbia University Press.

Regnier, V., & Pynoos, J. (eds.). 1987. *Housing the Aged: Design Directives and Policy Considerations.* New York: Elsevier.

Rowles, G. D. 1979. The last new home: Facilitating the older person's adjustment to institutional space. In S. M. Golant (ed.), *Location and Environment of Elderly Population.* Washington, DC: V. H. Winston & Sons.

Sloane, P. D., Long, K. M., Mitchell, C. M., Zimmerman, S. I., & Weisman, G. 2000. Therapeutic Environment Screening Survey for Nursing Homes (TESS-NH). <http://www.unc.edu/depts/tessnh/>, December 22, 2000.

Sloane, P. D., & Mathew, L. J. 1990. The Therapeutic Environment Screening Scale. *American Journal of Alzheimer's Care* 5 (6): 22–26.

Sloane, P. D., Mitchell, C. M., Long, K., & Lynn, M. 1995. TESS 2+ Instrument B: Unit observation Checklist—Physical Environment: A Report on the Psychometric Properties of Individual Items, and Initial Recommendations on Scaling. Chapel Hill: University of North Carolina.

Steinfeld, E. 1987. Adapting housing for older disabled people. In V. Regnier & J. Pynoos (eds.), *Housing for the Aged.* New York: Elsevier Science Publishing.

Thomas, W. 1994. *The Eden Alternative: Nature, Hope, and Nursing Homes.* Sherburne, NY: Eden Alternative Foundation.

Welch, B. L., & Welch, A. S. (eds.) 1970. *Physiological Effects of Noise.* New York: Plenum.

Wilson, K. B. 1996. *Assisted Living: Reconceptualizing Regulation to Meet Customers' Needs and Preferences.* Washington, DC: American Association of Retired Persons.

9 The Process of Care

Sheryl Zimmerman, Ph.D., J. Kevin Eckert, Ph.D., and Judith B. Wildfire, M.P.H.

A significant impetus to the growth of the field of residential care/assisted living (RC/AL) was to provide alternative residential options for persons who did not require or desire the medical care and medical model of care embodied by nursing homes. Consequently, the policies and services through which RC/AL is provided constitute its very essence, and the common philosophy underlying all care subsumed under the term *RC/AL* is that services are brought to residents in an effort to maintain their independence in a homelike environment (Regnier, 1993). Residents value privacy, control, and safety (Kane et al., 1998), and RC/AL aims to maximize these areas as well as resident dignity, autonomy, and independence. The Assisted Living Quality Coalition (1998) proposes specific policies in these areas, including to fully inform residents of their rights, to allow them to furnish their rooms as they desire and have visitors without restriction, and to facilitate the establishment and maintenance of a residents' council to provide a forum for communication. However, careful study has not examined whether and how the policies and practices across the broad field of RC/AL actually reflect these principles. Examining the process of care, as we do in this chapter, will clarify how closely care actually mirrors these tenets.

A second reason for examining processes of care is that they, along with structure, are considered when indicators of quality are sought (Donabedian, 1966). To the extent that the process of care is modifiable, understanding which components relate to better resident outcomes provides direction for intervention. In nursing home care, indicators of process have been examined, but there are inconsistent results as to whether select components relate to quality (Ramsay, Sainfort & Zimmerman, 1995). Searching for process-related indicators of quality is especially enticing in RC/AL: given structural differences across these settings and the heterogeneity of resident need, it can be expected that the process through which care is provided will exhibit variation. Examining the relationship between process and outcomes is beyond the scope of this chapter, but that will be the use to which these data are put in future analyses.

Here we explore individual and aggregate policies and services by type of RC/AL facility, make comparisons across facility types and with nursing homes, and identify some of the factors responsible for those differences. Data are used from the Collaborative Studies of Long-Term Care (CS-LTC), a four-state study of 233 stratified, randomly selected facilities and 2,839 randomly selected residents, funded by the National Institute on Aging. (See chapter 6 for a thorough description of the CS-LTC and its methods.) To facilitate cross-study comparisons, the CS-LTC collected process-related information with a modification of the Policy and Program Information Form (POLIF) of the Multiphasic Environmental Assessment Procedure (MEAP) (Moos & Lemke, 1996). As shown below, ten aggregated measures are organized by three process-of-care domains.

Requirements for Residents

1. *Acceptance of problem behavior* describes the extent to which aggressive, defiant, destructive, or eccentric behavior is tolerated within a facility.
2. *Overall admission policies* summarizes the admission expectations that a facility has for entering residents.
3. *Admission policies specific to activity of daily living (ADL) functioning* characterizes the facility's expectations for resident functioning in physical activities of daily living for entering residents.

Individual Freedom and Institutional Order

1. *Policy choice* describes the extent to which the facility allows the residents to individualize their routines.
2. *Policy clarity* captures the extent of formal and institutional mechanisms for defining expected behavior and communicating ideas.
3. *Resident control* reflects the degree to which residents are involved in facility administration and their influence on facility policy.
4. *Provision for privacy* summarizes the amount of privacy given to residents.

Provision of Services and Activities

1. *Availability of social and recreational activities* describes the organized activities available in the facility.
2. *Overall provision of services* summarizes the extent to which multiple services, including health and supportive services, are available to residents.
3. *Provision of health services* measures the prevalence and accessibility of health services for residents.

Component Items and Aggregate Measures of the Process of Care

Each measure listed above is an aggregate of multiple items. Six measures substantially follow the algorithms developed and tested by Moos and Lemke: acceptance of problem behavior, policy choice, policy clarity, resident control, provision for privacy, and availability of social and recreational activities. Since psychometric testing of these measures is extensive, it was not repeated for the CS-LTC. New measures were developed to capture the three POLIF areas of expectations for functioning (overall admission policies and admission policies specific to activity of daily living [ADL] functioning), availability of health services (provision of health services), and availability of daily living assistance (overall provision of services). The internal consistency and reliability of these measures were assessed and are presented below.

Each aggregate measure calculates the percentage of component items that are positively scored. The minimum possible value is 0 percent for a facility in which no item is positively scored. A facility with a score of 100 percent answered positively for all nonmissing component items. (If more than 25% of the items for a particular measure were missing, the measure was not calculated. For facilities missing some items but fewer than 25% of the items, a percentage of positively scored nonmissing items was calculated.) The component items for each measure are listed in tables 9.1 to 9.3.

The Requirements for Residents domain includes two newly created measures. The measure of overall admission policies sums the number of resident characteristics or conditions that are accepted for admission into a facility and calculates an overall percentage. The internal consistency of

Table 9.1. Component Items for the "Requirements for Residents" Domain

Acceptance of Problem Behavior	Overall Admission Policies	Admission Policies Specific to ADL Functioning
Facility policies with respect to:	Facility admits residents who:	Facility admits residents who are:
Refusing to participate in activities	Are unable to get out of bed	Unable to get out of bed
Refusing to take medicine	Are unable to walk	Unable to walk
Taking other than prescribed medicine	Are unable to feed self	Unable to feed self
Taking too much medicine	Are unable to dress self	Unable to dress self
Being drunk	Are unable to take care of appearance	Unable to take care of appearance
Wandering at night	Are unable to bathe or clean self	Unable to bathe or clean self
Leaving building during the evening without telling anyone	Are incontinent	Incontinent
Refusing to bathe regularly	Are unable to communicate needs	
Creating a disturbance	Are unable to handle money	
Pilfering or stealing	Are unable to make own bed	
Damaging property	Are unable to clean own room	
Verbally threatening another resident	Are confused or disoriented	
Physically attacking another resident	Are depressed	
Physically attacking staff	Are mentally retarded	
Attempting suicide	Are mentally ill	
Indecently exposing self	Are SSI recipients	
	Are Medicaid recipients	
	Have substance abuse problem	
	Need assistance taking medication	
	Require daily bandage change	
	Need assistance taking insulin or monitoring blood sugar	
	Need weekly BP monitoring	
	Require special diet	
	Exhibit problem behavior	

this index was very high, measured with an alpha of .84. The second newly created measure, admission policies specific to ADL functioning, focuses on a subset of resident conditions that are specific to residents who have impaired functioning in ADLs. The alpha for this measure was also high, .77, indicating good reliability. The remaining measure in this domain, acceptance of problem behavior, is based upon an existing measure developed and tested by Moos and Lemke.

All four measures that make up the Individual Freedom and Institutional Order domain (table 9.2) were derived from the POLIF; differences exist in only a few component items, and they are primarily minor wording changes. Of the three measures that define Provision of Services and Activities (table 9.3), two are similar to but a modification of those created by Moos and Lemke; specifically, several items were added that are not included in the original measures. Overall provision of services and provision of health services include six modified items to distinguish between on-site and off-site provision. The health services measure focuses on the subset of services specifically related to medical care. Cronbach's alphas for the overall services measure and the health services measure were high, .80 and .74, respectively.

Analytic Strategy

As discussed more thoroughly in chapter 6, data were collected in 193 RC/AL facilities and 40 nursing homes across Florida, Maryland, New Jersey, and North Carolina. RC/AL facilities were stratified into three main types under study, in order to capture the diversity of RC/AL: facilities with fewer than sixteen beds; facilities with sixteen or more beds that met criteria to constitute *new-model* RC/AL; and facilities with sixteen or more beds that did not meet these criteria (referred to as *traditional*). Data were collected by areas within a facility and ultimately aggregated into facility-level measures. The areas refer to specific sections that provide care primarily for residents with dementia. Facility administrators provided information separately for each area, and algorithms were developed to combine area items into the facility-level indicators that are described in this chapter. (Chapter 11 addresses process of care and other differences between dementia and nondementia care areas.)

Bivariate and multivariate statistics were used to examine the relationship between facility type (fewer than 16 beds, traditional, or new-model)

Table 9.2. Component Items for the "Individual Freedom and Institutional Order" Domain

Policy Choice	Policy Clarity	Resident Control	Provision for Privacy
Meal times flexible (breakfast, lunch, dinner)	Handbook for staff Handbook for residents	Residents have paid jobs in facility	Prevalence of private rooms
Dinner seating flexible	Orientation for new residents	Residents do unpaid chores	Prevalence of double rooms
Minimum of eleven hours for visitation	Formal staff meetings	Residents' council with regular meetings	Prevalence of private baths
Facility rules on:	Weekly staff meetings	Regular house meetings for residents	Prevalence of shared baths
Having own furniture	Orientation for volunteers	Resident committees	Prevalence of individual mailboxes
Moving furniture in own room	Newsletter	Newsletter written by residents	Dresser for every resident
Keeping fish or bird	Monthly newsletter	Bulletin board for residents	Locks on all bathroom doors
Keeping coffee maker or hot plate in room	Rules and regulations posted	*Residents involved in making policy on or planning:*	Residents can close own door
Doing some laundry in bathroom	Orientation for new staff	Entertainment	Residents can lock own door
Drinking glass of wine or beer at meals		Educational activities	
Skipping breakfast to sleep late		New activities	
Flexible wake time		Welcome activities	
Flexible bath or shower time		Menus	
Flexible bedtime		Mealtimes	
Curfew in facility		Visiting hours	
Background music playing		Public decor	
Some areas of building closed to residents		Dealing with safety hazards	
Drinking in own room		Dealing with residents' complaints	
		Making rules about use of alcohol	
		Selecting new residents	
		Moving residents' rooms	
		Deciding when a resident must leave	
		Changes in staff	
		Making rules about activity attendance	

Table 9.3. Component Items for the "Provision of Services and Activities" Domain

Availability of Social and Recreational Activities	Overall Provision of Services	Provision of Health Services
Exercise and physical fitness	Physician services on or off-site	Physician services on or off-site
Outside entertainment		
Discussion groups	Nursing services	Nursing services
Reality orientation groups	Medical clinic	Medical clinic
Self-help groups	Assistance in taking prescribed medication	Assistance in taking prescribed medication
Movies		
Club, drama, singing groups	Physical therapy on or off-site	Physical therapy on or off-site
Classes or lectures	Psychotherapy on or off-site	
Bingo, cards, other games	On-site X-rays	Psychotherapy on or off-site
Parties	On-site blood drawing	
Religious services	On-site defibrillator	On-site X-rays
Social hour	On-site CPR-trained staff	On-site blood drawing
Arts and crafts	Case management or social work	On-site defibrillator
	Religious services on or off-site	On-site CPR-trained staff
	Banking services on or off-site	
	Housekeeping or cleaning	
	Help residents cook meals	
	Barber or beautician on or off-site	
	Shopping services	
	Transportation	
	Assistance in handling money	
	Senior adult day care on or off-site	

and the process-of-care measures; all are unweighted. The bivariate measures describe individual and aggregate components of care, combining facilities of a like type across states. Using the aggregated measures, a process-of-care profile is presented for each facility type. Finally, the relationship between facility characteristics and process of care is examined using multivariate techniques that control for potential confounding by ownership, affiliation, facility age, and facility size. State is included in each model as an independent variable.

Results

Components Items of the Process of Care

Requirements for Residents. Table 9.4 shows the percentage of facilities that allow, tolerate, or discourage select problem behaviors. The remainder of the facilities find the behaviors intolerable, meaning that residents who persisted in those behaviors would likely be discharged. All or most facilities are tolerant of residents who do not participate in activities or will not take their medication; less than one-third are tolerant of residents who take too much medication, exhibit drunkenness, steal, damage property, attack others, or attempt suicide. Of all facility types, nursing homes are the most tolerant in five of sixteen (31%) areas: refusing medications, creating a disturbance, threatening verbally, attacking physically, and exposing oneself. Comparing RC/AL strata, on the whole, smaller fa-

Table 9.4. Proportion of Facilities That Will Not Discharge Residents for Select Problem Behaviors, by Facility Type (%)

| Problem Behavior | Residential Care/Assisted Living | | | Nursing Home |
	<16 Beds (N = 113)	Traditional (N = 40)	New-Model (N = 40)	(N = 40)
Won't participate in activities	100%	100%	100%	100%
Won't take medication	83	82	72	95
Takes nonprescribed medications	42	55	56	31
Takes too much medication	13	26	28	21
Exhibits drunkenness	10	26	26	21
Wanders at night	29	71	59	64
Exits building without notice	19	37	44	18
Refuses to bathe	65	87	67	77
Creates a disturbance	52	74	59	82
Steals from others	20	26	13	26
Damages property	26	24	18	26
Verbally threatens residents	29	29	23	36
Physically attacks residents	5	8	3	8
Physically attacks staff	5	13	10	20
Attempts suicide	14	11	21	10
Indecently exposes self	36	32	44	69

cilities are the least tolerant in one-half of the areas. Comparing traditional and new-model facilities, at least 10 percent more traditional facilities tolerate residents who will not take their medication, wander, refuse to bathe, create a disturbance, or steal; at least 10 percent more new-model facilities will tolerate residents who attempt suicide or expose themselves.

Table 9.5 indicates admission policies related to resident limitations in ADLs and resident characteristics. Nursing homes are the most lenient in their admission policies, having no ADL restrictions and restrictions in only a few areas (problem behavior, mental retardation or illness, drug or alcohol problems, being an SSI/Medicaid recipient). Residential care/assisted living facilities are also reticent to admit these residents, as well as some of those with ADL impairments. Comparing among these types, more new-model facilities report being likely to admit persons who cannot walk (90% of facilities will admit persons who are not ambulatory, as opposed to 43%–44% for small and traditional facilities). Small facilities are more likely than traditional ones to admit persons with ADL limitations in four areas: feeding, bathing, dressing, and grooming.

Individual Freedom and Institutional Order. Data for the four measures reflecting individual freedom and institutional order are presented in tables 9.6–9.9. The degree to which residents can establish their own daily routines is demonstrated through the items in table 9.6. These items include whether select policies are in force and the degree to which resident activities are allowed or tolerated. Facilities that do not allow or tolerate these activities discourage them or discharge residents who persist in them. It is evident that less autonomy is allowed in areas that might present harm, such as having a hot plate or coffee maker or drinking alcohol in individual rooms. In only one area are nursing homes noticeably less enabling than RC/AL: they do not allow residents to do laundry in the bathroom. In general, small RC/AL facilities seem least likely to enable resident choice. New-model facilities are the most accommodating: a larger proportion have no set time for bath, bed, or curfew, and they more often allow autonomy in drinking liquor, keeping a pet, and doing laundry.

Policy clarity, reflected in table 9.7, balances resident freedom with institutional order by providing opportunities to communicate about facility structures. Overall, handbooks and orientation for staff and formal staff meetings are more typical than are handbooks and orientation for

Table 9.5. Proportion of Facilities That Admit Residents with Select Characteristics, by Facility Type (%)

Resident Characteristic	Residential Care/Assisted Living			Nursing Home
	<16 Beds	Traditional	New-Model	
Activities of daily living				
Can't get out of bed	19%	54%	33%	100%
Can't walk	43	44	90	100
Can't feed self	48	23	43	100
Can't bathe or clean self	79	62	83	100
Can't dress self	81	69	88	100
Can't groom self	84	72	95	100
Incontinent	76	77	83	100
General				
Can't communicate needs	75	56	45	100
Can't handle money	91	97	100	100
Can't make bed	95	97	100	100
Can't clean room	96	97	100	100
Confused or disoriented	92	87	85	100
Depressed, sad, crying	91	92	90	100
Exhibits problem behavior	41	33	46	90
Mentally retarded	67	72	60	83
Mentally ill	72	67	68	80
Has drug or alcohol problem	38	49	49	65
Needs medication assistance	96	100	100	100
Needs daily bandage change	83	77	93	100
Needs insulin assistance	81	85	93	100
Needs blood pressure assistance	88	95	100	100
Needs special diet	90	95	85	100
SSI recipient	59	59	50	73
Medicaid recipient	55	53	38	80

Note: SSI = Supplemental Security Income.

residents. Except for the item related to posting rules and regulations, fewer small facilities have policies to facilitate clarity than does any other facility type, and more new-model facilities have policies in every category than do traditional facilities.

In addition to resident choice, facilities may have formal institutional structures through which residents are provided control. Table 9.8

Table 9.6. Proportion of Facilities That Have Policies Enabling Resident Choice, by Facility Type (%)

	Residential Care/Assisted Living			Nursing Home
	<16 Beds	Traditional	New-Model	
Policy in effect				
Breakfast time flexible	22%	24%	41%	21%
Lunch time flexible	4	24	26	15
Dinner time flexible	6	18	26	16
Can select seat at meals	64	53	80	80
Visitation ≥11 hours/day	87	95	100	87
No set time for awakening	29	37	41	23
No set time for baths	27	42	54	33
No set time for bed	68	82	95	85
No set time for curfew	67	82	92	85
No building areas closed	47	26	36	23
No background music playing	71	53	49	49
Allow or tolerate activity				
Drink liquor in own room	8	37	69	46
Have own furniture in room	95	100	100	100
Move furniture in own room	71	92	92	72
Fish or bird in room	53	68	84	64
Hot plate or coffee maker in room	3	11	26	0
Do some laundry in bathroom	50	58	72	36
Drink wine or beer at meals	40	58	77	77
Skip breakfast to sleep in	37	55	67	72

demonstrates resident involvement in multiple areas, by facility type. In only 4 of 23 (17%) discrete areas do more than three-quarters of any facility type have such policies (those four include having a residents' council and a resident-used bulletin board, and resident involvement in dealing with complaints and moving rooms). In these areas, fewer small facilities enable resident control, and nursing homes are either equal or superior to RC/AL. In fact, of all facility types, proportionately fewer small facilities enable resident control in almost every area. Traditional and new-model facilities differ by more than 10 percent in only three areas, with more traditional facilities allowing residents to have a paid job

Table 9.7. Proportion of Facilities That Have Policies to Facilitate Clarity, by Facility Type (%)

Policy in Effect	Residential Care/Assisted Living			Nursing Home
	<16 Beds	Traditional	New-Model	
Handbook for residents	55%	74%	85%	82%
Handbook for staff	72	97	100	95
Orientation for residents	60	68	74	82
Orientation for staff	74	95	97	100
Formal staff meetings	62	92	97	100
≥1 meeting/week	16	34	24	39
Orientation for volunteers	46	75	94	97
Newsletter	14	58	77	80
≥1 newsletter/month	100	100	100	100
Rules or regulations posted	77	68	72	90

(11% vs. 0%) and more new-model facilities having a residents' council (85% vs. 68%) and allowing resident input into rules about alcohol (33% vs. 13%). Fewer than 25 percent of all facility types have a resident-written newsletter or involve residents when planning entertainment, educational or orientation activities, selecting or discharging residents, and changing staff.

The final measure in the Individual Freedom and Institutional Order domain has to do with the provision of privacy. Table 9.9 illustrates that compared to RC/AL, fewer nursing homes have a majority of persons residing in private rooms or in rooms with two or fewer residents. (In calculating the proportion of residents who lived in private rooms, all apartments were categorized as private.) New-model facilities have more persons in private rooms and provide private baths for more residents than do traditional facilities, and traditional facilities have more privacy than small facilities. Finally, markedly more new-model facilities encourage or allow residents to lock their doors.

Provision of Services and Activities. In RC/AL, services are provided to attend to the health needs of residents, their need for support with ADLs, and their need for social and recreational stimulation. These services may be provided within the physical confines of the facility, or facility staff may assist in the use of community services, such as by transporting residents to off-site medical appointments. Data for the three measures constitut-

Table 9.8. Proportion of Facilities That Have Policies Enabling Resident Control, by Facility Type (%)

Resident Involvement	Residential Care/Assisted Living			Nursing Home
	<16 Beds	Traditional	New-Model	
Paid facility jobs	9%	11%	0%	5%
Unpaid facility jobs	38	61	59	64
≥10% do unpaid jobs	33	39	11	8
Residents' council	10	68	85	100
≥4% on residents' council	9	62	78	100
Council meets ≥2 times/month	9	4	3	5
House meetings	44	63	67	72
House meetings ≥1 time/month	66	72	69	79
Resident committees	2	29	36	58
Resident-written newsletter	7	14	13	10
Resident-used bulletin board	56	89	84	87
Planning entertainment	13	21	23	25
Planning educational activities	9	21	15	10
Planning orientation activities	7	11	13	0
Deciding new activities	8	21	28	23
Making attendance rules	33	47	51	69
Planning menus	36	55	56	74
Setting mealtimes	11	37	6	28
Setting visitation hours	29	42	46	36
Deciding public decor	37	55	54	44
Dealing with safety hazards	6	24	31	39
Dealing with complaints	29	66	62	77
Making rules about alcohol	7	13	33	23
Selecting new residents	2	3	5	5
Moving resident rooms	62	79	87	92
Discharging residents	10	16	18	28
Changing staff	9	13	10	15

ing provision of services and activities are presented in tables 9.10 and 9.11. Excluded from the presentation are services related to serving more than one meal per day, providing assistance in personal care or grooming, and providing laundry or linen service: virtually all facilities provided these services.

Table 9.9. Proportion of Facilities that Have Policies Enabling Resident Privacy, by Facility Type (%)

Policy in Effect	Residential Care/Assisted Living			Nursing Home
	<16 Beds	Traditional	New-Model	
≥50% of residents in private rooms	55%	61%	77%	11%
≤2 residents/room	87	83	96	56
≥50% of residents have private bath	8	45	72	8
≤2 residents/bath	12	58	61	43
Individual mailboxes	4	33	46	14
Individual dressers	95	94	82	89
Locks on all bathroom doors	48	58	64	43
Encourage or allow resident to close door	90	100	97	95
Encourage or allow resident to lock door	29	40	77	15

Except for small RC/AL, the majority of facilities provide weekly or more frequent nursing services, on-site psychotherapy, and physical therapy and are able to obtain X-rays and draw blood on-site. On-site physician services are common in these settings as well, with 41 percent of small RC/AL facilities and approximately 70 percent of other facilities providing weekly or monthly physician care. Most facilities also provide assistance for the off-site receipt of psychotherapy and physical therapy. In reference to daily-living and other services, very few facilities help residents cook their own meals or provide adult day care on-site. Most other services are provided by the majority of facilities, with smaller facilities being less likely and nursing homes being more likely to provide them on-site.

Exercise, games, and religious services are the most commonly reported social or recreational activities provided by facilities. Proportionately more nursing homes provide these activities, followed by new-model facilities (90%–95%), traditional facilities (79%–87%), and small facilities (47%–73%). In almost every comparison, proportionately fewer small facilities provide each activity.

Table 9.10. Proportion of Facilities That Provide Health and Daily Living Services, by Facility Type (%)

Service	Residential Care/Assisted Living			Nursing Home
	<16 Beds	Traditional	New-Model	
Health services				
Physician services				
On-site	42%	72%	70%	98%
Off-site	92	97	98	100
Nursing services ≥ weekly	26	82	85	100
Medical clinic on-site	6	28	28	20
Assistance with medications	96	100	98	100
Psychotherapy or counseling services				
On-site	25	74	78	98
Off-site	86	95	93	93
Physical therapy				
On-site	43	77	90	100
Off-site	86	85	73	80
X-rays obtained on-site	25	77	90	100
Blood drawing on-site	44	80	90	100
Defribrillator on-site	2	10	15	43
CPR-trained staff on-site	91	87	98	98
Daily-living and other services				
Case management or social work	36	62	64	100
Religious services				
On-site	51	72	70	88
Off-site	85	82	90	93
Banking or financial assistance				
On-site	13	64	50	85
Off-site	68	82	78	90
Housekeeping	99	100	100	100
Meals, helping residents cook	12	8	13	13
Barber or beautician				
On-site	77	87	100	98
Off-site	80	77	70	80
Shopping	83	85	80	88
Transportation, facility vehicle	70	82	78	53
Handling money	39	77	55	83
Adult day care				
On-site	11	5	18	5
Off-site	56	62	75	83

Table 9.11. Proportion of Facilities That Provide Social and Recreational Activities, by Facility Type (%)

	Residential Care/Assisted Living			Nursing Home
Frequency	<16 Beds	Traditional	New-Model	
Weekly or more often				
Exercise or physical fitness	73%	79%	95%	97%
Reality orientation groups	31	24	41	54
Bingo, cards, other games	58	87	92	100
Religious services	47	79	90	97
Social hour	44	53	82	67
Arts and crafts	30	57	62	54
Monthly or more often				
Outside entertainment	43	57	87	97
Discussion groups	54	84	90	92
Self-help groups	15	26	18	44
Movies	82	92	97	100
Clubs, drama, singing groups	19	58	64	72
Classes, lectures	12	42	26	56
Parties	53	90	92	100

Aggregate Measures of the Process of Care: Facility Profiles

Each of the ten measures presented in tables 9.4–9.11 generates an aggregated score, indicating the proportion of nonmissing items that are endorsed; scores can range from 0 to 100 percent, with higher scores being more favorable. In the case of service provision, facilities that did not provide or facilitate a service on- or off-site received a score of 0; those that did either one scored 1; and those that did both scored 2. Table 9.12 lists the mean scores and standard deviations for each measure by facility type. Figure 9.1 plots these mean scores.

Requirements for Residents. Overall, small facilities are least tolerant of problem behavior and nursing homes and traditional facilities are most tolerant. Nursing homes are most likely to admit residents, overall, including those with ADL impairments. Though RC/AL facilities are not markedly different in their overall admission policies (they all endorsed 70%–75% of items), new-model facilities are the most lenient, and traditional facilities are the least lenient, in their likelihood to admit persons

Table 9.12. Mean (SD) Scores for the Ten Aggregate Process of Care Measures, by Facility Type

	Residential Care/Assisted Living			Nursing Home
	<16 Beds	Traditional	New-Model	
Requirements for residents				
Acceptance of problem behaviors	30.6 (21.7)	41.8 (19.5)	34.9 (20.0)	42.3 (21.8)
Overall admission policies	72.5 (19.6)	69.7 (17.8)	75.6 (15.0)	94.6 (5.8)
ADL admission policies	61.4 (30.9)	51.6 (31.4)	73.2 (22.5)	100.0 (0.0)
Individual freedom, institutional order				
Policy choice	44.7 (13.0)	52.8 (15.4)	63.4 (14.7)	51.3 (14.2)
Policy clarity	47.9 (21.8)	69.9 (21.5)	78.1 (11.9)	81.7 (12.0)
Resident control	21.3 (14.5)	37.6 (15.2)	38.6 (11.0)	41.6 (12.0)
Provision for privacy	47.9 (14.8)	64.3 (24.0)	74.9 (22.1)	41.7 (19.8)
Provision of services and activities				
Social and recreational activities	41.4 (21.6)	61.4 (19.7)	66.7 (10.5)	72.3 (12.4)
Overall provision of services	51.0 (15.3)	67.7 (15.5)	69.6 (11.7)	77.4 (8.2)
Provision of health services	51.2 (18.1)	74.3 (17.0)	77.5 (11.7)	86.7 (7.0)

Notes: ADL = activity of daily living. Scores can range from 0% to 100%, with higher scores being more favorable.

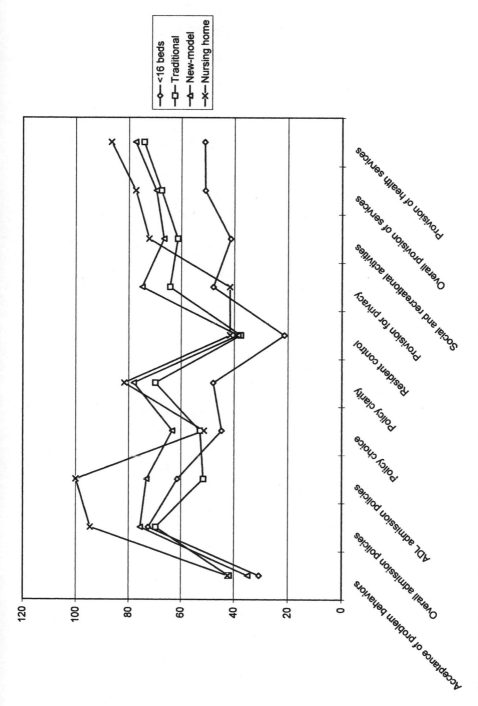

Fig. 9.1. Mean score of ten aggregated process of care measures, by facility type

with ADL impairments (mean score 73% vs. 52%). New-model facilities also have the least variation in this item than do small and traditional facilities.

Individual Freedom and Institutional Order. For all four measures in this domain, small facilities score least favorably and new-model facilities score as well as or better than traditional facilities. Nursing homes have only slightly clearer policies and resident control; they provide the least privacy. The greatest disparity among RC/AL types is in policy clarity and privacy, where there is a difference of almost 30 percent between small and new-model facilities. Compared to other RC/AL facility types, new-model facilities exhibit the least variation in policy clarity; small facilities exhibit the least variation in privacy.

Provision of Services and Activities. As with many measures in the previous domain, there was a consistent ordering with nursing homes having the highest scores, followed in order by new-model, traditional, and small RC/AL facilities. The differences between new-model and traditional facilities were not marked, ranging from 1 to 6 percent. New-model facilities exhibited the least variation of all RC/AL facility types.

The Relationship between Facility Characteristics and the Process of Care

Although differences across facility types are apparent in the preceding tables and figure, it is not clear whether the differences truly reflect differences related to facility type or whether they are due to other variables that are associated with facility type, such as size, ownership (profit or not-for-profit), age, and affiliation (with another facility). In this study, size ($p < .01$), ownership ($p < .001$), years in operation ($p < .01$), and affiliation ($p < .01$) were significantly related to facility type. Table 9.13 displays the direction and strength of results of separate regression analyses for each of the ten process-of-care measures. The following independent variables were included in all regressions: facility type, size, ownership, age, affiliation, and the state in which the facility is located. Only findings significant at $p < .05$ are displayed. Signs indicate the direction and the strength of the tested relationships, relative to the reference category or a one-unit increase in the measure of observation. For categorical variables, comparisons were made with facilities that are new-model, for-profit, have no affiliations, and are in North Carolina.

The multivariate analyses confirm some trends that were evident when

Table 9.13. Relationship between Facility Characteristics and the Process of Care: Results of Multivariate Linear Regression Analysis

	Direction and Strength of Unstandardized Regression Coefficients (p < .05)		
Requirements for Residents:	*Acceptance of Problem Behavior*	*Overall Admission Policies*	*ADL Admission Policies*
Facility type*			
<16 beds			
Traditional			−
Nursing home	+	+++	+++
Facility size			+
Not-for-profit ownership*		−	−
Age		−	
Some affiliation*			
State*			
Florida		−−	
Maryland	+		++
New Jersey		−−−	−−−
R-squared	0.09	0.38	0.37
Adjusted R-squared	0.05	0.35	0.34

Individual Freedom and Institutional Order:	*Policy Choice*	*Policy Clarity*	*Resident Control*	*Provision for Privacy*
Facility type*				
<16 beds	−−−	−−−	−−−	−−−
Traditional	−−−			−
Nursing home	−−−			−−−
Facility size				+
Not-for-profit ownership*	+++	+++		+++
Age				
Some affiliation*				
State*				
Florida				+
Maryland		−−		+++
New Jersey		−−−	−	++
R-squared	0.25	0.46	0.37	0.44
Adjusted R-squared	0.21	0.43	0.34	0.41

(continued)

218   S. Zimmerman, J. K. Eckert, and J. B. Wildfire

Table 9.13. (*Continued*)

Direction and Strength of Unstandardized Regression Coefficients (p < .05)			
Provision of Services and Activities:	*Social and Recreational Activities*	*Overall Provision of Services*	*Provision of Health Services*
Facility type*			
<16 beds	---	---	---
Traditional			
Nursing home			
Facility size			
Not-for-profit ownership*		+	++
Age			
Some affiliation*	++	+	++
State*			
Florida		--	
Maryland		---	
New Jersey	-	---	--
R-squared	0.40	0.50	0.53
Adjusted R-squared	0.38	0.47	0.50

* Reference category: new-model; for-profit; no affiliations; in North Carolina.

+ Positively associated, *p* < .05   – Negatively associated, *p* < .05
++ Positively associated, *p* < .01   -- Negatively associated, *p* < .01
+++ Positively associated, *p* < .001   --- Negatively associated, *p* < .001

reviewing the individual components of care (tables 9.4–9.11). Examining facility differences across all domains and making comparisons to new-model facilities, nursing homes are more lenient in their requirements for residents. The strongest facility-type differences are evidenced in the individual freedom and institutional order domain, where small facilities fare markedly less well than new-model facilities, and traditional facilities and nursing homes offer less opportunity for individualization and privacy than do new-model facilities. Small facilities also offer significantly fewer services than new-model facilities. Examining effects within each process-of-care domain, nursing homes and facilities in Maryland (compared to those in North Carolina) are more accepting of problem behavior. Overall admission policies are least restrictive in nursing homes and more restrictive in not-for-profit facilities, older facilities, and facilities located in Florida and New Jersey (when compared to North Carolina). ADL admission policies are more restrictive in traditional facilities, those that are not for profit, and those in New Jersey (compared to North Carolina); they are less restrictive in nursing homes, larger facilities, and facilities in Maryland (compared to North Carolina). Not-for-profit ownership has a strong positive relationship to policy choice, policy clarity, and provision for privacy, and small RC/AL facilities score comparatively worse in these areas. Facilities in Maryland and New Jersey have less clear policies, and facilities in all states other than North Carolina offer more privacy. Affiliation is related to more activities and services, and a strong state effect is evidenced in that facilities in North Carolina provide more overall services than those in other states.

Discussion

The data provided in this chapter focus on policies and services, but they do not capture all components of the process of care; other important domains of process include warmth, freedom from conflict, supportiveness, and relationships with residents and staff (Moos & Lemke, 1996). Other studies have shown, as the findings reported here do, that there is considerable variability across facilities in these domains and that they vary by facility size, ownership, and other variables (Timko & Moos, 1989). Another limitation of the information presented is that it is self-reported and may be subject to error; on more than one occasion, data collectors noted that they did not observe a service (e.g., a recreational activity) that was reported to exist. Such reporting errors would likely make a facility seem more favorable; alternatively, in cases in which the policy or practice stretches the limit of state regulation, the report might instead minimize actual service provision. The existence and extent of both of these tendencies is unknown, but is not expected to be great enough or consistent enough to invalidate the findings or the differences noted between RC/AL facility types.

Differences in the process of care across facility types are intriguing. In general (except for admission policies), small facilities (defined here as those with fewer than 16 beds) scored least favorably. It is thought, though, that small facilities are likely to excel in other components of process, such as fostering close relationships and individualizing care (Morgan, Eckert & Lyon, 1995). The relative importance of each of these areas in terms of resident satisfaction and outcomes is not known. A second intriguing conclusion is that traditional facilities do not differ dramatically from the new-model RC/AL examined in this chapter. Figure 9.1 graphically demonstrates similarities (within 10%) in acceptance of problem behavior, overall admission policies, policy clarity, resident control, provision for privacy, social and recreational activities, overall provision of services, and provision of health services. The largest differences are in relation to ADL admission policies, where the mean scores are 52 percent (traditional) and 73 percent (new-model). If the manner in which care is provided differs between traditional and new-model facilities, it is not evident through these domains.

Finally, it is worth noting that nursing homes are not as different from RC/AL settings as consumers might think; they differ from these settings by more than 10 percent only in overall and ADL admission policies. Some of the similarities across these settings may relate to the fact that providers are becoming more enlightened as to resident preferences and the importance of maximizing resident quality of life. Indeed, changes are evident when comparing these findings to those reported roughly twenty years ago (Moos, 1981). RC/AL facilities today have slightly less flexibility in terms of mealtimes and times for awakening, bathing, and bed, but they are slightly more likely to allow residents to move furniture in their rooms and have a fish, a bird, a hot plate, or a coffee maker; in general, nursing homes of today tend to allow more choice in all areas than they did twenty years ago. In terms of enabling resident control, today more RC/AL facilities involve residents in planning entertainment, orientation activities, and menus; making rules; and selecting other residents; nursing homes also enable more control in all of these areas than they did twenty years ago.

The process-of-care indicators reported in this chapter are important, as there is considerable evidence that variations in facility programs and policies relate to resident function. For example, the provision of structured programs relates to increased resident participation, as does the degree of choice, control, and privacy provided (Lemke & Moos, 1989b). Numerous studies demonstrate that depression, feelings of helplessness, and accelerated physical decline may be partly attributed to lack of environmental choice and control (Moos, 1981). Timko and Moos (1989) found that choice, control, and policy clarity are associated with better-rated resident well-being; less use of health services, daily living assistance, and social-recreational services; and better integration in the community;

apparently, clearly communicated policies improve psychological and physical well-being.

The relationship between the process of care and resident characteristics is not a simple one, however. For example, there are limits to resident control when a substantial proportion of residents are functionally impaired or have dementia; although these limits vary over time as individuals decline, the limits are widely believed to be an important indicator of quality care (Hawes et al., 1997). Functional ability and gender also may dictate the degree of choice and control that are considered desirable; Moos (1981) found that females and residents who were less functionally impaired were more likely to live in facilities high in choice and control. In essence, whether or not an environment constitutes a resource or a demand depends in part on the characteristics of the resident. Furthermore, the actual provision of services may differ across residents of similar ability because of personal preferences; the degree of benefit or challenge provided by a facility is intended to be one of negotiation, wherein residents are provided a choice of services and lifestyles, with the right to negotiate the risk associated with these choices (ALQC, 1998). Within this broad framework, there is nonetheless "bounded choice," which acknowledges that there are some absolute limits related to both the resident and the facility that limit the available options (Wilson, 1992).

Finally, as evidenced through the data provided in table 9.13, resident characteristics may relate to facility policies and services in a more global manner, and other effects are evident, as well. State differences are evident, for example, which likely reflect different regulatory constraints and differences in how RC/AL is used in different states. North Carolina's resident population is more impaired than those in other states (20% of North Carolinians receive assistance with three or more ADLs, compared to 10% in other states; 64% versus 40% have severe impairment; and more are incontinent [39% vs. 23%] [Hawes et al., 1995]), and this state provides more overall services and less privacy than the other three states under study. Also, as found in some other studies (Lemke & Moos, 1986), larger facilities and those that are not for profit tend to score more favorably on select process-of-care domains (although this relationship is not always consistent). Not-for-profit settings are typically considered to be superior in areas that are more difficult to regulate, which includes components of the social environment (Lemke & Moos, 1989a).

Conceptualizing the process of RC/AL is complex. Among other

222   *S. Zimmerman, J. K. Eckert, and J. B. Wildfire*

things, it requires consideration of differences across facility types (e.g., small, traditional, new-model), across states, across ownership, and within facility types (such as in relation to resident need). Aggregate constructs are useful for summarizing the many components that reflect process, but they mask the discrete components that constitute the residents' daily experiences: knowing that a facility cannot provide for a specified degree of need or will not allow residents an option when moving their rooms is what will matter to a prospective resident and his or her family. The information provided in this chapter can be a useful yardstick to help in considering, inch by inch or yard by yard, what is important in the provision of RC/AL services.

References

Assisted Living Quality Coalition. 1998. *Assisted Living Quality Initiative: Building a Structure That Promotes Quality.* Washington, DC: Public Policy Institute, American Association of Retired Persons.

Donabedian, A. 1966. Evaluating the quality of medical care. *Milbank Memorial Fund Quarterly* 44:166–96.

Hawes, C., Greene, A., Wood, M., & Woodsong C. 1997. *Family Members' Views: What Is Quality in Assisted Living Facilities Providing Care to People with Dementia?* Chicago: Alzheimer's Association.

Hawes, C., Lux, L., Wildfire, J., Green, R., Packer, L. E., Iannacchione, V., & Philips, C. 1995. *Study of North Carolina Domiciliary Care Home Residents.* Raleigh, NC: Research Triangle Institute.

Kane, R. A., Baker, M. O., Salmon, J., & Veazie, W. 1998. *Consumer Perspectives on Private versus Shared Accommodations in Assisted Living Settings.* Washington, DC: Public Policy Institute, American Association of Retired Persons.

Lemke, S., & Moos, R. H. 1986. Quality of residential settings for elderly adults. *Journal of Gerontology* 41 (2): 268–76.

———. 1989a. Ownership and quality of care in residential facilities for the elderly. *Gerontologist* 29 (2): 209–15.

———. 1989b. Personal and environmental determinants of activity involvement among elderly residents of congregate facilities. *Journal of Gerontology: Social Sciences* 44 (4): S139–48.

Moos, R. H. 1981. Environmental choice and control in community care settings for older people. *Journal of Applied Social Psychology* 11 (1): 23–43.

Moos, R. H., & Lemke, S. 1996. *Evaluating Residential Facilities: The Multiphasic Environmental Assessment Procedure.* Thousand Oaks, CA: Sage.

Morgan, L. A., Eckert, J. K., & Lyon, S. M. (eds.). 1995. *Small Board-and-Care*

Homes: Residential Care in Transition. Baltimore: Johns Hopkins University Press.

Ramsay, J. D., Sainfort, F., & Zimmerman, D. 1995. An empirical test of the structure, process, and outcome quality paradigm using resident-based, nursing facility assessment data. *American Journal of Medical Quality* 10 (2): 63–75.

Regnier, V. 1993. *Assisted Living Housing for the Elderly: Design Innovations from the United States and Europe.* New York: Wiley.

Timko, C., & Moos, R. H. 1989. Choice, control, and adaptation among elderly residents of sheltered care settings. *Journal of Applied Social Psychology* 19 (8): 636–55.

———. 1991. A typology of social climates in group residential facilities for older people. *Journal of Gerontology: Social Sciences* 46 (3): S160–69.

Wilson, K. W. 1992. Management philosophy: A critical element in implementing assisted living. In National Eldercare Institute on Housing and Supportive Services, *Supportive Housing Options.* Los Angeles: University of Southern California, Andrus Gerontology Center.

10 Aging in Place

Shulamit L. Bernard, Ph.D., R.N., Sheryl Zimmerman, Ph.D., and J. Kevin Eckert, Ph.D.

A growing number of older adults who have physical or mental disabilities are turning to residential care/assisted living (RC/AL) facilities when they can no longer live independently and require a supportive environment. Many who enter RC/AL settings do so with significant deficits in their ability to perform activities of daily living; they often wish to remain in these settings as their frailties increase. *Aging in place* is the term that describes the phenomenon of growing older within a specific environmental setting. Whereas early definitions of aging in place focused on older persons' preference to remain, or age in place, in their own home, increasingly the term has expanded to include RC/AL environments (Silverstone & Horowitz, 1993).

Aging in place is a complex concept, one that requires an interaction between the aging individual and the residential setting. This interaction is characterized by changes in the person's function or cognition with complementary accommodations in the setting over time (Lawton, 1990; Pynoos, 1990). However, there is no uniform RC/AL model, and considerable variation exists in the ability of these settings to meet residents' scheduled and unscheduled needs for assistance (US GAO, 1999). RC/AL settings that enable residents to age in place require an accommodating model of care (Lawton, 1980), with an emphasis on an environment that is capable of providing supportive services to the extent permitted by state regulations (MacDonald, Remus & Liang, 1994). To accommodate changing needs, this model requires that services be made available to residents in the RC/AL setting rather than moving residents to more institutional setting as their needs change (Mollica, 1995).

Whether residents of RC/AL are able to age in place is dependent on the ability and willingness of owners, administrators, and operators to provide the needed support; whether the environment is sufficiently flexible to accommodate increasing frailty (particularly mobility deficits); and whether the resident, or regulatory payment systems, can pay for the additional required services (Moos & Lemke, 1994). Facilities that promote aging in place have been described as ascribing to a "retention model" as opposed to a "transfer model" (Heumann, 1993). A facility that ascribes to a retention model is, by implication, tolerant of residents who have difficulty performing tasks related to activities of daily living, who have multiple needs resulting from cognitive or physical impairments, and who require community- or facility-provided services to address these needs. In this chapter we present a conceptual model of aging in place with specific factors that are hypothesized to influence the likelihood of individual aging in place. In addition, discharge policies related to specific resident characteristics are explored among a sample of RC/AL facilities.

A Model of Aging in Place in Residential Care/Assisted Living

Community-Level Factors

Regulatory Environment. Few federal standards or guidelines govern RC/AL; individual states have the primary responsibility for setting policies that oversee the licensure of such facilities and the care provided to residents in RC/AL settings (US GAO, 1999). Consequently, the ability to age in place is, in large part, a function of local and state policies and guidelines and how they are implemented. As discussed in chapter 1, as of 2000, twenty-nine states had RC/AL regulations and another twelve were drafting or revising assisted living or general board-and-care regulations (Mollica, 2000).

State policies that enable the provision of a variety or an array of services to a person in RC/AL facilities promote aging-in-place goals. States have adopted one of two approaches related to these goals: (1) licensure of a program or a facility that combines housing and services and (2) licensure or certification of services provided in RC/AL (Mollica, 1995). Although several states have constructed lists of levels of disability and medical conditions that may or may not be addressed in RC/AL, the most flexible policy conditions residency in a facility on the expertise of the facility's staff. In these cases, residents can remain in a RC/AL setting if care for unstable conditions is provided by a certified home health agency or an appropriately qualified facility staff.

Community Resources. Additional community-level characteristics that may influence facility retention policies include geographic location, competition, the availability of nursing home beds in the community, and the availability of community resources such as home health or hospice care. It is expected that facilities located in states that are less restrictive about admissions or discharge criteria and facilities in communities that have community-based long-term-care services with which the RC/AL facility could contract for additional services would be more likely to enable residents to remain in the facility until near the end of their lives. In addition, market forces, such as the nursing-home-bed-to-older-adult ratio or a proliferation of newly built RC/AL facilities could influence the availability of long-term-care options and the willingness of operators to retain frail residents in order to maintain or increase occupancy rates.

Facility-Level Factors

RC/AL facilities, particularly the newer, purpose-built models, often claim to promote the concept of aging in place. Such claims often lead residents and family members to expect that the resident will remain in the facility as health conditions decline or as needs for assistance progress. However, the ability to age in place is more clearly reflected in the range of services offered by the facility and in the facility's expressed rules governing who will be permitted to move in and when residents will be required to leave (US GAO, 1999). The facility's choice of whom to serve and the particular services it chooses to provide or make available will have a direct bearing on whether a resident is able to age in place. Although state regulations include requirements for the types and levels of services that RC/AL facilities may and may not provide (e.g., in addition to basic accommodations that include room, board, and housekeeping, RC/AL facilities may be required to provide additional services such as assistance with activities of daily living or ongoing health monitoring, and they may also be expected to either provide or arrange for medical services, including transportation to these services), a number of facility characteristics influence whether or not a facility is willing to tolerate particular resident needs and provide the additional services that would allow a resident to age in place. These characteristics include the facility type, size, ownership, staff resources and training, relationship with community health care providers, and age.

   Facility Characteristics. Small facilities offer several theoretical advantages as aging-in-place sites. First of all, small settings with less formal organizational structures may be more flexible in the provision of care and less likely to have formal policies regarding departures. The owner or operator of a small, independently owned facility is often the primary caregiver as well and tends to develop a close relationship with residents (Morgan, Eckert & Lyon, 1995). Therefore, small settings with less formal organizational structures may better attend to the pace and complexity of resident tasks and may also provide a more flexible and individualized approach to caring for residents. There may be greater reluctance on the part of the operator for the resident to move to a nursing home. Nonetheless, smaller homes were built as residences; many of the homes are older and lack the flexibility to change the physical structure as the needs of residents change. This limitation may result in the resident's needing to move if mobility becomes impaired.

Larger facilities, particularly the new-model RC/AL facilities, may have environmental supports, such as rails or wide doorways, and a menu of services in addition to the basic services that can be purchased by the resident to meet increasing demands (Kane & Wilson, 1993; Mollica, 1995). However, these settings may not provide the meaningful social relationships between residents and operators that can develop in smaller homes. Also, some facilities are owned by corporations that have a variety of facilities. Such organizations may have a financial incentive to move residents to their more institutional, higher-reimbursement facilities rather than to allow them to age in place.

Aging-in-Place Capacity. Facilities vary in the extent to which they are willing or able to admit residents with certain care needs and retain residents as their needs change over time. The numbers and kinds of services available in RC/AL settings may be dependent on the philosophy of care of the facility or the operator and the residents' ability to pay (Kane & Wilson, 1993; Lybrand, 1993). Also, the availability of services to residents can vary significantly by the RC/AL settings: some settings have formal arrangements with home health agencies, whereas others use outside agencies to provide episodic nursing care; some small settings use agencies to provide assistance with daily activities, and in others, residents leave the facility to attend day activity programs (Hawes, Wildfire & Lux, 1993). When asked to list the services they provide, operators typically list meals, housekeeping, transportation, laundry and linen service, activities, medication monitoring, and assistance with bathing and dressing (Kane & Wilson, 1993). In many settings, add-on levels of care can be purchased separately. For example, medication monitoring is typically included in

the basic fee, but medication dispensing may require an extra charge; po-
diatrists' and physicians' visits can be obtained on a fee-for-service basis.
Skilled nursing and ancillary care can often be obtained through third-
party providers.

Individual-Level Factors

Health and Functional Status. Resident factors influence the ability to
age in place. For example, a resident who wanders or becomes combative
or presents other problem behaviors that are difficult for facility staff to
manage may not be well tolerated in RC/AL settings. Alternatively, a resident who has multiple, complex medical conditions, even if there are no
behavior difficulties, presents a different type of challenge that an RC/AL
facility may not be prepared to manage. The facility operator may be reluctant or unable to provide the monitoring and skilled services that such
residents require and therefore may transfer the resident to a more medicalized or institutional setting.

Social and Economic Resources. A resident's income level or insurance
status may also determine the ability to age in place. Facilities vary in their
willingness to accept public payment; residents who receive Medicaid or
other public funding either may not be admitted or may be discharged
once private resources are depleted. The resident who has private insurance or is otherwise able to purchase services in addition to the basic services offered by the facility may be able to remain in RC/AL as the need
for more intensive services increases. Lower-income residents, however,
may not be able to afford additional services and may be discharged to
nursing home settings where public funding can finance their stay.

The Interplay of Community, Facility, and Individual Factors

Figure 10.1 expands on the preceding examples and illustrates the interplay of factors that influence the ability of a resident to age in place in
RC/AL settings. Aging in place, as this model implies, is influenced by a
constellation of variables, both mutable and immutable. Aspects of the
regulatory environment, such as state admission and retention policies,
dictate the resident's ability to age in place by influencing the range of services that may be offered in RC/AL. If the regulatory environment is supportive, and the facility willing, residents may be able to remain in these
settings. However, a facility may not choose to provide all allowable services; for example, a facility owned by a corporation that also manages

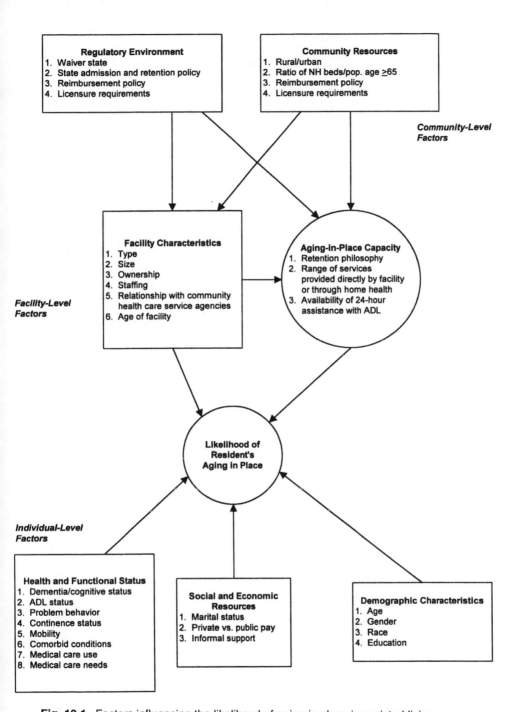

Fig. 10.1. Factors influencing the likelihood of aging in place in assisted living facilities

nursing homes may choose to move the resident to one of its more med-icalized settings as the resident becomes more frail. Finally, despite the most permissive regulations and facility policies, some residents may pre-sent challenges that exceed the scope of RC/AL. The remainder of this chapter examines individual-level factors for discharge in a sample of RC/AL facilities, with consideration of the interplay of community- and facility-level factors.

Aging in Place in Residential Care/Assisted Living in Four States

Data for the remainder of this chapter derive from the Collaborative Stud-ies of Long-Term Care (CS-LTC), a study of 193 RC/AL facilities in Florida, Maryland, New Jersey, and North Carolina. In the CS-LTC, fa-cilities were stratified to reflect three types of care: facilities with fewer than sixteen beds; facilities with sixteen or more beds that were built after 1987 and fit a new-model philosophy (defined as meeting at least one of the following criteria: at least two different private pay monthly rates; 20% or more of its resident population requiring assistance in transfer; 25% or more of its resident population incontinent daily; or an RN or LPN on duty at all times); and facilities with sixteen or more beds that do not meet new-model criteria. (Chapter 6 provides additional information about the methods of the CS-LTC.)

Operators of the CS-LTC facilities were asked whether they would discharge residents because of payment source or disabilities or needs in a number of areas, including an inability to perform activities of daily liv-ing or instrumental activities of daily living; affective, cognitive, or men-tal disorders; and select medical monitoring needs. The results, shown by facility type, are displayed in table 10.1. The table displays the proportion of facilities, by type, where the administrator indicated that the facility would discharge a resident who had a given characteristic or disability. The results suggest that there are differences in tolerance of these char-acteristics by facility type as well as differences in rates of tolerance by the particular resident need or characteristic.

Individual-Level Factors

Residents Who Are Unable to Perform Activities of Daily Living. Disabil-ity in the performance of seven activities of daily living (ADLs) were as-

Table 10.1. Proportion of Residential Care/Assisted Living Facilities That Discharge Residents with Select Characteristics, by Facility Type (%)

Resident Characteristic	<16 Beds	Traditional	New-Model
Activities of daily living (ADLs)			
Unable to get out of bed	56.6%	73.0%	47.9%
Unable to walk (confined to chair or wheelchair)	40.2	55.0	10.4
Unable to feed themselves	34.0	60.5	33.3
Unable to bathe or clean themselves	14.0	23.1	12.5
Unable to dress themselves	13.1	25.0	6.3
Unable to take care of their own appearance (e.g., comb hair, shave)	11.2	15.4	2.1
Incontinent (of urine or feces)	15.9	25.0	12.5
Instrumental ADLs			
Unable to handle their own money	1.9	2.5	0
Unable to make their own bed	2.8	0	0
Unable to clean their own room	0.9	0	0
Affective, cognitive, or mental needs			
Unable to make their needs or wishes understood	16.2	27.5	29.2
Confused or disoriented	4.7	10.0	12.5
Depressed	6.7	5.0	8.3
Mentally retarded	19.8	13.5	17.4
Mentally ill	20.4	29.0	21.3
Exhibit problem behaviors (e.g., wandering, being noisy, threatening)	60.6	61.5	58.3
Have drug or alcohol abuse problem	54.4	37.5	40.9
Insurance and payment source			
SSI recipients	22.3	27.8	36.2
Medicaid recipients	25.7	39.0	44.7
Medical needs			
Need assistance taking medication	1.2	0	0
Require bandages to be changed daily	14.3	12.8	10.4
Need assistance taking insulin or monitoring blood sugar	13.3	10.3	4.2
Need blood pressure or pulse monitored at least weekly	5.7	0	0
Require a special diet, such as pureed food	6.7	5.0	10.4

Note: SSI = Supplemental Security Income.

sessed: getting out of bed, walking (confined to chair or wheelchair), feeding oneself, bathing or cleaning oneself, dressing oneself, taking care of one's own appearance (e.g., combing hair, shaving), and managing continence (of urine or feces). The resident characteristic least tolerated in RC/AL is the inability to get out of bed. The proportion of facilities willing to discharge a resident for this reason ranges from a high of 73 percent for the traditional RC/AL to 57 percent for a small facility and 48 percent for the new-model facility. An inability to care for one's appearance is better tolerated, with discharge percentages ranging from 2 percent of new-model facilities to 15 percent of traditional ones. It is interesting that only 10 percent of new-model facilities would discharge a resident who is unable to walk or is confined to a chair, whereas 40 percent of small facilities and 55 percent of traditional RC/AL would do so. This difference may be partly explained by the inclusion criteria for the new-model facilities, one of which requires that 20 percent or more of the resident population need assistance in transfer. However, this finding may also be attributed to the ability of new-model facilities to accommodate wheelchairs whereas older facilities, particularly small settings that may be converted private homes, cannot.

Approximately 13–25 percent of facilities would discharge a resident because of incontinence. Since incontinence is a major determinant of nursing home placement, these results suggest that the majority of RC/AL facilities are willing to care for the incontinent resident. These results also imply that incontinence may be less of a barrier to aging in place than mobility impairment. Another disability that seems to present a barrier to aging in place is the inability to feed oneself. There are marked differences by facility type in the willingness to retain this type of resident. Among the traditional facilities, 61 percent of administrators reported that an inability to feed oneself would be a cause for discharge, whereas one-half as many small and new-model facilities would discharge these residents.

Residents Who Are Unable to Perform Instrumental Activities of Daily Living. Nearly all the RC/AL facilities in this study would retain residents who were unable to handle their own money, make their own bed, or clean their own room. This suggests that the RC/AL facilities studied viewed these types of needs to be within the range of services provided. Only six small RC/AL facilities would discharge residents for one of these three reasons; only one traditional facility would discharge a resident who was unable to manage money; and no new-model facility would discharge a resident for any of these reasons.

Residents with Affective Disorders, Cognitive Impairment, or Mental Illness. There is little variation by facility type in discharge policies related to mental illness or mental retardation. The proportions of facilities that would discharge residents for these reasons range between 20 and 29 percent for mental illness and between 14 and 20 percent for mental retardation. Confusion, disorientation, and depression are well tolerated in these settings; problem behaviors are not well tolerated. The proportion of facilities that would discharge a resident who was exhibiting problem behaviors ranges from 58 to 62 percent. This finding is consistent with other studies, both qualitative and quantitative, that have found that operators have difficulty coping with problem behaviors (Morgan, Eckert & Lyon, 1995). Facilities also seem to have less tolerance for residents who have drug or alcohol abuse problems, with discharge proportions ranging between 38 and 54 percent.

Insurance and Payment Source. A larger proportion of the new-model facilities have a policy that would support the discharge of a resident who required Supplemental Security Income (SSI) benefits or Medicaid. The presence of a discharge policy related to SSI eligibility ranged from a low of 22 percent among small facilities to 28 percent among traditional facilities and 36 percent among new-model facilities. The trend is similar for Medicaid eligibility, ranging from a low of 26 percent for the small facilities to 39 percent for the traditional and 45 percent for the new-model. These findings support the observed trend that new-model facilities are typically built and marketed for a higher-income population, whereas smaller facilities, which may often be family owned and operated, may be more willing to retain residents as their resources become depleted and the resident spends down to public funding eligibility.

Residents with Medical Care Needs. The medical care needs referred to in this study include activities related to the monitoring or supervision of interventions to manage chronic illness, including assistance in taking medications, daily bandage changes, assistance in taking insulin or monitoring blood sugar, weekly blood-pressure or pulse monitoring, and the need for a special diet. As shown in table 10.1, these medical care needs are well tolerated in RC/AL facilities. Only 2 facilities (small RC/AL facilities) would discharge a resident who required assistance taking medications, and only 6 facilities (small RC/AL) would discharge a resident who required weekly monitoring of blood pressure or pulse. There is less tolerance of the need for daily bandage change or diabetic monitoring, but the discharge rate for any facility type does not exceed 14 percent for either of these needs.

Facility- and Community-Level Factors

The association between facility- and community-level factors and the propensity to discharge residents with a given characteristics was examined by the use of multivariable analysis. A series of models were estimated using each of the resident characteristics as a dependent variable, including in the model variables such as the state in which the facility was located, the facility type, the ownership (for-profit vs. not-for-profit), facility size, and facility age. The significant findings are displayed in table 10.2.

When the multivariable model includes the influence of state, ownership, facility size, and facility age, the importance of facility type in explaining differences in discharge policies related to disabilities having to do with activities of daily living is minimal. In other words, with the exception of a discharge policy related to the inability to walk, it makes no difference whether residents are in small, traditional, or new-model facilities in terms of whether the facility is likely to discharge them based on resident characteristics. Factors that do seem to make a considerable difference are the state in which the facility is located, who owns the facility, and the age of the facility. With North Carolina as the reference category, facilities located in Florida and New Jersey are much more likely to have a discharge policy related to resident disability. Compared with facilities located in North Carolina, facilities in Florida are more likely to have a discharge policy for residents who are unable to get out of bed, who are unable to feed themselves, or who are unable to care for their appearance. Facilities located in New Jersey are more likely than those located in North Carolina to have a discharge policy related to an inability to feed oneself, to bathe, dress, or care for one's appearance. For-profit status is also associated with a greater tendency to discharge for ADL-related reasons, particularly an inability to bathe, dress, or maintain continence. Finally, as the age of the facility increases, so does the propensity to discharge residents who are unable to walk, eat independently, or maintain urinary or fecal continence.

None of the multivariable models for characteristics related to instru-

Table 10.2. Community and Facility Factors Associated with Discharging Residents with Select Characteristics

Resident Characteristic	State[a]			Facility Type[a]		Ownership*	Facility Size	Facility Age	p Value[b]
	MD	FL	NJ	Traditional	New-Model				
Activities of daily living									
Unable to get out of bed		++							p < .001
Unable to walk		++	++		−			+	p < .001
Unable to feed self		++						+	p < .001
Unable to bathe or clean self		++				+			p < .001
Unable to dress self		++				++			p < .001
Unable to care for appearance		++	++						p < .001
Incontinent (of urine or feces)						+		+	p < .005
Affective, cognitive, or mental									
Unable to make needs understood			++			++			p < .001
Confused or disoriented								+	p < .005
Mentally retarded	+	++	+	−		++			p < .001

(continued)

Table 10.2. (Continued)

Resident Characteristic	State[a]			Facility Type[a]		Ownership*	Facility Size	Facility Age	p Value[b]
	MD	FL	NJ	Traditional	New-Model				
Insurance and payment source									
SSI recipient		+	++						$p < .01$
Medicaid recipient			+						$p < .10$
Medical needs									
Assistance with insulin or monitoring blood sugar								+	$p < .05$
Require a special diet								+	$p < .05$

Note: SSI = Supplemental Security Income.

[a]Reference category: in North Carolina; <16 beds; not-for-profit.

[b]Determined by chi-square statistic.

+ Positively associated, $p < .05$

++ Positively associated, $p < .01$

− Negatively associated, $p < .05$

mental activities of daily living were significant, which is to be expected because the number of facilities that discharge residents for these reasons is minimal. However, there is significantly more variation among the resident characteristics that are related to affective, cognitive, or mental disabilities. A resident who is unable to make her or his needs understood is more likely to be in a facility that would discharge for this reason if that facility is located in the state of New Jersey or if the facility is for-profit. Also, older facilities are associated with an increase in the likelihood of having a discharge policy related to residents who are confused or disoriented. Compared with facilities located in North Carolina, RC/AL facilities located in Maryland, Florida, and New Jersey are more likely to have a discharge policy related to mental retardation. For-profit ownership is also associated with a discharge policy for this reason, whereas traditional facilities are less likely to have a discharge policy related to mental retardation as compared with small facilities. None of these facility- or community-level factors were found to influence whether a facility had a discharge policy related to residents' being depressed, being mentally ill, exhibiting problem behaviors, or having drug or alcohol problems. This finding is somewhat surprising, since more than one-half of the administrators interviewed stated that the facility would discharge a resident who had behavior problems or alcohol or drug problems. Perhaps behavior problems are difficult for all facilities to manage and it does not matter where the facility is located or what type it is. With the exception of discharge policies related to mental retardation, which often depend on state regulations, the willingness and ability of a facility to tolerate affective or cognitive disorders may be driven by the severity of a combination of resident-level factors.

The only factor that is associated with discharge policies related to public insurance and payment source is facility location. Relative to North Carolina, facilities located in New Jersey or Florida are more likely to say they discharge residents who receive SSI benefits. In addition, facilities located in New Jersey are more likely to have a discharge policy related to residents' receiving Medicaid insurance.

Increased facility age is associated with an increase in the likelihood of having a policy to discharge residents requiring assistance with and monitoring of insulin injections and blood sugar and of residents requiring a special diet. Discharge policies for the remaining medical needs, medication assistance, daily bandage change, and weekly blood-pressure or pulse monitoring, did not vary by these facility- or community-level factors.

Conclusion

The belief that individuals should be moved progressively to elderly housing, RC/AL facilities, nursing homes, and hospitals as their level of dependency increases is not shared by most older people (MacDonald, Remus & Liang, 1994). Older adults desire to remain in familiar surroundings or in the least restrictive setting, with needed services brought to them where they live (D'Angelo, 1996; Sheehan, 1992). It has been argued that older people should be able to enter a residential setting, such as RC/AL, with light to moderate needs for care and remain in that setting for as long as they wish (Kane, 1993). Accordingly, involuntary departure from a residential facility would be justified only if the resident's medical condition was so unstable that hospital-like care would be warranted or if the resident ceased to be able to interact with the environment and could not obtain benefit from its privacy and autonomy-enhancing features (Kane, 1995–96).

Indeed, aging in place highlights the importance of person-environment fit (Kahana, 1982; Lawton, Windley & Byerts, 1982) and requires continuous reassessment and evaluation of the fit between the needs and abilities of the older person and the capability of the setting to address those needs (Silverstone & Horowitz, 1993; Callahan, 1993). It has been suggested that facilities that function in an aging-in-place model include residents with a range of service needs along a continuum of care (Lewin-VHI, 1996). Clearly, aging in place in any setting requires a flexible, supportive environment and a range of services to compensate for limitations or disabilities. Such a model of care in RC/AL can potentially result in more appropriate care at less cost than providing similar services in more institutionalized or medicalized settings, such as nursing homes. Alternatively, aging in place can be detrimental to the well-being of residents if it means that frail people are retained in environments that cannot properly support their needs. Whether one advocates for or against aging in place in RC/AL may depend upon one's perspective. For example, state policy decisions regarding aging in place often reflect political compromises with constituency groups such as nursing home associations and home health agencies, who view RC/AL facilities as either competition or a market opportunity for their services (Mollica, 1995; Mollica & Snow, 1996).

Although the findings from the CS-LTC suggest that there are certain resident characteristics that place a resident at higher risk for discharge from a RC/AL facility, these findings are inconclusive because they are based on cross-sectional data. Longitudinal studies are needed to confirm whether the stated discharge policies are associated with lower retention rates for residents with particular characteristics. However, these findings do suggest that residents with needs related to immobility, an inability to feed oneself, and problem behaviors such as wandering or becoming noisy or threatening are less likely to be retained in RC/AL facilities. These three characteristics have in common a need for staff availability, training, and close monitoring and have implications for the resident with dementia who presents unique care challenges. Nursing homes are the most commonly used institutional settings for persons with dementia, but over the past decade and a half, RC/AL facilities have emerged as important care providers for persons with cognitive disorders; families are turning increasingly to these settings because they often appear less costly and may offer a more homelike environment (Lybrand, 1993).

Community-level factors influence the ability to age in place either positively or negatively depending upon whether the facility is located in a state that encourages or discourages aging in place by regulations such as admission and retention policies, state licensure requirements, and waiver status regarding public reimbursement. State policy does influence aging in place. Some states, such as Oregon, promote programs that allow residents to choose to age in place rather than to enter nursing homes (Kane & Wilson, 1993; Folkemer et al., 1996); others have regulations that carefully define eligibility for residence and for remaining in such facilities. Some states set general criteria for the type of resident who can be served and the level of care that can be provided, whereas other states set very specific regulations regarding the extent of services provided (US GAO, 1999). Within this variation, regulations typically address components of the living unit, admission and retention criteria, and the types and level of services that the facility may provide. State policy is currently in flux, and many states are reexamining policies that prohibit those needing a nursing home level of services from being served in RC/AL (Lewin-VHI, 1996).

Meeting the challenge of residential care for older adults with minimal care needs is not difficult, particularly if they have the private means to procure services (Heumann & Boldy, 1993). As RC/AL facilities proliferate, the challenge is to develop affordable, supportive, residential care settings that allow people with severely compromised physical or cognitive functioning, such as residents with dementia, to remain in these settings over time. Much of the innovation and debate regarding long-term-care issues that directly impact aging in place occur on the state level. There are a number of stakeholders that influence the shape of state policy, including residents and their families who wish to remain in RC/AL settings if the level of care is appropriate and RC/AL and nursing home administrators and other professionals who believe that aging in place can be a viable alternative to nursing homes—again, if the level of care is appropriate. Addressing and continually reassessing person-environment fit is the crux of appropriate aging in place.

References

Callahan, J. J. 1993. *Aging in Place.* Amityville, NY: Baywood Publishing.

D'Angelo, H. 1996. Caring in Place. *Assisted Living Today* 3:29–31.

Folkemer, D., Jensen, A., Lipson, L., Stauffer, M., & Fox-Grage, W. 1996. *Adult Foster-Care for the Elderly: A Review of State Regulatory and Funding Strategies.* Vol. 1. Washington, DC: Public Policy Institute, American Association of Retired Persons.

Hawes, C., Wildfire, J. B., & Lux, L. J. 1993. *The Regulation of Board and Care Homes: Results of a Survey in the 50 States and the District of Columbia: National Summary.* Washington, DC: American Association of Retired Persons.

Heumann, L. F. 1993. Aging in place in housing designed for independent living: The case of the U.S. Section 202 Program. In L. F. Heumann & D. P. Boldy (eds.), *Aging in Place with Dignity: International Solutions Relating to the Low-Income and Frail Elderly.* Westport, CT: Praeger.

Heumann, L. F., & Boldy, D. P. (eds.). 1993. *Aging in Place with Dignity: International Solutions Relating to the Low-Income and Frail Elderly.* Westport, CT: Praeger.

Kahana, E. 1982. A congruence model of person-environment interaction. In M. P. Lawton, P. G. Windley, & T. O. Byerts (eds.), *Aging and the Environment: Theoretical Approaches.* New York: Springer.

Kane, R. A. 1993. Dangers lurking in the continuum of care: Repertoire of services is a better goal. *Journal of Aging and Social Policy* 5:1–7.

————. 1995–96. Transforming care institutions for the frail elderly: Out of one shall be many. *Generations* 19:52–68.

Kane, R. A., & Wilson, K. B. 1993. *Assisted Living in the United States: A New Paradigm for Residential Care for Frail Older Persons?* Washington, DC: American Association of Retired Persons.

Lawton, M. P. 1980. Housing the elderly: Residential quality and residential satisfaction. *Research on Aging* 2:309–28.

————. 1990. Knowledge resources and gaps in housing for the aged. In D. Tilson (ed.), *Aging in Place: Supporting the Frail Elderly in Residential Environments.* Glenview, IL: Scott Foresman.

Lawton, M. P., Windley, P. G., & Byerts, T. O. 1982. *Aging and the Environment: Theoretical Approaches.* New York: Springer.

Lewin-VHI. 1996. National study of assisted living for the frail elderly: Literature review update. U.S. Department of Health and Human Services, Washington, DC.

Lybrand, C. 1993. An overview of the assisted living industry. Assisted Living Facilities Association of America, Fairfax, VA.

MacDonald, M., Remus, G., & Liang, G. 1994. Research considerations: The link between housing and health in the elderly. *Journal of Gerontological Nursing* 16:5–10.

Mollica, R. L. 1995. *Guide to Assisted Living and State Policy.* U.S. Department of Health and Human Services. No. HHS-100-94-0024.

————. 2000. State Assisted Living Policy, 2000. Portland, ME: National Academy for State Health Policy.

Mollica, R. L., & Snow, K. I. 1996. *State Assisted Living Policy, 1996.* Portland, ME: National Academy for State Health Policy.

Moos, R. H., & Lemke, S. 1994. *Group Residences for Older Adults: Physical Features, Policies, and Social Climate.* Oxford: Oxford University Press.

Morgan, L. A., Eckert, J. K., & Lyon, S. M. (eds.). 1995. *Small Board-and-Care Homes: Residential Care in Transition.* Baltimore: Johns Hopkins University Press.

Pynoos, J. 1990. Public policy and aging in place: Identifying the problems and potential solutions. In D. Tilson (ed.), *Aging in Place: Supporting the Frail Elderly in Residential Environments.* Glenview, IL: Scott Foresman.

Sheehan, N. W. 1992. *Successful Administration of Senior Housing: Working with Elderly Residents.* Newbury Park, CA: Sage.

Silverstone, B. M., & Horowitz, A. 1993. Aging in place: The role of families. In J. J. Callahan (ed.), *Aging in Place.* Amityville, NY: Baywood Publishing.

U.S. Congress, General Accounting Office. 1999. *Assisted Living: Quality-of-Care and Consumer Protection Issues in Four States.* GAO/HEHS-99-27. Washington, DC: Government Printing Office.

11 Care for Persons with Dementia

*Philip D. Sloane, M.D., M.P.H., Sheryl Zimmerman, Ph.D.,
and Marcia G. Ory, Ph.D., M.P.H.*

Alzheimer disease and related dementias are among the most common diseases and conditions leading to placement in a residential care/assisted living (RC/AL) facility or nursing home. Persons with dementia now constitute the majority of nursing home residents (Teresi et al., 2000). As is demonstrated in this chapter, the number of residents with dementia in RC/AL has been growing as well. Therefore, owners, operators, and staff of all types of long-term-care facilities should be familiar with the unique needs of persons with dementia and direct care toward those needs.

In this chapter we present an overview of dementia care in RC/AL facilities in the United States, beginning with an overview of the common types of dementia seen in older persons in long-term care and emphasizing how the disease results in unique patient behaviors and needs. We discuss the prevalence and characteristics of persons with dementia in RC/AL, drawing on data from the four-state Collaborative Studies of Long-Term Care (CS-LTC), and present issues unique to the provision of quality care for persons with dementia, using data from the CS-LTC on the prevalence of certain indicators of dementia-sensitive care in both non-dementia-specific areas and dementia-specific care areas. We conclude with a brief discussion of the relationship between the quality of care and the quality of life for persons with dementia and the challenges of providing both.

The Challenge of Alzheimer Disease and Related Dementias

The terms *cognitive impairment, dementia,* and *Alzheimer disease* are often used interchangeably in long-term care; however, they have somewhat different meanings. *Cognitive impairment* is the broadest term, implying a reduction in brain performance in one or more domains, such as memory, abstraction, language, visuospatial ability, and attention (Emery & Oxman, 1994). It may or may not be reversible. Mild cognitive impairment can be confirmed only with sophisticated neuropsychological tests; more severe impairment can be identified using screening tests such as the Mini-Mental State Examination (Folstein, Folstein & McHugh, 1975). *Dementia* is by far the most common cause of moderate or severe cognitive impairment. Dementia is a progressive, irreversible, organic brain condition (Weiner, 1996). A variety of diseases cause dementia, the most common of which are Alzheimer disease and cerebrovascular disease. Dementia involves a reduction in multiple categories of cognitive ability, including memory, and the impairment is sufficient to interfere with self-maintenance, work, and social relationships.

A diagnosis of dementia must be made by a physician or other health professional; it implies that certain diagnostic criteria have been met and that depression and delirium have been ruled out (APA, 1994). Making a dementia diagnosis is challenging, especially in early stages of the illness or when other problems (e.g., a stroke) interfere with communication; one study of twenty-four hundred new admissions to a nursing home found that medical experts agreed only 76–81 percent of the time as to whether a person had dementia, was not demented, or had an indeterminate diagnosis (Magaziner et al., 1996). *Alzheimer disease* is by far the most common cause of dementia, affecting between 2 and 4 million persons in the United States (US GAO, 1998). Its cause is unknown, but it appears to have a strong genetic component; the current thinking is that Alzheimer disease results from an abnormal buildup of certain substances in the brain, most likely as a result of genetic factors. It can be diagnosed with certainty only by brain biopsy or autopsy, so virtually every living case of "Alzheimer disease" has a diagnosis that is preceded by the word *probable* or *possible*. Therefore, though Alzheimer disease is usually the condition being treated in long-term care, it is more correct to use the term *dementia* or, if a medical diagnosis is not present, *cognitive impairment*.

Alzheimer disease affects primarily older persons, becoming increasingly common after age 80 (US GAO, 1998). The disease begins insidiously and progresses gradually; the type and timing of disease manifestations vary from person to person. There is, however, a general pattern of progression, and this has been depicted using a variety of staging systems (Berg, 1988; Reisberg et al., 1982). Table 11.1 presents a composite staging system that is useful in long-term care. It describes four stages of dementia: mild, moderate, severe, and very severe. As indicated by table

Table 11.1. Characteristics of Persons with Dementia, by Disease Stage

Stage of Dementia	Common Resident Characteristics
Mild	Cognition and language: Unreliable memory for recent events; lack of initiative for healthy daily tasks; inability to reliably manage finances, meal planning, or shopping; inability to carry on a good conversation. MMSE[a] score 18+. ADLs[b]: Walks, eats, and toilets independently; may need supervision with dressing and bathing. Behaviors: Confusion, frustration, depression, mood swings.
Moderate	Cognition and language: Very poor memory for recent events; easily confused or upset by changes in routine, new places, or unfamiliar people; needs 24-hour supervision because of poor judgment and confusion; converses in sentences but has difficulty following a line of thought or understanding complex ideas. MMSE score 11–17. ADLs: Needs assistance with bathing, dressing, and grooming; walks, transfers, and eats independently; may need reminders to go to the toilet; may be partially or totally incontinent. Behaviors: Confusion, repetitive questions, disorientation, mood swings, exiting behavior, delusions, wandering.
Severe	Cognition and language: Poor memory for both recent and past events; little understanding of daily schedule and events; communicates in short sentences; inability to follow complex commands; recognizes only persons seen very regularly. MMSE score 1–10. ADLs: Developing gait instability and falls; can feed self but may forget to eat or drink regularly, or may hold food in mouth. Behaviors: Resists caregiving; delusions; physical abusiveness; repetitive vocalization (words); socially inappropriate behaviors.
Very severe	Cognition and language: Aware of little other than immediate surroundings; speaks in a few words or unintelligible sounds; rarely recognizes individuals but does respond to the way in which he or she is approached. MMSE score 0. ADLs: Needs total or near-total assistance; shuffles short distance with assistance or is nonambulatory; is incontinent of urine and stool; often feeds poorly. Behaviors: Resists caregiving; screaming.

Note: This table applies generally to persons with Alzheimer disease and related dementias. Considerable variation is present from person to person in the manifestation of these diseases, however.
[a]Mini-Mental State Examination (Folstein, Folstein & McHugh, 1975).
[b]Activities of daily living.

11.1, dementia's effects can be grouped into three general domains: thinking (cognition), activities of daily living, and behaviors. Such a system can be useful in long-term-care settings, because it helps care providers understand how problems and needs vary over the course of the disease and why individuals with the same diagnosis can be so diverse.

Care for Persons with Alzheimer Disease and Related Dementias

The care of persons with dementia largely consists of attending to everyday needs and managing behavioral problems (Small et al., 1997). Medical management, though important, focuses on identifying and treating other diseases such as depression, visual impairment, and arthritis and preventing complications such as infections, hip fractures, and medication side effects (Ham, 1997). Behavioral problems are the most pervasive care issue; these require constant supervision because the person may be disoriented, may be unable to express his or her wants and needs, and may exhibit a host of agitated and disruptive behaviors, ranging from repeatedly asking the same question to hitting, biting, and screaming. Although major behavioral disturbances do not occur in every patient with dementia, the disorder results in a vulnerability to such problems as disinhibition, low frustration tolerance, lability, impaired judgment, apathy, and the inability to initiate tasks.

Several factors make Alzheimer disease and related dementias particularly challenging for caregivers. The illness typically lasts for many years (sometimes ten or more years), during which time care needs increase. Because persons with dementia rarely understand the nature of their illness, they often do not appreciate their needs; as a result they tend to argue with, insult, or fight with persons who are trying to provide care. They also often engage in behaviors that are embarrassing to others (e.g., saying inappropriate things, taking their clothes off in public) or hazardous (e.g., wandering outside and getting lost, starting fights). Also, they rarely express interest in, empathy for, or appreciation to caregivers; indeed, in late stages of the disease they often do not even recognize close family members. The long-time course, the need for twenty-four-hour supervision and care in later stages of illness, the frequent development of medical or functional complications (e.g., incontinence, feeding problems), and the prevalence of disruptive behaviors (e.g., wandering, paranoia, assaultiveness) cause the vast majority of persons with dementia to eventually be placed in long-term-care facilities (Epping & Poisal, 1997), where they constitute an increasingly large proportion of the population. Thus, dementia care is more and more the future of institutional long-term care in the United States, and the provision of quality care to this population has attracted increasing attention.

Dementia Care in Nursing Homes

Nursing homes have been until recently the major source of institutional care for persons with dementia, and currently they remain the most frequently used institutional setting for dementia care (Epping & Poisal, 1997). The majority of nursing home residents have cognitive impairment; the 1985 National Nursing Home Survey found that 63 percent of all nursing home residents were disoriented or memory impaired to an extent that regularly hindered performance of basic activities of daily living (NCHS, 1987). Recently, 48 percent (746,100) of the nearly 1.56 million nursing home residents in the United States were identified as having an active diagnosis of dementia documented on the Minimum Data Set, a standardized reporting form in use in all federally certified nursing homes (US DHHS, 1998). Given that diagnostic reporting of dementia is often incomplete, the true proportion of nursing home residents with dementia is probably higher.

Whether nursing homes are the optimal care setting for persons with dementia is controversial. There are some clear benefits: twenty-four-hour supervision, emotional relief for families, safety and few restrictions on wanderers, and increased opportunities for social stimulation (US OTA, 1987). However, it is argued that medical and skilled nursing needs are minor for many such residents until late in the disease process and that nursing home care has been associated with problems such as premature death, permanent injury, increased disability, unnecessary fear and suffering, inadequate food and food service, and the lack of proper therapies (IM, 1986; Zimmerman & Sloane, 1999). For these reasons, the quality of this care is under ongoing study.

One alternative to traditional nursing home care for persons with Alzheimer disease and related disorders has been special-care units (SCUs). These specialized units first began several decades ago as locked units created by large facilities to care for older persons with severe behavioral problems, the vast majority of whom had advanced dementia.

More recently, SCUs have tended to be activity-focused environments, targeted toward early and midstage disease. By 1996 approximately one-fourth of nursing homes had at least one organized dementia care unit, wing, or program (Leon, Cheng & Alvarez, 1997; Teresi et al., 1998).

SCUs claim to do a better job than traditional nursing home units in selecting, training, and supervising their staff; in providing activities designed for the cognitively impaired; in involving the family in treatment; and in offering physical environments that enhance safety, provide better orientation, and more appropriately stimulate persons with dementia. However, these components of special care are not always evidenced, nor do they necessarily translate to better outcomes (Grant, 1998). Indeed, research findings on the efficacy of SCUs have been inconclusive. Comparative outcome studies have found positive, negative, and neutral effects of SCUs on outcomes related to resident function (e.g., cognitive, physical, behavioral, and affective), staff and cost outcomes (e.g., stress, burnout, and utilization), and family outcomes (e.g., depression and satisfaction) (Grant & Ory, 2000; Sloane et al., 1995; Zimmerman & Sloane, 1999).

Dementia Care in Residential Care/Assisted Living

Residential care/assisted living (RC/AL) refers to an extremely varied group of facilities that are certified by the states at non-nursing-home levels of care, often under several separate licensure categories. Designations for such homes vary as well and include rest homes, domiciliary care, personal care homes, foster-care homes, homes for the aged, adult homes, group homes, board and care, residential-care homes for the elderly, and assisted living. Across the nation, as many as 1.5 million elderly and disabled individuals are housed in more than 36,000 licensed and an unknown number of unlicensed RC/AL homes (Hawes et al., 1993). RC/AL facilities do not require a certificate of need, are subject to fewer regulations, and offer more opportunities to experiment than traditional nursing homes do; they constitute the fastest-growing segment of institutional care nationwide.

Available data indicate that these facilities have a significant and growing population of residents who evidence disorientation, memory impairment, and confusion. Hawes and associates (1995), in a study of board-and-care homes in ten states, estimated the prevalence of cognitive impairment at 40 percent. They also concluded that cognitive impairment had increased since the 1980s. There is considerable evidence of behavior problems, including verbal abuse, wandering, and being difficult to control, bathe, and change, among residents in RC/AL facilities (Avorn et al., 1989; Eckert, Namazi & Kahana, 1987; Mor, Sherwood & Gutkin, 1986). Families of persons with Alzheimer disease and related dementias are turning increasingly to RC/AL settings. In part this represents a search for superior care alternatives, and in part it occurs because such homes often appear less costly (Rajecki, 1992).

Specialized Dementia Units. The recent growth of RC/AL facilities has been paralleled by the development of specialized dementia programs and units within these settings (Alzheimer's Association, 1994). Much of this growth was due to new knowledge and techniques of care that developed in the 1980s and 1990s, which were best implemented not in the highly regulated nursing home setting but rather in "dementia-specific assisted living residences" (Cohen & Day, 1994; Coons, 1987; Faunce & Brunette, 1986; Zeisel, 1995). The number and proportion of RC/AL homes with specialized dementia units is unknown; the highest reported estimate is from a survey of facilities in Massachusetts, among which 18 percent offered dementia SCUs (Stocker & Silverstein, 1996).

The variety of specialized dementia units parallels the diversity of RC/AL homes. Davis and associates (2000) proposed that such units could be separated into five types: small (10 beds or fewer), freestanding, independently operated dementia-specific homes; two or more small (generally with 10 or fewer beds), freestanding dementia-specific homes that share a central administration; larger (more than 10 beds) freestanding homes operated as dementia-specific facilities; a distinct dementia unit that is adjacent to and operated in conjunction with a larger assisted living facility; and a distinct dementia unit that is adjacent to and operated in conjunction with a skilled nursing unit.

The Quality of Dementia Care. Many questions exist about dementia care in RC/AL facilities. To what extent are current homes providing dementia care? Who is being served? What are the characteristics of the services? To what extent is specialized care present, and what is it like? The remainder of this chapter seeks to address these questions, using data from a large, four-state study of RC/AL homes, the Collaborative Studies of Long-Term Care.

The Scope of Dementia in Residential Care/Assisted Living: Data from the Collaborative Studies of Long-Term Care

The Collaborative Studies of Long-Term Care (CS-LTC) is a study of residential long-term care across four states: Florida, Maryland, New Jersey, and North Carolina. These states have well-developed residential-care industries yet exhibit variability to provide a broad perspective of the field. Within each of these states, residential-care facilities were sampled in three strata, to further capture the existing variation: facilities with fewer than 16 beds ($N = 113$); new-model homes (facilities with 16 or more beds that reflect components of purpose-built, new-model assisted living [i.e., built after January 1, 1987, and (1) having at least two private pay rates or (2) having 20% or more of the residents requiring assistance in transfer or (3) having 25% or more of residents incontinent daily or (4) having either an RN or an LPN on duty at all times] [$N = 40$]); and traditional facilities with 16 or more beds that do not meet the new-model definition ($N = 40$).

Data were collected between October 1997 and November 1998 on randomly selected facilities ($N = 193$) and residents over the age of 65 ($N = 2,078$) and derived from interviews with residents, administrators, and care providers. All residents of small facilities and approximately twenty residents from each of the larger facilities were recruited. Facility data were collected separately for those areas of a facility that were "dementia-specific": designated as an Alzheimer's or dementia unit, where 75 percent or more of residents had a diagnosis of Alzheimer disease or a related disorder. In total there were only 22 of these dementia-specific care areas (9, 3, and 10 in the small, traditional, and new-model strata, respectively). Further details on the goals and methods of the CS-LTC are provided in chapter 6 of this book.

Data from the RC/AL homes in the CS-LTC were analyzed to begin to understand the scope and characteristics of dementia care in the RC/AL setting. Among the issues addressed in these analyses were the prevalence of dementia, the characteristics of persons with dementia, the presence of markers of dementia-sensitive care, and the number and characteristics of specialized care areas in the facilities participating in that study.

The Prevalence of Dementia

The CS-LTC study obtained three measures of cognitive status. The first was the Mini-Mental State Examination (MMSE), a thirty-item face-to-face interview that is well-established as a screen for dementia (Tombaugh & McIntyre, 1992). MMSE scores were available for 59 percent of the CS-LTC subjects; the majority of the missing scores were due to the inability of the subject to communicate or cooperate with an examiner, resulting in over 25 percent of items being coded as missing. The second source was the Minimum Data Set Cognition Scale (MDS-COGS), a ten-point measure of cognition that uses reported data from staff (Hartmaier et al., 1994). MDS-COGS scores were available for 97 percent of the CS-LTC subjects in RC/AL facilities. Finally, information was obtained on the existence of a dementia diagnosis in the subject's history or medical record. These data were less standardized, as is true generally for diagnostic data from long-term-care facilities.

All these data sources were used to estimate the prevalence of "probable moderate or severe dementia" in the three RC/AL strata of the CS-LTC study. The designation of "probable moderate or severe dementia" was assigned using the MMSE of 0–16 when the MMSE was available. This cutoff was 90 percent predictive of an expert-panel diagnosis of dementia in a prior study of 2,285 new nursing home admissions (Magaziner et al., 2000). If an MMSE score was not available, an MDS-COGS score of 4–10 was used to designate probable moderate or severe dementia. This criterion was selected using data from the same prior study, which found that an MDS-COGS score of 4 was equivalent to a mean MMSE of 15, whereas an MDS-COGS of 3 was equivalent to a mean MMSE of 17. For the twenty-four subjects with neither an MMSE or a MDS-COGS, the diagnosis of dementia was used. These data sources disagreed in only one instance, and in that case the subject was designated as not demented because other notes indicated that the resident was well oriented.

Table 11.2 displays the estimated prevalence of cognitive impairment in CS-LTC subjects in RC/AL facilities, by stratum. Using the MDS-COGS, 63 percent of the residents in smaller homes have cognitive impairment. The figures for larger, traditional facilities and larger, new-model facilities are 46 and 52 percent, respectively. The estimates based on the MMSE are lower; however, many of the nearly 40 percent of subjects who could not be tested are likely to have had cognitive impairment.

Table 11.2. Number and Proportion (%) of Residents with Cognitive Impairment and Dementia in Residential Care/Assisted Living, by Facility Type

Cognitive Status	<16 Beds	Traditional	New-Model
Minimum Data Set Cognition Scale (MDS-COGS)[a]			
Normal	237 (37%)	343 (55%)	363 (48%)
Mild–moderate impairment	204 (32)	184 (30)	191 (25)
Severe impairment	151 (23)	74 (12)	156 (21)
Very severe impairment	51 (8)	22 (4)	46 (6)
Mini-Mental State Examination (MMSE)[b]			
Normal	180 (47)	295 (68)	221 (53)
Mild impairment	106 (28)	87 (20)	111 (27)
Moderate impairment	59 (15)	41 (9)	53 (13)
Severe–very severe impairment	37 (9)	14 (3)	28 (7)
Prevalence of moderate or severe dementia,[c] *by location*			
No dementia–mild dementia	386 (58)	498 (77)	499 (65)
Probable moderate or severe dementia			
In non-dementia-specific care area	222 (33)	133 (21)	182 (24)
In dementia-specific care area	57 (9)	17 (3)	84 (11)

Notes: There were 2,078 subjects in the study. Of these, 56 subjects were not assessed using the MDS-COGS; 843 were not assessed using the MMSE (usually because of the inability to communicate or to cooperate); and 24 were missing both measures.
[a]Hartmaier et al., 1994. Cognitive status was determined as follows: 0–1 = normal; 2–4 = mild–moderate impairment; 5–8 = severe impairment; 9–10 = very severe impairment.
[b]Folstein, Folstein & McHugh, 1975. Cognitive status was determined as follows: 24–30 = normal; 17–23 = mild impairment; 11–16 = moderate impairment; 0–10 = severe impairment.
[c]MMSE was used if available; if unavailable, MDS-COGS was used; if both were unavailable, reported diagnosis of dementia was used. Cutoffs: MMSE <17 or MDS-COGS >3.

Using data from the MMSE, the MDS-COGS, and diagnoses, the estimated prevalence of moderate or severe dementia was 42 percent in small facilities, 24 percent in larger, traditional facilities, and 35 percent in larger, new-model facilities. Thus, the entire spectrum of dementia, and of dementia care needs, is represented by residents of these facilities.

These results suggest that approximately one-half of the residents in

RC/AL facilities have significant cognitive impairment and that approximately one-third have moderate or severe dementia. This figure is higher than that reported previously (Hawes et al., 1995). However, it has long been suspected that the rate of cognitive impairment in these facilities has been increasing, so the observed figures may represent a true increase rather than a difference in sampling. It should be noted that the prevalence reported here was based on subjects in the CS-LTC study who were age 65 and older; because the vast majority of RC/AL residents are elderly, the figures for facilities overall (including all residents) would be likely to differ no more than a few percentage points from those reported here.

Characteristics of Persons with Dementia

The CS-LTC study gathered a variety of data on the demographic, functional, and behavioral characteristics of the study subjects. Table 11.3 displays selected resident-level data on subjects who did not have moderate or severe dementia (referred to as nondemented, although this group also includes individuals with mild dementia) and on those with "probable moderate or severe dementia" who resided in non-dementia-specific care areas (NDSCAs) and dementia-specific care areas (DSCAs). In general, persons with dementia residing in NDSCAs did not differ markedly from persons who were nondemented in terms of their gender, race, marital, or payment status (except in new-model facilities, where somewhat more persons with dementia were married and fewer were on welfare or Medicaid). Marked differences were evident, however, in the prevalence of activity of daily living (ADL) dependency and behavioral problems. Persons with dementia markedly and consistently required more assistance with personal hygiene, transferring, locomotion, eating, and continence—indeed all ADLs were markedly more impaired among persons with dementia. These findings suggest that a significant proportion of the persons requiring ADL assistance in RC/AL have dementia. Not surprisingly, the same is true for behavioral problems: persons with dementia were reported to have a higher prevalence of constant requests for attention, resisting care, physical aggression, wandering or pacing, and physical restlessness. These trends were evident across all three strata.

The data in table 11.3 further suggest that DSCAs are attracting residents with somewhat different characteristics than those found in NDSCAs. Residents of DSCAs tended to be more physically impaired

Table 11.3. Characteristics of Residential Care/Assisted Living Residents with and without Dementia, per Location, by Facility Type (%)

Characteristic	Dementia Status[a]	<16 Beds	Traditional	New-Model
Demographics				
Female gender	Nondemented	74%	77%	72%
	Demented, NDSCA	79	76	79
	Demented, DSCA	80	77	82
White race or ethnicity	Nondemented	88	93	94
	Demented, NDSCA	77	90	95
	Demented, DSCA	98	88	100
Married, spouse alive	Nondemented	8	10	11
	Demented, NDSCA	10	9	20
	Demented, DSCA	26	12	17
On welfare or Medicaid	Nondemented	16	14	12
	Demented, NDSCA	19	14	6
	Demented, DSCA	0	12	5
ADL dependency[b]				
Personal hygiene	Nondemented	27	13	18
	Demented, NDSCA	66	53	58
	Demented, DSCA	89	47	74
Transfer to bed or	Nondemented	14	4	12
chair	Demented, NDSCA	29	23	33
	Demented, DSCA	54	12	23
Locomotion on unit	Nondemented	12	5	8
	Demented, NDSCA	25	22	28
	Demented, DSCA	52	6	17
Eating	Nondemented	3	1	1
	Demented, NDSCA	22	19	16
	Demented, DSCA	38	12	24
Incontinence daily,	Nondemented	16	8	18
urine	Demented, NDSCA	51	39	52
	Demented, DSCA	77	24	57
Behavioral problems[c]				
Constant requests	Nondemented	12	5	6
for attention	Demented, NDSCA	16	17	14
	Demented, DSCA	18	29	20

(*continued*)

Table 11.3. (*Continued*)

Characteristic	Dementia Status[a]	<16 Beds	Traditional	New-Model
Resists staff	Nondemented	5	4	5
assistance	Demented, NDSCA	11	10	20
	Demented, DSCA	33	24	33
Physical aggression	Nondemented	2	1	2
	Demented, NDSCA	5	9	9
	Demented, DSCA	30	6	21
Wandering or pacing	Nondemented	5	4	5
	Demented, NDSCA	19	21	26
	Demented, DSCA	28	29	44
Physical restlessness	Nondemented	4	2	3
	Demented, NDSCA	18	18	16
	Demented, DSCA	30	29	26

Note: NDSCA = non-dementia-specific care area; DSCA = dementia-specific care area; ADL = activity of daily living.
[a]See table 11.2 and the text for the method of determining dementia status.
[b]Regularly requiring at least limited physical assistance in activities of daily living.
[c]Occurring at least once a week.

(e.g., to be incontinent, to have difficulty eating), although this was not true in all ADLs or all strata. DSCA residents also tended to have higher prevalences of behavioral problems such as resistiveness, physical aggression, wandering or pacing, and restlessness. These findings are generally true for both the small (fewer than 16-bed) and the new-model facilities; though they are not as evident in the traditional facilities, it should be noted that only 3 such facilities in the CS-LTC sample had DSCAs.

Dementia-Sensitive Care

Because a significant proportion of persons in RC/AL facilities have dementia, it follows that these facilities should provide care that is sensitive to their needs. Defining the elements of quality care for persons with dementia in long-term care is challenging, however. Since these facilities serve as the homes for their residents, quality care must attend to mental, social, and physical well-being and provide for such needs as autonomy, human interaction, and a sense of meaning in life.

As is evident from their characteristics, persons with dementia vary widely. Consequently, care needs and goals for care vary as well. For example, the goals and elements of quality care for a person with early dementia are likely to be quite different from those that would apply to someone with end-stage disease. Furthermore, persons with dementia often have multiple other diseases and disabilities, including both acute and chronic problems. They can often benefit from efforts to improve, maintain, or prevent decline in function; but because of their cognitive impairment, they are not likely to initiate such efforts. All these factors point to the fact that dementia-sensitive care is multidimensional and varies according to individual needs and preferences (US OTA, 1987).

Conceptualizing Quality

One popular method of viewing quality is in terms of three aspects—structure, process, and outcome (Donabedian, 1966). Structure (inputs) refers to the personnel, facilities, policies, and other elements that characterize the environment in which care is provided; examples include physical features such as the configuration of the room, the use of space, access to the outdoors, lighting, and noise. Process refers to the activities or procedures that constitute the actual provision of care; care planning, the act of administering medications, and the provision of activities are examples of the process of care. Outcome refers to characteristics of the residents that can be considered to have been impacted by care; examples include the rate and degree of recovery after a hip fracture, the incidence of complications such as dehydration or decubitus ulcers, and resident satisfaction with the facility and the care it provides (US OTA, 1987).

Much of "good dementia care" is also good care for any resident. For example, most older persons—demented or not—are better served by an environment that is clean and in good repair. In this chapter the term *dementia-sensitive care* is used to refer to elements that are particularly important to persons with dementia. For example, exit control is a dementia-specific element of care. When compared with someone who is cognitively intact, a person with dementia is at far greater risk if he or she walks unescorted off the grounds of a facility; therefore, exit control is a structural element of dementia-sensitive care. Another example is policies and procedures that actively offer water to residents. Since persons with dementia are prone to dehydration (in part because they do not initiate self-maintenance behaviors such as drinking water), provision of hydration would be a process measure of dementia-sensitive care. The elements of dementia-sensitive care presented here were based on two manuals of dementia care, *Guidelines for Dignity: Goals of Specialized Alzheimer/Dementia Care in Residential Settings* (AA, 1992) and *Key Elements of Dementia Care* (AA, 1997). These elements and their CS-LTC measures are listed in table 11.4.

Measures of Quality Used in This Chapter

The dementia-sensitive measures presented in table 11.4 and discussed in greater detail later in this chapter involve the structure and process of care. They are not outcomes. Whether it is appropriate to define quality in this manner is debatable, because outcomes are the ultimate goal of care, and the relationships between structure and process on the one hand and outcomes on the other is as yet unproven in this population. Therefore, the term *dementia-sensitive care* is used to indicate the elements discussed in

Table 11.4. Selected Components of Dementia-Sensitive Care and Related Measures Available in the Collaborative Studies of Long-Term Care (CS-LTC)

Component of Care	Measures from the CS-LTC
Structure of care	
A philosophy that addresses dementia-related needs	Admission and discharge policies that tolerate dementia-related needs and problems
Appropriate staff resources and training to address dementia needs	Self-reported requirement for dementia training for staff
A physical environment that attends to dementia	Provision for safety, orientation, continuity with the past, minimization of adverse stimuli, and availability of pleasant and engaging stimuli
Process of care	
Respect for the residents' autonomy and individuality	Provision of flexible wake-up times and bedtimes
Provision of a variety of activities to address dementia needs and contribute to life satisfaction	Availability of and participation in activities involving gardening, children, and exercise or fitness
Provision of safety with minimization of restrictions and restraints	Use of physical restraints and psychotropic medications

this chapter, and it must be understood that their influence on resident outcomes is largely theoretical. However, an equally cogent argument is that, since persons with dementia have a terminal disease and by the nature of their illness live in the present with little sense of a past or future, the minute-to-minute experience of such individuals should be an important consideration. This being the case, the elements of the resident's immediate environment—the structure and process—may indeed be valid measures of quality.

Dementia Care in the Collaborative Studies of Long-Term Care

Nonspecialized Settings

Because dementia is so prevalent in the RC/AL population, nearly every facility that cares for older adults houses persons with significant cognitive impairment. It is therefore both reasonable and prudent to examine the extent to which these settings provide dementia-sensitive care. This section presents data from the CS-LTC study on nonspecialized settings, where the majority of persons with dementia reside.

The Structure of Care. Table 11.5 presents CS-LTC data on selected structural measures of dementia-sensitive care for NDSCAs, by type of facility. It indicates that the vast majority of facilities will admit persons who suffer from confusion but that only a minority of facilities in all three strata will admit persons with behavioral problems. The retention of persons with behavioral problems appears somewhat greater among the larger homes, although very few facilities will tolerate physically assaultive behavior.

The CS-LTC gathered very little data about specific staffing and training issues related to dementia. A single question to administrators asked about requirements for dementia training. It indicated a slightly lower rate among small homes (74%, compared to 85%–95%), which is consistent with a general trend for the smaller homes to require less formal training.

Among the many physical environmental measures gathered in the CS-LTC study, five domains were chosen as particularly important for dementia care over and above what is needed by all long-term-care residents: safety, orientation, continuity with the past, minimization of adverse stimuli, and provision of favorable stimuli. In general, safety as measured by controlled exits was superior in larger facilities (42%–56% vs.

Table 11.5. Proportion of Residential Care/Assisted Living Non-Dementia-Specific Care Areas Exhibiting Selected Structural Measures of Dementia-Sensitive Care, by Facility Type (%)

	<16 Beds	Traditional	New-Model
Admission and discharge policies			
Will admit if			
Confused or disoriented	91%	84%	84%
Problem behaviors present	37	32	41
Will tolerate			
Wandering at night	35	70	60
Creating a disturbance	51	73	57
Verbal threats to residents	28	27	22
Physical attacks on residents	5	8	3
Staffing and training			
Require staff to have dementia training	74	85	95
Physical environmental features[a]			
Safety			
Exits controlled	34	42	56
Orientation			
Short or absent hallways	91	26	13
Resident rooms with			
Personal objects outside	14	28	37
Door open to hallway	73	51	36
Toilet visible from bed	20	15	2
Sign or graphic on bathroom door	3	1	1
Continuity with the past			
Resident living areas with 3 or more			
personal pictures or mementos	81	82	92
Public areas rated as "very homelike"	84	28	58
Minimization of adverse stimuli			
Areas in which the following were			
not heard			
Staff calling out	94	85	76
TV or radio noise	21	41	24
Loudspeaker	94	80	76
Alarms or call bells	92	85	76

(*continued*)

Table 11.5. *(Continued)*

	<16 Beds	Traditional	New-Model
Provision of pleasant or engaging stimuli			
Areas rated as having extensive			
or "quite a bit" of			
Tactile stimuli	53	41	74
Visual stimuli in public areas	66	59	92

aEnvironmental features were measured by direct observation during a structured 30 to 60-minute midafternoon walk through the area using the TESS-RC (see chapter 6 for details about the TESS-RC).

34%), but larger facilities were not superior in providing for continuity; smaller homes tended to have less noise (with the exception of television and radio); and new-model homes tended to provide more pleasant or engaging stimuli and to have more consistent exit control. In many instances, larger, traditional homes tended to be intermediate between the other two types, except that their public areas tended to be quite institutional and to be relatively devoid of visual and tactile stimuli.

The Process of Care. Table 11.6 presents CS-LTC data on selected dementia-relevant measures of the process of care for NDSCAs, by facility type. The domains evaluated include provision for flexibility in bedtimes, the availability of and participation in activities, the use of physical restraints, and the use of pharmacologic restraints. Results indicate that across all strata, greater flexibility was reported in evening bedtimes than in morning wake-up times (68%–95% compared to 24%–38%). Larger homes tended to report more formal activities than smaller homes, but rates of participation in formal activities during an afternoon observation were quite low (less than 20%), even among residents without dementia; they were slightly higher among residents in the traditional homes. Observed physical restraint was low among residents with dementia who were out of bed (1%–6%) but moderate among those in bed (bedrails included; 15%–33%). Physical restraint use was higher in the new-model facilities (11%) compared with the other two strata (4%). Finally, psychotropic medications were frequently prescribed to persons with dementia. Depending on the stratum, between 19 and 35 percent of residents with dementia regularly received antipsychotics, and between 15 and 27 percent received anxioltyics, sedatives, or hypnotics. The rate of

Table 11.6. Proportion of Residential Care/Assisted Living Non-Dementia-Specific Care Areas Exhibiting Selected Process Measures of Dementia-Sensitive Care, by Facility Type (%)

	<16 Beds	Traditional	New-Model
Provision for flexibility			
Flexible wake-up time	24%	35%	38%
Flexible bedtime	68	81	95
Provision of activities			
Areas offering			
Gardening ≥ once/month	32	36	30
Activities involving children ≥ once/month	38	62	68
Exercise or fitness ≥ once/week	71	78	95
Residents observed in formal group activity during afternoon			
All residents	4	13	9
Residents with moderate–severe dementia	3	14	7
Use of physical restraints for residents with moderate–severe dementia[a]			
Residents reported to be restrained at times	14	23	26
Residents observed to be restrained[b]	4	4	11
Residents observed			
In bed	13	22	21
Of these, % restrained	25	15	33
Out of bed	86	78	77
Of these, % restrained	1	1	6
Residents with moderate–severe dementia on psychotropic medication at least 4 days a week			
Antipsychotics	35	25	19
Anxiolytics, sedatives, hypnotics	27	15	18
Either of the above	50	33	35

[a]Includes geriatric chair with fixed lapboard, trunk restraint, postural chair, wrist or ankle restraints. For persons in bed, includes use of full bedrail.
[b]These residents and the time of observation are not meant to necessarily correspond with those residents reported to be restrained.

use was highest in the small homes. Comparison data from nursing homes suggests that the rates in RC/AL are somewhat lower; although the studies are limited and not entirely comparable, between 43 and 77 percent of nursing home residents with dementia have been reported to be on psychotropic medication (Rovner et al., 1996; Koopmens et al., 1996).

Dementia-Specific Settings

As noted earlier, specialized dementia care is a growing trend throughout long-term care. One of the goals of the CS-LTC was to gather data on the prevalence of specialized dementia care in RC/AL and to study aspects of the structure and process of care in those settings.

The Prevalence of Specialized Dementia Care Settings. In the CS-LTC, DSCAs were defined as geographic regions of a facility (or the whole facility) that presented themselves to the public as specializing in the care of Alzheimer disease and related disorders and had a population in which at least 75 percent had a diagnosis of a dementing disorder. Table 11.7 presents data on the prevalence of DSCAs in RC/AL facilities in the CS-

Table 11.7. Prevalence of Specialized Dementia Care in Residential Care/Assisted Living Facilities, by Facility Type

	<16 Beds	Traditional	New-Model
Total number of facilities sampled	113	40	40
Number of DSCAs identified[a]	9	3	10
Proportion of facilities with DSCAs	8%	8%	25%
That have only residents with dementia	100%	33%	20%
With both DSCAs and NDSCAs[b]	0%	67%	80%
Proportion of all residents with moderate or severe dementia who			
Reside in DSCAs	20%	11%	32%
Reside in NDSCAs	80%	89%	68%

Notes: Data from a stratified random sample of licensed facilities in Florida, Maryland, New Jersey, and North Carolina. Data collection conducted between September 1997 and October 1998.

[a]DCSAs are dementia-specific care areas. They are defined as a portion of a facility, or an entire facility, that presents itself to the public as specializing in the care of persons with Alzheimer disease or a related diagnosis and in which at least 75% of residents have a diagnosis of a dementing disorder.

[b]NDSCAs are non-dementia-specific care areas.

LTC. It is evident that DSCAs were found most commonly in larger, new-model facilities. A quarter of these facilities had specialized dementia care areas, and 32 percent of residents with moderate or severe dementia in new-model facilities resided in DSCAs. Almost 10 percent of small homes had DSCAs, and 20 percent of persons with moderate or severe dementia residing in small facilities were in DSCAs; furthermore, in all small facilities with DSCAs, the entire facility was dementia-specific. A similar percentage of traditional-style homes had DSCAs, but only 11 percent of residents with moderate or severe dementia were located in DSCAs.

Thus, dementia-specific care settings are not uncommon in RC/AL, particularly in the new-model homes. In the next section, data from the CS-LTC present dementia-sensitive indicators of the structure and process of care in DSCAs and compare them with the NDSCAs among the same types of homes. In reviewing these data, it is important to remember that the sample sizes are small (9 DSCAs in small homes, 3 in traditional homes, and 10 in new-model homes); therefore any conclusions drawn from these data are extremely tentative.

The Structure of Care. Table 11.8 displays selected structural measures

Table 11.8. Proportion of Residential Care/Assisted Living Dementia-Specific Care Areas Exhibiting Selected Structural Measures of Dementia-Sensitive Care, by Facility Type (%)

	<16 Beds	Traditional	New-Model
Admission and discharge policies			
Will admit if			
Confused or disoriented	100%	100%	100%
Problem behaviors present	89	33	70
Will tolerate			
Wandering at night	89	33	38
Creating a disturbance	67	100	67
Verbal threats to residents	44	100	44
Physical attacks on residents	0	67	0
Staffing and training			
Require staff to have dementia training	100	100	100

(continued)

Table 11.8. *(Continued)*

	<16 Beds	Traditional	New-Model
Physical environmental features[a]			
Safety			
Exits controlled	75	93	73
Orientation			
Short or absent hallways	100	0	30
Resident rooms with			
Personal objects outside	4	22	44
Door open to hallway	88	59	12
Toilet visible from bed	3	50	2
Sign or graphic on bathroom door	0	37	0
Continuity with the past			
Resident living areas with three or more			
personal pictures or mementos	69	61	86
Public areas rated as "very homelike"	44	67	60
Minimization of adverse stimuli			
Areas in which the following			
were not heard			
Staff calling out	100	100	80
TV or radio noise	22	0	0
Loudspeaker	89	67	80
Alarms or call bells	78	33	90
Provision of pleasant or engaging stimuli			
Areas rated as having extensive			
or "quite a bit" of			
Tactile stimuli	22	33	60
Visual stimuli in public areas	56	100	89

[a]Environmental features were measured by direct observation during a structured 30 to 60-minute midafternoon walk through the area using the TESS-RC (see chapter 6 for details about the TESS-RC).

of dementia-sensitive care in the DSCAs within the CS-LTC. Not surprisingly, all DSCAs admit persons with confusion and disorientation and require staff to have dementia training. At least one DSCA in each stratum did not admit persons with problem behaviors, and many would discharge persons with certain difficult behaviors such as physical aggressiveness. When table 11.8 is compared with table 11.5, it can be seen that

DSCA were generally, but not always, more receptive than NDSCAs in terms of admitting and retaining persons with dementia symptoms.

With respect to environmental features that are thought to be dementia-sensitive, DSCAs did not appear to be markedly better than NDSCAs. The single exception was the provision of exits controlled by a lock, alarm, or constant monitoring, which, in each stratum, was more common in DSCAs than in NDSCAs (tables 11.5 and 11.8). In many other features—orientation cues, continuity with the past, minimization of adverse stimuli, and provision of pleasant or engaging stimuli— DSCAs did not provide more dementia-sensitive environments than NDSCAs. Comparing across strata, no type of DSCA consistently provided a more dementia-sensitive environment.

The Process of Care. Table 11.9 displays selected measures of the process of care in DSCAs in the CS-LTC study. When these are compared with the findings for NDSCAs (table 11.6) they indicate that, as for structure, the process of care in DSCAs does not appear markedly more dementia-sensitive than in NDSCAs. The provision for flexible wake-up times and bedtimes appears increased in DSCAs, and activity participation for persons with dementia may be slightly greater; however, other dementia-specific measures of the process of care—provision of selected activities, limitation of physical restraints, and restricted use of psychotropic medication—differ little between DSCAs and NDSCAs. Indeed, if anything, physical restraints and psychotropic medications will be used more frequently in the study DSCAs.

Discussion

What constitutes quality of life for institutionalized persons with dementia? The answer to this question should serve as the basis for developing, conducting, and evaluating long-term-care settings for persons with dementia. Yet this question is frustratingly difficult to answer. Indeed, the field of dementia research is plagued by an absence of measures and accepted standards for quality of life in the later stages of the disease—the precise time at which individuals are most likely to reside in RC/AL facilities.

The best answer is an unhelpful one: quality of life depends on the individual and should express individual desires and preferences. It is un-

Table 11.9. Proportion of Residential Care/Assisted Living Dementia-Specific Care Areas Exhibiting Selected Process Measures of Dementia-Sensitive Care, by Facility Type (%)

	<16 Beds	Traditional	New-Model
Provision for flexibility			
Flexible wake-up time	67%	33%	67%
Flexible bedtime	100	33	100
Provision of activities			
Areas offering			
Gardening ≥ once/month	22	67	44
Activities involving children ≥ once/month	0	67	67
Exercise or fitness ≥ once/week	89	100	100
Residents observed in formal group activity during afternoon			
All residents	11	20	10
Residents with moderate–severe dementia	11	24	11
Use of physical restraints for residents with moderate–severe dementia[a]			
Residents reported to be restrained at times	40	0	11
Residents observed to be restrained[b]	16	0	6
Residents observed			
In bed	15	35	17
Of these, % restrained	38	0	14
Out of bed	82	65	82
Of these, % restrained	9	0	5
Residents with moderate–severe dementia on psychotropic medication at least 4 days a week			
Antipsychotics	32	29	30
Anxiolytics, sedatives, hypnotics	25	18	26
Either of the above	49	41	43

[a]Includes geriatric chair with fixed lapboard, trunk restraint, postural chair, wrist or ankle restraints. For persons in bed, includes use of full bedrail.
[b]These residents and the time of observation are not meant to necessarily correspond with those residents reported to be restrained.

helpful because what is right for the individual is virtually impossible to measure in a research study such as the CS-LTC. For example, though in general physical restraint use is believed to be harmful for older persons, and the modest increase in physical restraint use observed in DSCAs compared with NDSCAs does not provide support for DSCAs as superior care settings, there is no way of knowing from these data whether the specific residents who received restraints had peculiar circumstances that made restraint use appropriate. Similarly, involvement in activities is generally considered therapeutic; however, it is therapeutic only if the right activities are provided to the right person at a time when the individual is receptive to them. Such a degree of individualization is necessary in long-term care and is difficult to assess in research.

Despite these caveats, the data in this chapter do provide a rich and informative profile of dementia care in RC/AL facilities. They suggest that the prevalence of cognitive impairment may now approach 50 percent in these facilities and that approximately one-third of residents in these homes have moderate or severe dementia. They also indicate that the persons with dementia have not only cognitive and behavioral needs but also great ADL care needs. Thus, the major care challenge in RC/AL is increasingly the care of persons with dementia.

How good is the care provided to the hundreds of thousands of persons with dementia in RC/AL facilities? The easy answer is that it is not optimal; perhaps this is the best answer. The finding that programs that specialize in dementia care appear quite similar to those that do not, in terms of the structure-and-process measures reviewed, indicates that the typical dementia unit in RC/AL cannot be looked on as an innovative care model. Alternatively, it could mean that to the extent that it is innovative, such innovations are being embraced by the RC/AL field in general, not just those settings that purportedly specialize in dementia care.

Probably the most accurate conclusion that can be drawn is that the CS-LTC data provide a benchmark against which future progress can be measured and from which future directions can be charted. These data indicate that the majority of persons with dementia in RC/AL are in non-specialized areas and that the specialized areas differ little from the non-specialized ones. Also, because they house many persons with dementia, recommended changes in care should be directed at facilities in general, not just at dementia units. The data also indicate that dementia care must be multidimensional, addressing medical, functional, and psychosocial needs simultaneously, and that individualization of care is required.

References

Alzheimer's Association. 1992. *Guidelines for Dignity: Goals of Specialized Alzheimer/Dementia Care in Residential Settings*. Chicago: Alzheimer disease and Related Disorders Association.

————. 1994. *Residential Settings: An Examination of Alzheimer Issues*. Chicago: Alzheimer disease and Related Disorders Association.

————. 1997. *Key Elements of Dementia Care*. Chicago: Alzheimer disease and Related Disorders Association.

American Psychiatric Association. 1994. *Diagnostic and Statistical Manual of Mental Disorders (DSM-IV)*. 4th ed. Washington, DC: American Psychiatric Press.

Avorn, J., Dryer, P., Connelly, K., & Soumerai, S. 1989. Use of psychoactive medication and the quality of care in rest homes: Findings and policy implications of a statewide study. *New England Journal of Medicine* 320 (4): 227–32.

Berg, L. 1988. Clinical Dementia Rating (CDR). *Psychopharmacology Bulletin* 24:637–39.

Chen, A. 1989. The cost of operation in board and care homes. In M. Moon, G. Gaberlavage & S. J. Newman (eds.), *Preserving Independence, Supporting Needs: The Role of Board and Care Homes*. Washington, DC: Public Policy Institute, American Association of Retired Persons.

Cohen, U., & Day, K. 1994. *Contemporary Environments for People with Dementia*. Baltimore: Johns Hopkins University Press.

Coons, D. 1987. *Designing a Residential Care Unit for Persons with Dementia*. Washington, DC: U.S. Congress, Office of Technology Assessment.

Davis, K. J., Sloane, P. D., Mitchell, C. M., Preisser, J., Grant, L., Hawes, M. C., Lindeman, D., Montgomery, R., Long, K., Phillips, C., and Koch, G. 2000. Specialized dementia programs in residential settings. *Gerontologist* 40 (1): 32–42.

Donabedian, A. 1966. Evaluating the quality of medical care. *Milbank Memorial Fund Quarterly* 44:166–206.

Eckert, J. K., Namazi, K. H., & Kahana, E. 1987. Unlicensed board and care homes: An extra-familial living arrangement for the elderly. *Journal of Cross-Cultural Gerontology* 2:377–93.

Emery, V. O., & Oxman, T. E. 1994. *Dementia: Presentations, Differences, and Nosology*. Baltimore: Johns Hopkins University Press.

Epping, F. J., & Poisal, J. A. 1997. Mental health of Medicare beneficiaries, 1995. *Health Care Financing Review* 15:207–10.

Faunce, I., & Brunette, M. 1986. The Alzheimer's project of Kennebec Valley: A national model. *American Journal of Alzheimer's Care*, fall.

Folstein, M. F., Folstein, S. E., & McHugh, P. R. 1975. Mini-mental state: A practical method for grading the cognitive state of patients for the clinician. *Journal of Psychiatric Research* 12:189–98.

Grant, L. A. 1998. Beyond the dichotomy: An empirical typology of Alzheimer's care in nursing homes. *Research on Aging* 20:569–92.

Grant, L. A., & Ory, M. G. 2000. Alzheimer's special care units in the United States. *Research and Practice in Alzheimer's Disease* 4:19–43.

Gwyther, L. 1990. Assisted living: Unique advantages for older adults with Alzheimer's and their families. *Long Term Care Advances* 1 (4): 8–11.

Ham, R. J. 1997. Confusion, dementia, and delirium. In R. J. Ham & P. D. Sloane (eds.), *Primary Care Geriatrics: A Case-Based Approach*. 3d ed. Chicago: Mosby-Yearbook.

Hartmaier, S., Sloane, P. D., Guess, H., & Koch, G. 1994. The MDS Cognition Scale: A valid instrument for identifying and staging nursing home residents with dementia using the Minimum Data Set. *Journal of the American Geriatrics Society* 42:1173–79.

Hawes, C., Mor, V., Wildfire, J., Lux, L., Green, R., Iannacchione, V., & Phillips, C. D. 1995. *Executive Summary: Analysis of the Effects of Regulation on the Quality of Care in Board and Care Homes*. Research Triangle Park, NC: Research Triangle Institute.

Hawes, C., Wildfire, J. B., & Lux, J. L. 1993. *The Regulation of Board and Care Homes: Results of a Survey in the 50 States and the District of Columbia: National Summary*. Washington, DC: American Association of Retired Persons.

Institute of Medicine. 1986. *Improving the Quality of Care in Nursing Homes*. Washington, DC: National Academy Press.

Kane, R., & Wilson, K. B. 1993. *Assisted Living in the United States: A New Paradigm for Residential Care for Frail Older Persons?* Washington, DC: American Association of Retired Persons.

Koopmens, R. T., Van Rossum, S. M., Van den Hoogen, H. S., Heksler, Y. A., Willekens-Bogaers, M. A., & Van Weel, C. 1996. Psychotropic drug use in a group of Dutch nursing home patients with dementia: Many users, long term use, but low doses. *Pharmacy World and Science* 18:42–47.

Leon, J., Cheng, M., & Alvarez, R. 1997. Trends in special care: Changes in SCU from 1991 to 1995. *Journal of Mental Health and Aging* 3:149–68.

Magaziner, J., German, P., Zimmerman, S. I., Hebel, J. R., Burton, L., Gruber-Baldini, A. L., May, C., & Kittner, S. 2000. The prevalence of dementia in a statewide sample of new nursing home admissions age 65 and older: Diagnosis by expert panel. *Gerontologist* 40:663–72.

Magaziner, J., Zimmerman, S. I., German, P. S., Kuhn, K., May, C., Hooper, F., Cox, D., Hebel, J. R., Kittner, S., Burton, L., Fishman, P., Kaup, B., Rosario, J., & Cody, M. 1996. Ascertaining dementia by expert panel in epidemiologic studies of nursing home residents. *Annals of Epidemiology* 6:431–37.

Mor, V., Sherwood, S., & Gutkin, C. 1986. A national study of residential care for the aged. *Gerontologist* 26:405–17.

Morgan, L. A., Eckert, J. K., & Lyon, S. M. (eds.). 1995. *Small Board-and-Care Homes: Residential Care in Transition.* Baltimore: Johns Hopkins University Press.

National Center for Health Statistics. 1987. *Use of Nursing Homes by the Elderly: Preliminary Data from the National Nursing Home Survey.* Advance data from Vital and Health Statistics, no. 135. DHHS pub. no. (PHS) 87-1250. Hyattsville, MD: Public Health Service.

Rajecki, R. 1992. Charting a new course in Alzheimer care. *Contemporary Long Term Care*, August.

Reisberg, B., Ferris, S. H., de Leon, M. J., & Crook, T. 1982. The global deterioration scale for assessment of primary degenerative dementia. *American Journal of Psychiatry* 139 (9): 1136–39.

Rovner, B. W., Steele, C. D., Shmuely, V., & Folstein, M. F. 1996. A randomized trial of dementia care in nursing homes. *Journal of the American Geriatrics Society* 44:7–13.

Sloane, P. D. 1998. Advances in the treatment of Alzheimer disease. *American Family Physician* 58:1577–86.

Sloane, P., Lindeman, D., Phillips, C., Moritz, D., & Koch, G. 1995. Evaluating Alzheimer's special care units: Reviewing the evidence and identifying potential sources of study bias. *Gerontologist* 35 (1): 103–11.

Small, G. W., Rabins, P. R., Barry, P. P., Buckholtz, N. S., DeKosky, S. T., Ferris, S. H., Finkel, S. I., Gwyther, L. P., Khachaturian, Z. S., Lebowitz, B. D., McRae, T. D., Morris, J. C., Oakley, F., Schneider, L. S., Streim, J. E., Sunderland, T., Teri, L. A., & Tune, L. E. 1997. Diagnosis and treatment of Alzheimer disease and related disorders: Consensus statement of the American Association for Geriatric Psychiatry, the Alzheimer's Association, and the American Geriatrics Society. *Journal of the American Medical Association* 278:1363–71.

Stocker, K. B., & Silverstein, N. M. 1996. Assisted living residences in Massachusetts: How ready and willing are they to serve people with Alzheimer disease or a related disorder? *American Journal of Alzheimer disease*, March–April, 28–38.

Teresi, J., Grant, L. A., Holmes, D., & Ory, M. G. 1998. Staffing in traditional and special dementia care units: Preliminary findings from the National Institute on Aging collaborative studies. *Journal of Gerontological Nursing* 24 (1): 49–53.

Teresi, J., Morris, J. N., Mattis, S., & Reisberg, B. 2000. Cognitive impairment among SCU and non-SCU residents in the United States: Prevalence estimates from the National Institute on Aging collaborative studies of special care units for Alzheimer disease. *Research and Practice in Alzheimer disease* 4:117–38.

Tombaugh, T. N., & McIntyre, N. J. 1992. The Mini-Mental State Examination: A comprehensive review. *Journal of the American Geriatrics Society* 40:922–35.

U.S. Congress, General Accounting Office. 1998. *Alzheimer disease: Estimates of Prevalence in the United States.* Washington, DC: General Accounting Office. Report GAO/HEHS-98-16.

U.S. Congress, Office of Technological Assessment. 1987. *Losing a Million Minds: Confronting the Tragedy of Alzheimer disease and Other Dementias.* Washington, DC: Government Printing Office.

U.S. Department of Health and Human Services. 1998. *Characteristics of Nursing Home Residents, 1996.* Pub. no. 99 0006. Rockville, MD: Agency for Health Care Policy and Research.

Weiner, M. F. 1996. *The Dementias: Diagnosis, Management, and Research.* 2d ed. Washington, DC: American Psychiatric Press.

Zeisel. J. 1995. Dementia-specific assisted living residences. *American Journal of Alzheimer disease and Related Disorders Care and Research* 10 (3): 40–41.

Zimmerman, S. I., & Sloane, P. D. 1999. Optimum residential care for persons with dementia. *Generations* 23 (3): 62–68.

12 Economics and Financing

Sally C. Stearns, Ph.D., and Leslie A. Morgan, Ph.D.

Economic forces play a major role in the structure and viability of the residential care/assisted living (RC/AL) industry. Conceptually, the issues relevant to the economics and financing of RC/AL facilities may be divided into two levels, as indicated in table 12.1: industry domains and individual firm (facility) domains. Key industry domains include current and future demand, financing and investment resources, and the regulatory environment. Key firm (facility) domains include aspects of ownership, staffing, expenses, and revenues. These issues, both at the firm level and in aggregate at the industry level, will determine the effectiveness and growth of the RC/AL industry.

We begin this chapter by reviewing background information related to the industry and firm domains. A descriptive exploration of the firm domains is then presented, using data from the Collaborative Studies of Long-Term Care (CS-LTC), a study of RC/AL in four states (Florida, Maryland, New Jersey, and North Carolina). We conclude with a discussion of the issues identified as most central to the growth of RC/AL facilities.

The Industry Environment

The industry domains shape the environment for RC/AL facilities. Four major demographic trends result in predictions of substantial increases in future demand for formal RC/AL services: the aging of the baby boomers, the increasing longevity of the elderly population, the greater participation by women in the labor force, and the increasing geographic dispersion of adult children from their parents. Policy plays a central role in demand, as well.

There is an important distinction between public and private demand in the demand projections. Historically, much of the demand for RC/AL

Table 12.1. Key Economics and Financing Domains

Industry Domains	Firm (Facility) Domains
Market demand and supply	Ownership
Demographics	Type
Public versus private demand	Owner involvement
Growth and competition	Staffing
Financing and investment	Per resident by type
Revenue sources	Turnover
Access to capital	Expenses
Regulatory environment	Revenue
Facility licensure	Charges
Medicaid waivers and payment	Sources
Quality	Profit or loss

(also called board and care) came from individuals without sufficient health and resources (family or financial) to live independently. Many of these individuals relied on federal and state programs, primarily Supplemental Security Income (SSI) or State Supplemental Payments (SSP), for funds to pay for their care. Mor, Gutkin, and Sherwood (1985) reported that 43 percent of residents were SSI recipients, and Hawes, Wildfire, and Lux (1993) cited data indicating that approximately 50 percent of residents depend on some type of public payment (SSP, Medicaid, Medicaid 2176 Home and Community-Based Care Waivers, or other state or county funds). Yet the public programs had little control over the service providers or users because the industry, especially smaller facilities, was unregulated in many states. Capitman (1989) predicted that public payers would be reluctant to increase involvement through such programs as Medicaid unless those individuals who could be cared for most appropriately and efficiently could be identified. The fact that many users were low-income and reliant on public sources for income also meant that many RC/AL providers (particularly smaller operations) were at best marginally profitable (Mor, Gutkin & Sherwood, 1985; Chen 1989). Much of the motivation for provision of the services may have come from nonfinancial considerations or the family economy model (Morgan, Eckert & Lyon, 1995).

Over the past decade, however, both public payers and people with substantial private resources have become increasingly interested in RC/AL. As a result of the evolution of the industry, more and different options are available, especially for private pay clients. States see RC/AL as a way to reduce the growth in nursing home utilization. In 1996, 22 state Medicaid programs provided reimbursement for assisted living (AL), with the number increasing to 39 by 2000; other states were planning for Medicaid reimbursement (Mollica, 2000). All four of the CS-LTC states provide some Medicaid reimbursement for RC/AL. Although the greatest demand for senior housing is still from people with lower incomes (NIC, 1997), many middle- or upper-income individuals or their children see RC/AL as a desirable way to support older adults during a period of increasing functional dependency.

The result has been a burgeoning RC/AL industry. Construction of housing for seniors increased dramatically during the 1990s, and the growth has not yet abated. Construction increased 11 percent from 1997 to 1998 (ASHA, 1998) and the number of AL facilities operating in 1998 increased by 49 percent (Croswell, 1999). Although much of the financing for acquisition and start-up costs was previously patchy or nonexistent, *Fortune* magazine identified RC/AL as one of the top three potential growth industries in 1997 (US GAO, 1999). The tenure and implications of this period of growth remain uncertain, however, as some market analysts express concern that the industry is overbuilt; others worry that insufficient oversight exists to ensure quality care (NJG, 1999).

The affordability of RC/AL may be defined as prices relative to the financial resources of the residents. The average monthly cost to live in a RC/AL residence is $1,807 (NCAL, 1998). Reported monthly rates range from less than $1,000 to more than $4,000 (US GAO, 1999), and many facilities vary their price according to the level of services required. A majority of facilities are for-profit, but the percent of facilities that are not-for-profit can vary considerably across states. (A majority of facilities also serve only the private pay market [US GAO, 1999]). In 1998 SSI programs paid aged poor persons $494 a month; supplemental payments are available to persons in RC/AL in most states. Waiver states usually use SSI payments for room and board and Medicaid payments for services, and the combination covers most of the total costs. Public payments also vary according to whether they are made to the resident or the home, and rates are often adjusted for case mix. For example, in 1990 Connecticut's total monthly payment ranged as high as $2,000 a month (Hawes, Wildfire & Lux, 1993). Even adjusted for case mix, however, public payments are likely to fall considerably below rates that are set in a market that competes for private pay patients.

Not surprisingly, increased regulatory oversight has accompanied the growth within the industry. The General Accounting Office recently reported that information provided to prospective residents is insufficient in many cases, and it cited evidence of violations of a range of consumer protections (US GAO, 1999). As of 2000, twenty-nine states had licensing regulations using the term *assisted living,* and nineteen states had created task forces or processes to make recommendations for developing assisted living rules (Mollica, 2000). (See chapter 1 of this volume for more information about policy and regulations.) Some states are implementing cost-reporting processes in order to set Medicaid payment rates. These processes and other regulations or guidelines will affect a range of issues from quality to payment.

Prior Studies of Residential Care/Assisted Living Facilities

All RC/AL facilities are similar in that they provide accommodations and some supportive services including assistance with activities of daily living. The main categories of operating expenses include salaries, food, and room expenses (including utilities, mortgages, etc.). There is substantial variation, however, in the type and intensity of care provided, both within and across facilities. Hypothesized sources of variation are multiple. Smaller facilities may be more likely to use unpaid owner or volunteer time. Larger facilities may be more likely to offer a broader range of personal care or support services, yet the rates of staff hours per resident day may be lower in larger facilities because of economies of scale. The rates of staff turnover, which are potentially an indicator of quality of care, may also differ in relation to facility characteristics or local labor market conditions. In addition to variation in expenses, charges to residents and sources of revenue vary considerably. Some facilities rely solely on private sources of revenue to cover their costs; others make extensive use of public funds such as Medicaid (NCAL, 1998).

With a few exceptions, the results from prior studies cannot be generalized, either because of the limited number of facilities involved, the age of the data, restrictions of the types of facilities studied, or survey nonresponse. Table 12.2 provides selected information about several studies conducted since 1985. Some are case studies, whereas others involve more extensive primary data collection. Some focus on small homes; others address a broader spectrum of facility size. Selected points relevant to the RC/AL facility domains are described below.

Mor, Gutkin, and Sherwood (1985) surveyed a random sample of 269 homes with one hundred or fewer beds in five states. Following exclusions for nonresponse and multilevel affiliation, data were available for 164 facilities. The focus of the analysis was on the variation in average cost per month for three expenditure categories (total, food, and staffing) in relation to resident case mix and the regulatory environment. Overall, food expenses accounted for more than a third of expenses per resident month, whereas salaries accounted for slightly less than a third. Bivariate analysis showed that food expenses per resident month declined with size (possibly representing economics of scale) but that staffing expenses per resident month increased with size (most likely a result of nonassignment of expenses for owner-contributed hours by small homes but also possibly caused by differences in specialization). Food expenses per resident month did not vary with size in a multiple regression analysis; instead, they varied with selected case-mix measures. Staffing expenses did not vary with case mix but were significantly lower in facilities where the owner co-resided or had other income. Staffing expenses were significantly higher in facilities governed by federal administration of SSI, and facilities governed by state programs in which regulatory agencies had closed facilities in the previous two years had lower total and staffing costs. The latter finding may reflect geographic clustering of low-cost homes because of differences in either cost of living or regulatory standards.

Chen (1989) characterized three categories of costs: acquisition, start-up, and operating, examining the income statements of 13 board and care homes, ranging in size up to fifty beds. Staffing accounted for more than 40 percent of expenses in most facilities and as much as 70–80 percent of expenses in a few facilities. Room expenses generally accounted for less than 20 percent of expenses, as did food expenses. As noted by Chen, these data describe only the 13 homes that were willing to provide income statements and cannot be used to characterize the broader population of

Table 12.2. Selected Facility-Level Studies Related to Economics and Financing Facility Domains since 1985

Study	Sample	Domains Covered	Findings and Comments
Mor, Gutkin & Sherwood, 1985	164 facilities with <100 beds in 5 states	Ownership type, owner involvement, staffing, expenses	Ownership role had a substantial effect on average expenditures (in total and staff) per resident month. Food expenses varied with case-mix measures, but staffing expenses did not.
Chen, 1989	13 facilities with <50 beds	Expenses, revenue sources, profit	Staff expenses predominated and resulted in economics of scale. Careful control of expenses could lead to modest profit margins.
Morgan, Eckert & Lyon, 1995	108 facilities with <16 beds in Maryland	Ownership, expenses, revenues, profit	Slim profit margins for many small homes converted to losses if adjusted for a salary for owners. Profitability was dependent on owner status and orientation toward private versus public market.

Source	Sample	Variables	Notes
Bratesman et al., 1998	519 facilities with >9 beds in North Carolina	Ownership, expenses, revenue, profit	Direct-service costs were higher for facilities that were nonprofit, older, affiliated with nursing homes, or oriented toward the private market.
ASHA, NIC & PWC, 1998	73 assisted living facilities	Staffing, expenses, revenue	Provides comparisons on a series of data for assisted living facilities to congregate and continuing-care retirement communities.
NCAL, 1998	366 facilities in 44 states (228 facilities for staffing)	Staffing, expenses, revenue	Provides information on a series of facts and trends, including residents, operations, financing, and supply and demand. Survey represents a 10% response rate, although there is no known bias in response.
US GAO, 1999	622 facilities in 4 states (CA, FL, OR, OH)	Ownership, charges, revenues	Wide variation in ownership type (for-profit) by state. Wide variation in monthly rates, and a majority of facilities served only a private pay market.

homes. His conclusions, however, that economies of scale are likely to exist and that smaller facilities must be able to respond to labor cost increases in order to survive are undoubtedly still relevant.

Morgan, Eckert, and Lyon (1995) analyzed interview data for a sample of 108 small homes, mostly ranging from one to fifteen beds. As in other studies, staffing and food accounted for roughly two-thirds of monthly expenses. Expenses were largely constrained by work contributions by nonsalaried owners, and the high cost of more intensive care was driven by the salaries of specialized or skilled personnel. The homes were primarily for-profit, and the family economy model confounded charges to residents and expenses with other costs and income to the home. A dichotomy was identified between elite homes catering to the private market and more economically marginal homes serving a large proportion of low-income residents receiving formal public support or income.

In 1995 North Carolina became one of the first states to require RC/AL facilities to submit audited cost-report data for reimbursements by Medicaid. Bratesman and associates (1998) analyzed data with a focus on direct service costs for 519 facilities (out of 2,367 in the cost-report database) that met certain criteria (i.e., they had 10 or more beds, were oriented toward elderly population, and were single homes rather than part of a chain). They found that direct services (e.g., food, staff providing care, etc.) to the patient accounted for less than one-half of total costs, with the rest going to facility-related expenses, administration, and ancillary services. The variation among facilities was considerable, however. Direct service costs were higher for not-for-profit facilities, facilities with a greater proportion of private pay clients, older facilities, and facilities affiliated with nursing homes. The inability to control for case mix limited the ability to draw firm conclusions pertaining to these factors.

Two recent surveys (ASHA, NIC & PWC, 1998; NCAL, 1998) provide a wealth of interesting data on staffing, expenses, and revenue in RC/AL facilities around the country. The main limitation of the surveys is a high nonresponse rate; for example, the 366 facilities responding to the survey by the National Center for Assisted Living represent only a 10 percent response rate. Therefore, the representativeness of the surveys is not guaranteed. The survey by the American Senior Housing Association provides comparisons of AL facilities to alternative residential arrangements for the elderly (congregate housing and continuing-care retirement communities). The survey by the National Center for Assisted Living provides a much broader assessment, including information on case mix and detailed staffing and turnover data. A key point of interest in this survey is the high turnover rates (from 30% to 60%) reported for most employee categories in RC/AL. The study defined turnover, however, as the ratio of staff hired during the previous year to the average number of staff positions during the year. This approach would overstate turnover in any facility that was growing in size during the year.

A survey conducted by the General Accounting Office assessed the quality of care and consumer protection in four states, but the survey also obtained some limited information pertinent to economics and financing. The percentage of facilities that were for-profit ranged from 45 percent in Ohio to 86 percent in Oregon. The survey also found that the majority of facilities served only a private pay market (albeit with some residents using SSI funds and supplementing with other resources). Forty percent of the facilities reported receiving Medicaid or other public funds to care for one or more residents (US GAO, 1999).

The existing studies provide some useful information, but data on several important facility domains are limited. For example, though the more recent surveys provide some descriptive data on the staffing composition and turnover, the variation in these data in relation to key facility characteristics is not described or analyzed. The information on owner involvement is also quite limited. Data from the CS-LTC are used in the next section to provide further insights into the RC/AL facility domains and to confirm and expand on previously reported domains.

Facility Domains: Residential Care/Assisted Living Facilities in the Collaborative Studies of Long-Term Care

The Collaborative Studies of Long-Term Care (CS-LTC) is a study of RC/AL across four states: Florida, Maryland, New Jersey, and North Carolina. These states have RC/AL industries that are relatively well developed but also vary on a number of factors. Facilities were sampled in three strata within each state to ensure variation in size, age, and case mix. The three strata are facilities with fewer than sixteen beds ($N = 113$); facilities with sixteen or more beds that reflect components of purpose-built, new-model assisted living promoting aging in place ($N = 40$); and facilities with sixteen or more beds that are more traditional and do not meet the new-model definition ($N = 40$). Specifically, the new-model facilities were built after January 1, 1987 and have at least one of the following characteristics: two private-pay rates, 20 percent or more of residents requiring assistance in transfer, 25 percent or more of residents incontinent daily, or either an RN or LPN on duty at all times. Data were collected from the 193 randomly selected facilities between October 1997 and November 1998. (For additional information about the CS-LTC design and methods, see chapter 6.)

This section provides a descriptive assessment of the firm/facility domains pertaining to economics and financing for the RC/AL facilities in the CS-LTC. Four topics are considered: ownership issues, staffing (including hours per resident by type of service and personal care aide turnover), facility expenses, and facility revenues. The analysis focuses on variation across facilities in these factors by CS-LTC strata, which reflect intrinsic differences such as size or facility orientation. Additional breakdowns are provided in some cases according to facility ownership (for-profit or not-for-profit) and service type.

Data Sources and Completeness

The data presented in this section come primarily from a survey completed by facility administrators. The first half of the survey addressed issues of staffing and turnover; the second half collected information on facility expenses and revenues. The staffing data included owner involvement in facility work, hours worked by staff (paid, contract, and unpaid) according to six task types (administration, registered nursing tasks, licensed practical nursing tasks, personal care, planned activities, and other tasks), turnover during the previous six months according to staff classification (administration, nursing, personal care, and activities workers), and personal care aide wages and benefits. For facilities in North Carolina, data on expenses and revenues were obtained from cost reports submitted to the state for Medicaid reimbursement in lieu of the second half of the administrator survey. The expense and revenue components of the survey were modeled after the North Carolina cost-reporting form and the National Nursing Home Survey, although more aggregate expense categories were used to reduce respondent burden.

After follow-up data collection for nonrespondents, the survey had a high response (submission) rate of 95 percent (183 out of 193 facilities). Four returned surveys that listed zero or missing hours for all tasks were excluded from the analysis, and two other facilities were missing data on policies and procedures. Data from 177 facilities are used in the analyses that follow. The 16 excluded facilities are small (11 facilities) or from Maryland (6 facilities). A number of surveys with complete staffing information did not have reliable information on costs (expenses or revenues). The implications of the missing cost data are addressed later in the chapter.

Ownership Issues: Profit Status and Owner Involvement

Ownership roles in RC/AL range from shareholders who have little involvement in day-to-day facility operations to owners who operate the facility, either in their own residence or at a separate location. Table 12.3 shows that facilities with fewer than sixteen beds were most likely (61%) and new-model facilities were least likely (8%) to report that owners performed facility-related work. Since by definition surplus revenues in not-for-profit facilities cannot accrue to owners, it is more relevant to assess owner involvement according to for-profit status. The RC/AL facilities in the four CS-LTC study states are predominantly for-profit within each stratum, ranging from 68 percent for traditional homes to 92 percent for facilities with fewer than sixteen beds. Roughly 65 percent of both small and traditional for-profit facilities have owners who report working within the facility. The relatively low likelihood of having owners perform

Table 12.3. Residential Care/Assisted Living Ownership and Owner Involvement, by Facility Type

	<16 Beds	*Traditional*	*New-Model*
Number of facilities	101	37	39
Percent of facilities in which			
owner works in facility	61.4%	43.2%	7.7%
Ownership type: proportion for-profit	92.1%	67.6%	71.8%
Percent of facilities in which owner			
works in facility, by ownership type			
For-profit	65.6%	64.0%	10.7%
Not-for-profit or governmental[a]	12.5%	0%	0%
Average hours worked last week by			
owners who work in for-profit facilities	58.2	55.9	60.0
Average hours on call last week by			
owners who work in for-profit facilities	59.3	77.3	0

[a]The one CS-LTC facility owned by the government is grouped with not-for-profit facilities.

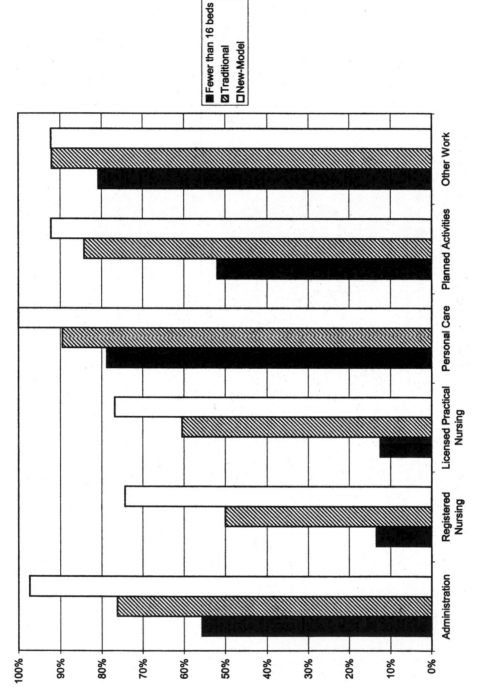

Fig. 12.1. Percentage of facilities using paid staff, by type of facility and type of task

facility-related work in new-model facilities (11 percent of facilities) may reflect a different orientation or ownership structure for these facilities. Small and traditional facilities may be more likely to have a resident owner dependent on residual revenue in excess of facility expenses, whereas new-model facilities may be much more likely to be owned by shareholders. In fact, out of the 39 new-model facilities, only 3 for-profit facilities (all in Florida) reported that the owner worked within the facility. None of the traditional or new-model not-for-profit facilities reported any owners doing facility-related work. Among the 8 not-for-profit facilities with fewer than sixteen beds, only 1 facility (12.5%) reported an owner doing facility-related work; this report may be a data error or may reflect an unusual situation such as a facility run by a religious organization.

To avoid excessively high reports of hours worked by resident owners, the survey differentiated between hours of work and hours on call. Table 12.3 indicates that owners of for-profit facilities who reported working in their facilities also reported similar average hours worked per week by stratum, ranging from 56 hours for traditional facilities to 60 hours per week for owners of new-model facilities. Reported hours on call by owners of these facilities were 59 hours for small facilities and 77 hours for traditional facilities, on average. Owners of the for-profit new-model facilities did not report any on-call hours; this finding might be expected since these facilities may be less likely to have an owner in residence, although it is important to remember that this category comprised only 3 facilities, all in Florida.

Staffing

In addition to work done by owners, RC/AL facilities may hire their own paid staff, use contract staff, or rely on unpaid labor. Figure 12.1 shows the proportion of facilities in each stratum using paid staff by tasks performed. The categories of tasks include administration, registered nursing, licensed practical nursing, personal care, planned activities, and other work (such as food service, maintenance, transportation, etc.). Facilities with fewer than sixteen beds are least likely and new-model facilities are most likely to use paid staff in each task category. The difference is particularly striking for the two nursing tasks, with only 13 percent of the smaller facilities having paid nursing staff but roughly 75 percent of the new-model facilities having paid nursing staff. The absence of nursing staff paid by a facility does not mean that residents are not receiving any

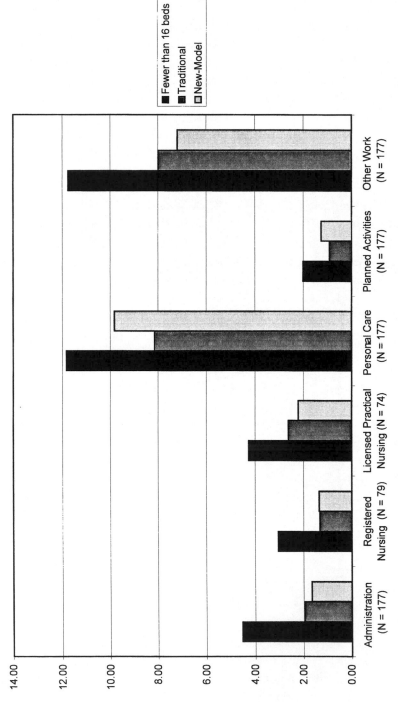

Fig. 12.2. Total hours spent per resident per week in residential care/assisted living facilities, by facility type and type of task

nursing services, though, because such services may be obtained from external providers and reimbursed directly through Medicare or private sources.

Fewer than 10 percent of facilities use contract staff for most tasks. Sixteen percent of traditional facilities reported using contract registered nursing staff. Within each stratum, facilities are most likely to use contract staff to perform "other" facility work, with the amount for other work ranging from 13 percent of small facilities to 28 percent of new-model facilities. The survey also collected information on unpaid staff hours by task in addition to paid hours. The survey did not distinguish between unpaid hours by owners' families, unpaid overtime by paid staff, and volunteer hours. Few facilities reported unpaid hours for registered nursing, licensed practical nursing, or personal care tasks. Facilities reporting unpaid hours for administration ranged from 24 percent for small facilities to 46 percent for new-model facilities, and facilities reporting unpaid hours for planned activities ranged from 24 percent for small facilities to 69 percent for new-model.

Figure 12.2 displays information on the total reported hours per resident per week by facility type and task. Total hours include all hours worked during the previous week reported by owners, paid facility staff, contract staff, and unpaid staff. On-call hours by owners are excluded. The registered nursing and licensed practical nursing hours are calculated using data only for facilities that reported providing these services by owners, paid staff, or contract staff. (Recall that residents may receive additional nursing services reimbursed directly by other payers [e.g., private pay, Medicare, etc.] that would not be reflected in the facility's reported nursing hours.) Compared to traditional or new-model facilities, small homes reported significantly more hours spent per resident ($p < 0.05$) for all tasks. These differences in hours per resident for administration, planned activities, or other tasks (e.g., dietary preparation, facility maintenance) may be attributable to economies of scale enjoyed by the larger traditional or new-model facilities. The differences in the tasks related to resident care, however, are less straightforward. The significance of the difference in personal care hours disappeared once for-profit status and facility case-mix measures related to incontinence and mobility were controlled for in regression analyses (not shown). Small homes continued to report significantly more registered and licensed practical nursing hours even after controlling for ownership and case mix, although it is impor-

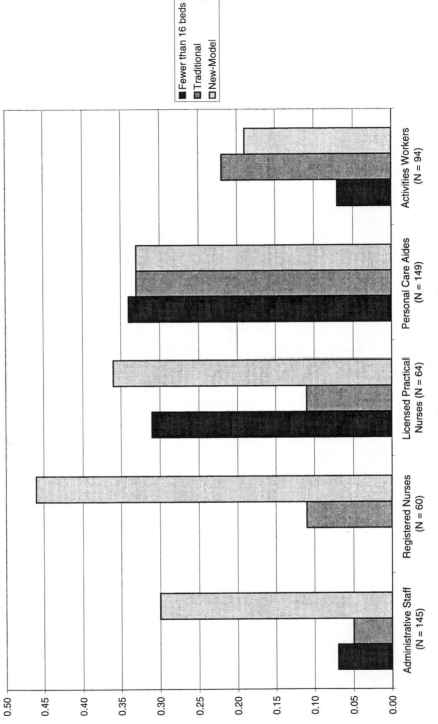

Fig. 12.3. Paid staff turnover during past six months, by facility type and type of staff

tant to remember that less than 15 percent of small homes reported paid facility staff for nursing tasks. These findings could reflect reporting bias (e.g., small homes owned by nurses may have more nursing hours reported by owners) or real differences in service intensity among facility types. Further analyses are required to determine whether the reported variation in hours per resident relate to differences in resident outcomes once such data are available from the CS-LTC.

Staff Turnover

The continuity and quality of care provided to persons in RC/AL facilities may be compromised if turnover is frequent among paid staff. Figure 12.3 shows reported turnover during the previous six months by facility stratum for five types of staff: administrative staff, registered nurses, licensed practical nurses, personal care aides, and activities workers. Turnover is calculated as the number of staff who quit during that period divided by the total number of staff in that category, where the number of staff is the sum of full-time and part-time workers, with part-time workers weighted at one-half. Data are displayed only for facilities that use paid staff of each type.

Two aspects of the figure are striking. First, reported turnover in new-model facilities is higher or roughly as high as turnover in small or traditional facilities for each staff type. Second, turnover among personal care aides is high across all three types of facilities. Given the importance of personal care services for RC/AL facility residents, further explorations of the reasons for turnover among personal care aides and of any associations of turnover with resident outcomes will be important components of future CS-LTC analyses.

Two factors that may affect turnover are salary and benefits. Roughly 130 facilities responded to questions on these policies for their personal care aides. Small facilities reported average salaries (not adjusted for regional cost differences) of $6.50 per hour; traditional and new-model facilities reported averages of $7.00. Only 35 percent of small facilities said they provided health insurance benefits for personal care aides, compared to 73 and 82 percent for traditional and new-model facilities, respectively. Regression analyses did not reveal a significant relationship between personal care aide turnover and salary and benefits, indicating that other factors such as case mix, facility management style, or working relationships may be stronger determinants of turnover.

Expenses and Revenues

As noted earlier, response rates regarding information on facility expenses were lower than for questions on facility staffing. Table 12.4 shows that response rates were nearly identical across facility strata at approximately 50 percent within each stratum. Response rates were relatively higher in North Carolina and Florida (70% and 63%, respectively) and lower in Maryland and New Jersey (32% and 37%, respectively). Response rates were somewhat higher for expenses than for revenues, as shown by the table, with small facilities being relatively more reluctant or less able to provide revenue information. With the exception of cost-report data from facilities with more than nine beds in North Carolina, none of the expense or revenue information was audited; the data presented in this section are therefore subject to reporting errors.

Not surprisingly, average annual reported expenses per bed were lowest for small facilities (at $10,902) and highest for new-model facilities (at

Table 12.4. Reported Residential Care/Assisted Living Facility Expenses and Revenues, by Facility Type

	<16 Beds	Traditional	New-Model
Original sample facilities	113	40	40
Facilities reporting expenses	56	21	21
Annual expenses per bed	$10,902	$13,959	$19,355
Composition of expenses			
Salaries and benefits	39.7%	58.4%	52.6%
Food	15.7%	12.0%	12.2%
Capital financing	20.8%	13.4%	24.8%
Facilities reporting revenues	49	20	19
Annual revenues per bed	$14,047	$15,339	$21,593
Percent of revenues that are public	33.4%	19.4%	13.3%
Percent of facilities reporting positive residual revenue (profit)	83.7%	65.0%	68.4%
Average profit per bed among facilities making profits	$3,347	$4,933	$7,036
Median profit per bed among facilities making profits	$1,941	$2,648	$3,504

Note: Most data were not audited.

$19,355). Some of this difference is probably due to greater use of unpaid owner or staff time in the small facilities. As shown in the data on composition of expenses, small facilities reported that only 40 percent of total expenses were attributable on average to salaries, wages, and benefits, whereas traditional and new-model facilities reported 58 and 53 percent of expenses in this category. Small facilities spent a larger proportion of total expenses on food and capital financing (including rent, interest and financing charges, amortization of improvements, and depreciation charges) than did traditional facilities. Capital financing expenses as a percent of total expenses may have been relatively high on average in new-model facilities (25% of total expenses) because of the recent construction of many of these facilities.

Across all settings, basic monthly rates range from $453 to $4,050. Forty-five percent of facilities charge differing rates depending on the level of services a resident receives. As shown in table 12.4, small facilities reported lower average annual revenues per bed ($14,047) relative to traditional facilities ($15,339) or new-model facilities ($21,593). Median revenues per bed (not shown) were close to average revenues per bed. The small facilities drew a greater proportion of their total revenues from public sources (defined to include Medicaid, SSI, SSI state supplements, and other state or county special assistance) at 33 percent than did traditional facilities (19%) or new-model facilities (19%).

Small facilities were significantly more likely to report "profits" (measured as positive residual revenue, or the difference between reported expenses and revenues) than were traditional facilities or new-model facilities. The greater likelihood of profit at small facilities does not necessarily indicate financial health for these facilities, however, since owners of smaller facilities often are unpaid and rely on residual revenues in excess of expenses (e.g., "profit") as their only source of return from the venture. The distribution of profits per bed among facilities making profits was highly skewed within each stratum. The average and median profits per bed among facilities making profits were lowest at small facilities ($3,347 on average, with a median of $1,941) and highest at new-model facilities ($7,036 on average, with a median of $3,504). Subtracting payments that approximate the market opportunity cost for unpaid owners would further reduce the amount of profits accruing to the small facilities in this analysis.

Discussion

The analyses in this chapter provide three contributions to the literature on the economics and financing of RC/AL. First, though the sampling design does not allow generalization to the RC/AL industry as a whole, the descriptive analyses confirm and extend our awareness of some of the variations that exist between small, traditional, and new-model facilities with respect to owner involvement, staffing, and expenses and revenues. Second, the analyses raise some interesting questions for further empirical exploration in the CS-LTC longitudinal data on resident outcomes. In particular, does variation in staffing intensity per resident or in measures such as turnover correlate to observed differences in resident outcomes? If so, then the quality and appropriateness of care provided in RC/AL settings might be enhanced by developing guidelines for staffing intensity and innovations to reduce turnover. If not, then greater efficiency in the provision of RC/AL might be attained by concentrating or consolidating resource use, such as by expanding the use of shared contract services across facilities.

The third contribution pertains to the broader framework for developing policy recommendations related to the growth of the industry. The competing interests of public and private demand will undoubtedly confront the evolving RC/AL industry with substantial challenges. Small homes are being forced to undertake the costs to implement processes necessary to function in a regulated environment. Facilities that target the private market are being forced to reconcile their original goals with the realities of stiff competition from other facilities and a resident population that will necessarily become poorer and less functional as it ages. Affordability and the likely event of spend-down of assets by residents over time are issues of substantial future importance. Quality and appropriateness of care at reasonable cost will remain as central challenges for the industry.

References

American Seniors Housing Association. 1998. *Seniors Housing Construction Report, 1998.* Washington, DC: American Seniors Housing Association.

American Seniors Housing Association, National Investment Center, and Price Waterhouse Coopers. 1998. The state of seniors housing. American Seniors Housing Association, Washington, DC.

Bratesman, S., Leak, S. C., Prince, J. H., Maddox, G. L., & Hermanson, S. 1998. *Tracking the Cost of Assisted Living: The Initial Experience of Cost Reporting in North Carolina.* GSA 1998 Poster Presentation. <qww.geri.duke .edu/ltc/ltc2.html>, November 5, 2000.

Capitman, J. A. 1989. Present and future roles of SSI and Medicaid in funding board and care homes. In M. Moon, G. Gaberlavage, & S. J. Newman (eds.), *Preserving Independence, Supporting Needs: The Role of Board and Care Homes.* Washington, DC: Public Policy Institute, American Association of Retired Persons.

Chen, A. 1989. The cost of operation in board and care homes. In M. Moon, G. Gaberlavage, & S. J. Newman (eds.), *Preserving Independence, Supporting Needs: The Role of Board and Care Homes.* Washington, DC: Public Policy Institute, American Association of Retired Persons.

Croswell, C. L. 1999. Better, not bigger: Construction costs soar on wings of patient demand, construction and design survey finds. *Modern Healthcare* 29 (12): 23–26, 28–34, 36–38.

Hawes, C., Wildfire, J. & Lux, L. 1993. *The Regulation of Board and Care Homes: Results of a Survey in the 50 States and the District of Columbia: National Summary.* Washington, DC: American Association of Retired Persons.

Mollica, R. L. 2000. *State Assisted Living Policy, 2000.* Portland, ME: National Academy for State Health Policy.

Mor, V., Gutkin, C. E., & Sherwood, S. 1985. The cost of residential care homes serving elderly adults. *Journal of Gerontology* 40 (2): 164–71.

Morgan, L. A., Eckert, J. K., & Lyon, S. M. (eds.). 1995. *Small Board-and-Care Homes: Residential Care in Transition.* Baltimore: Johns Hopkins University Press.

National Center for Assisted Living. 1998. *Facts and Trends: The Assisted Living Sourcebook, 1998.* Washington, DC: American Health Care Association.

National Investment Conference for the Senior Living and Long Term Care Industries. 1997. *National Housing Survey of Adults Age 60+:* Opinions, Attitudes, Perceptions, and Behaviors. Annapolis, MD: National Investment Conference for the Senior Living and Long Term Care Industries.

National Journal Group. 1999. Assisted Living: Boom and Bust or Trend of Future? *Healthline*, March 30.

U.S. Congress, General Accounting Office. 1999. *Assisted Living: Quality of Care and Consumer Protection Issues in Four States.* GAO HEHS-99-27. Washington, DC: General Accounting Office.

13 Connectedness in Residential Care
A Qualitative Perspective

J. Kevin Eckert, Ph.D., Sheryl Zimmerman, Ph.D., and Leslie A. Morgan, Ph.D.

This chapter is about the nature of the connections in residential long-term care: connections between residents and staff, residents and residents, residents and the facilities in which they live, and residents and the larger community. Its goal is to view residents as people, living life within the range of residential care/assisted living settings (RC/AL). In lieu of interviewing residents directly about their quality of life or satisfaction, field evaluators who were trained to observe residents in their diverse settings acted as key informants. From their perspective, what emerged as most important while observing residents in situ was the nature and style of their interactions with people and place, a theme referred to as connectedness.

The field evaluators were collecting data for the Collaborative Studies of Long-Term Care (CS-LTC), a four-state study of residential care provided in 193 facilities in Florida, Maryland, New Jersey, and North Carolina. The facilities were stratified to include those with fewer than sixteen beds; those with sixteen or more beds that reflected newer, purpose-built assisted living (new-model); and other facilities with sixteen or more beds (traditional). (See chapter 6 for details of the methods of the CS-LTC.) To further the understanding of life in such facilities, the CS-LTC evaluators were asked to observe and record what was going on around them as they performed their structured observational, evaluative, and interviewing tasks. Since many of the evaluators conducted interviews in more than one state and across a range of RC/AL facilities and nursing homes, they were exposed to various dimensions of life. By virtue of their extensive exposure to facilities, residents, and staff, they constituted an important information resource. Although not key informants in the traditional sense (i.e., they were not members of the group or culture under study), they possessed important information on life within facilities that could not be captured by standard quantitative methods.

Design

The qualities of a good informant include having knowledge of the subject, understanding the information required by the investigator, and being willing and able to communicate. As noted by Bernard (1994), if an investigator is willing to become a "student," a good informant can educate. Moreover, trustworthy informants who are observant, reflective, articulate, and know how to tell a good story are central to qualitative research. CS-LTC evaluators met these and other important criteria: they were trained, observant, articulate, and interested; they conducted interviews across the range of actors in RC/AL facilities and nursing homes (i.e., residents, caregivers, administrators, and families); they were in the facilities on multiple days and at different times of day; they were sensitized to making careful observation of the physical and social environment; and they were eager to tell a story about what they saw and elaborate on their experiences while in the field. As multiple observers with systematic exposure to a wide range of facilities within a concentrated time frame, the evaluators were able to corroborate observations and subjective interpretations, thereby increasing the trustworthiness of their observations.

Evaluator Characteristics

The fourteen field evaluators for the CS-LTC had multiple experiences visiting RC/AL facilities and nursing homes. All of the evaluators had visited at least 50 long-term-care facilities in relationship to this and related studies of long-term care; nine evaluators had visited over 100 facilities. Twelve of the fourteen evaluators were female, thirteen were Caucasian, and one was African American. All of the evaluators had at least some college education. Seven evaluators were trained as nurses. Taken together, the evaluators' extensive field experience and professional training increased the comparative value of their observations.

Data Sources

Questions of validity are often difficult to define in qualitative research because of its nonlinear design and its dependence on the investigator(s) as the central instrument of research. In this study, validity or, more appropriately, the trustworthiness of the data, is enhanced through triangulation of observers and methods (Gilchrist, 1992). First, in many instances more than one evaluator made multiple visits to the same facility. Second, in most cases evaluators spent multiple days within the same facility. Third, multiple methods were used to gather the observations and experiences of the evaluators. Specifically, three types of qualitative data were collected from evaluators: field journals, personal interviews, and structured debriefing sessions.

Field Journals. The evaluators maintained field journals designed to gather and record impressions, reactions, events, and incidents observed in the field. To structure their observations and note-taking, they were asked to comment on six broad features: the physical environment, the staff, the residents, social interactions, the caregiving philosophy, and the community setting. For convenience, preformatted journal pages and three-ring binders were provided. In addition to the six characteristic codes, each page provided space for the interviewer ID, the facility ID, the facility type, the state, and the date and time of the observation.

Personal Interviews with Evaluators. Face-to-face interviews approximately one hour in length were conducted with the evaluators. The interviews were tape recorded and transcribed. Each interview began with the evaluator responding to the general question "What were your most memorable experiences while conducting interviews for this study?" The interviews were reflexive, allowing evaluators to elaborate on their responses, tell stories, and reflect on themes inherent to the overall study, such as the quality of care, social interactions, the community setting, and physical characteristics of the facilities.

Structured Debriefing Sessions. Two debriefing sessions were conducted with the evaluators. After baseline data collection in North Carolina and Florida was completed, a four-hour debriefing session was conducted with seven evaluators, the principal investigators, the project staff, and a consultant. A second two-hour debriefing session with seven evaluators was conducted at the completion of baseline data collection in the remaining two states. In each session, evaluators were encouraged to share experiences, impressions, and stories about what they had observed while in the field. Both sessions were tape recorded and transcribed.

Analysis Plan

The three sources of data were entered into an analytic database for qualitative analysis using Qualitative Solutions and Research's NUD*IST (Non-numerical Unstructured Data Indexing Searching and Theorizing) software (Scolari, 1997). The software facilitates coding data in an index system, searching text or searching patterns of coding, and theorizing about the data. The coding scheme for this analysis was developed through an iterative process that incorporated a priori coding categories reflecting the interest of the investigators as well as categories emerging from the text. The process began by reading the text of the first debriefing session and applying codes for components of the process-and-structure-of-care paradigm that helped focus the CS-LTC (Donabedian, 1966). This activity resulted in twenty-six indexing (or content) codes. The investigators then reread the coded texts, collapsing and combining related and overlapping categories and creating new ones to reflect the content.

The indexing system comprised twenty possible content codes and subcodes that included philosophy of care (subcodes: small RC/AL, large RC/AL, nursing home), dementia care, staff-resident interactions, resident-resident interactions, facility-community integration, resident recruitment, selecting a home, dislocation from family and friends, family involvement concerns, resident-facility congruence, caregiver ethnicity (subcode: religion), quality (subcodes: positive dimensions, negative dimensions), aging in place, and research in RC/AL. The three sources of data were then recoded using the indexing system. As the panel of investigators read and discussed the coded texts, the strength and quantity of the evaluators' comments on residents' interactions with people and place emerged as a central theme. This central theme is referred to as connectedness. Eight of the twenty content codes directly addressed the theme of connectedness: staff-resident interaction, resident-resident interaction, facility-community integration, resident recruitment, dislocation from family and friends, family involvement and concerns, resident-facility congruence, and selecting a home. These eight coding categories associated with connectedness accounted for over one-quarter of the coded texts and ran through each of the three types of data collected. The pervasiveness of the connectedness theme is illustrated in table 13.1.

The Importance of Connectedness

The literature on the quality of life in long-term-care settings has identified the physical environment, the organizational structure (including facility policies, staffing, and financing), recreational activities, and the so-

Table 13.1. Pervasiveness of Connectedness Theme as a Proportion of Total Text Units (%)

Connectedness-Related Codes	Percentage of All Coded Text Units[a]
Staff-resident interaction	8.6%
Resident-resident interaction	4.5
Facility-community integration	2.8
Resident recruitment	1.7
Dislocation from family and friends	0.3
Family involvement and concerns	7.1
Resident-facility congruence	4.4
Selecting a home	1.8

[a]One text unit = one sentence. Field journals, debriefing sessions, and face-to-face interviews contained 8,442 total text units.

cial environment as main factors affecting residents' quality of life (Clark & Bowling, 1990; Cox et al., 1991; Kahana, 1982; Moos, 1980). Although these factors have been shown to be important, several studies indicate that human relationships and social contact with others are more crucial in determining quality of life (Kayser-Jones, 1990; Ross, 1990; Walker & Rosser, 1988). The theme of connectedness illustrates the salience of human relationships and connections as observed by the evaluators in the field.

Connections with Staff

From any perspective (that of regulators, policymakers, administrators, residents, or residents' families), the role of staff, especially direct-care staff, is crucial, not only in meeting residents' physical needs but in meeting their emotional needs as well. Research in a range of care settings considers the quantity and quality of staff-resident interaction as a key element in measuring quality (Moos and Lemke, 1985). Typically, staff-resident interactions are assessed by recording behaviors such as eating together or meeting residents' needs for assistance with functional activities or social and recreational activities. The importance of staff, however, extends beyond tending to residents' physical needs to dealing with their psychological and emotional needs as well. The ability of staff to show empathy, kindness, and affection toward residents is illustrated in evaluators' descriptions of quality:

> For good quality the staff should be attentive both to the physical and emotional needs of residents. Staff need to make time for them. To sit down and talk to them. To sit down and have tea with them. To know when their family hasn't been in to see them and they are upset. This makes it seem like family too. The human part of it is by far most important.

> The main ingredient [of quality] is being concerned about mother as a person. Knowing what she likes and what is good for her and knowing her correct name. I've been in facilities where I've called a family member and referred to Helen and the family member says, "it's Ellen." The family says, "I got this form from the nursing home about your study and they spelled her name wrong. I've told them several times over the past several months that this is my mother's name and they still have it wrong." Personalization is very important.

> I think that quality depends on people being there who really care so it is not like a warehouse situation. One nurse said to me, "my title means nothing, we all work together. I help whenever I can and they help me whenever they can."

Intersecting the central theme of connectedness was facility size. Across the three types of data (personal interviews, field journals, and debriefing sessions) approximately 9 percent of the evaluators' narratives referred to the benefits of small homes compared to 2.5 percent for larger homes. Although the evaluators were aware of the CS-LTC designation of small as fewer than sixteen beds, there is no specific cutoff point for small versus large in evaluators' comments. Smaller homes have been characterized as unique in that they may provide an environment more conducive to the development of close personal relationships, individualized care, or a family-like atmosphere (Sherman & Newman, 1988; Morgan, Eckert & Lyon, 1995). Moreover, Silverstone (1978) suggests that smaller environments can offer relatively permanent primary group relations, wherein needs for individualized attention, including the need for affection, can be met and realized. This relationship is not surprising, because research on the formation and maintenance of successful communities of all types, ones that foster interaction and a sense of belonging, stresses the importance of size. Small groups are thought to possess special qualities, known collectively as the "small group effect," that facilitate high levels of communication, emotional involvement, sharing, and commitment (Olson, 1965). Small facility size seems an important consideration in this dynamic, because although small groups were observed as forming within larger facilities, evaluators spoke of such groups as "cliques" and interpreted their presence negatively, since they included some people and excluded others.

Several studies report on the relationship between facility size and staff-resident interaction. For example, Reschovsky and Ruchlin (1993) found that very small homes (four to six residents) outperformed larger homes with respect to measures of resident and staff interaction, showing an inverse relationship between size of the home and the quality of social interaction. Staff roles have also been found to differ in small and large homes. Although the tenure of home operators was longer in smaller homes, their duties encompassed most of the major activities, such as housekeeping, cooking, medical supervision, and personal care (Morgan, Eckert & Lyon, 1995; Newcomer, Breuer & Zhang, 1993); in larger facilities these roles are parceled out to many people. Evaluators' comments illustrate how they perceived the effect of the size of a facility on the nature and quality of staff-resident interactions. As shown in table 13.2, evaluators contrasted small and large homes along several dimensions.

The home-versus-institution theme linked small size with being like a family and with caregivers having more personal knowledge of residents and deeper personal relationships with them. The following two narratives illustrate these themes.

> In smaller homes, the people always looked like they were in a family. The large homes were institutions. No matter how nice the nurses were, which they were, it was more like "I have a patient, and these are my nurses." The small homes were homier, more like a family.

> My impression is that small facilities have staff who really know the residents. A larger facility with a lot of privacy does not allow for as much staff-resident contact. For example, when interviewing a nurse for the study, she said, "No one reads." I had just interviewed a resident who put down his Eric Segal novel to talk to me.

Table 13.2. Staff-Resident Relations in Small versus Large Facilities

Small Facilities	Large Facilities
Like a home	Like an institution
Part of a family	Residents as isolated individuals
Line between residents and staff blurred	Clear distinction between residents and staff
Simple, easy to understand, quiet	Overwhelming, confusing
Time for the individual	Too busy for the individual
Person-focused	Task-focused

Smaller size fosters primary group relationships in which the line between the resident and staff becomes blurred. Such settings can be characterized by members living in close proximity and being bound together by expressive functions, relatedness, and a long-term commitment (Johnson & Grant, 1985). In the first narrative below, the style of care extended to the resident and the commitment to caring for the resident are similar to what might be expected among close kin. The second narrative illustrates the family-like atmosphere found in some small homes and the attentiveness of the caregiver.

In a Jewish Orthodox home, the operator moved a 90-year-old resident into her side of the house, her personal home. The lady lives in her bedroom. She takes care of her just like she would her mother. She had been taking care of her for ten or eleven years. This was a home with five people, all orthodox Jews. The day that I was there she had nurses coming in since the lady was in her final weeks. She had been caring for this lady in her bedroom for over a year. She sleeps with her at night. She had known her for a long time.

I remember a small independent home with about six or seven residents. What impressed me most about that home was that it was very much a family. The German woman who ran it was in her late sixties or early seventies and was a good cook. She took very good care of her residents and felt that they were very much her family. She had two students living in the basement who helped her out on a voluntary basis when she really needed it. It was like a family because of her attitude toward the residents. She knew them very well; she knew their idiosyncrasies. She was very attentive.

Evaluators perceived that staff-resident interactions and connections were limited in larger facilities by the scale of the environment (e.g., long hallways), too many residents and staff to know personally, and staff turnover. The first narrative that follows addresses the question of scale and also makes a point expressed by several evaluators that medium-size homes may combine the best qualities of both small and large homes.

> In the large homes, there is the problem of people not knowing people and the caregivers changing all the time. The system is overwhelming. You'd go down the hall and residents would ask for help in finding their room. In the medium size homes, about 16 to 25 residents, it seemed like you were getting the best of both worlds. You had more access to activities and larger accommodations, the staffing was more intimate and it was less overwhelming in terms of not knowing anybody or the staff or residents changing.

> I really feel there is a need and desire for small homes among families. This comes from talking to families on the telephone. One woman said to me that her mother was in a large chain home where she had no idea where she was. She took her out of there. She is in a small home, they have seven people, and she absolutely loves it. She doesn't get lost, she knows where her room is, she knows the other people by name, and she can function in this small, confined area where there are routines. There is not as much to wonder about and get lost in.

Connections with Other Residents

Remarkably little has been written about the quality of life in care settings from the point of view of residents (Aller & Van Ess Coeling, 1995; Abt Associates, 1996; Eckert & Morgan, 2001). As a result, little is known about the social and emotional connections between residents living in either nursing homes or RC/AL facilities. This lack of attention among researchers is probably due to the focus on the resident as a patient, or a consumer of services. In one of the few studies in this area, Morgan, Eckert, and Lyon (1995) found that nearly 80 percent of residents in small homes reported very close or somewhat close relationships with other residents.

As the size of the homes increased, the degree of closeness among residents decreased. The board-and-care residents mentioned friendliness, shared background, kindness, helpfulness, trust, and dependability as reasons for their sense of comfort with others living in the homes. Aller and Van Ess Coeling (1995), in a qualitative study, identified three themes that long-term-care residents believe contribute to their quality of life: the ability to communicate with other residents and staff within the facility, the ability to care for oneself, and the ability to care for and help others in more need than themselves. In viewing residents as people living life within in a facility, the evaluators suggest that the connections (or their absence) between residents are an important dimension of quality of life in a home. Three themes emerge related to the connections between residents: the effects of the physical layout and size of the facility, facility policies and practices, and shared interests and backgrounds of residents.

Physical Layout and Size. Not surprisingly, as with resident-staff interaction, facility size was mentioned as a factor affecting the relationships and connections between residents. Evaluators associate the lack of interactions with physical layout as well as with policies that govern what might be termed *institutional* seating arrangements at meals.

> In homes where residents were separated into little apartment units, they were not as interactive. In most places residents eat at least one meal together. In many instances I think people sat where they did because that is where they were put. I can't think of many interactions while people were eating. I think in many cases being in a smaller home caused residents to interact more with each other.

Most field journal entries commenting on resident-to-resident interaction were in reference to smaller homes; 80 percent addressed the positive aspects of such interactions. The following selections give a sense of the connections between residents observed in smaller homes.

Very high levels of resident interaction.

Residents are male and female and interact nicely.

Residents were upbeat and happy, even the one in hospice care. One resident isolated by language was constantly hugged and stroked by others.

The house was very homey. The one male resident seemed very happy and was helping us identify the other residents.

The residents really care about one another. If one needs a napkin or more seasoning for her food they pass it over.

In only a few instances were positive comments made concerning large RC/AL facilities. In a facility in Florida, an evaluator observed that a group of residents got together each morning to have coffee and watch the sun rise, engage in games, and exercise. However, in other instances, a lack of interaction between residents was noted.

The retarded man watched TV all day in his room. Interaction was only from staff to resident and resident to staff. Since the 92-year-old mother was very ill in bed, the others did not interact with each other, that I saw.

Policies and Physical Design. As the comments above indicate, size, physical layout, and seating arrangements at mealtime may influence patterns of interactions between residents. These effects are not deterministic, however; they may be influenced by other factors. Policies, practices, and physical design can attenuate the potentially alienating effects of size or newness to the environment and can facilitate connections between residents and contribute to their quality of life. The following three narratives illustrate how new residents can be integrated into a facility, how flexible physical design can facilitate and maintain connections, and how residents helping other residents can sustain meaning and satisfaction (Aller & Van Ess Coeling, 1995).

When the new resident moves in, the staff arrange to have the new resident matched up with a buddy (resident) who they think will make a compatible companion. The administrator thinks that this has been the best thing they have done. The staff encourages the two people to get together. Moving relatives to a place where they don't know anyone can be a traumatic experience, this can ease the transition to the new place.

The facility had several sets of sisters living next door to each other. Adjoining doors could be left open making them into a two bedroom suite.

There was this one little lady who just wanted to go home. And she wanted to go for a walk and she was going to walk home. Well, the aide took her for a little walk, down the hall. And then the aide had to do something else, so she came back. She wanted someone to walk her down there. One of the other residents, another little old lady, just came along and took her by the hand, held her hand and they walked. They walked down the hall and they came back; she walked that lady for a half-hour. Both of them were just as happy as could be. One was walking and the other one was taking care of her. And I just sat there and cried almost, because it was so . . . But they were taking care of each other.

Shared Characteristics and Background. Evaluators observed the powerful influences of shared religious beliefs and ethnicity in amplifying resident connections and interaction. They also noted that the ethnic background of staff sometimes facilitated interaction, especially among ethnic groups with a "cultural bias" toward the elderly. The first example below illustrates how sharing religious beliefs and experiences transcends the potentially alienating effects of large size and different physical abilities of residents.

One of the most memorable places was a large church home. They really made you feel welcome. They were admitted there because they worked as missionaries for years out in the field. That was one of the requirements for them to be admitted. It was a particular religious group. It was Protestant. You could have worked as a janitor all your life if you were part of the religion. They all had this in common. They were quite friendly with one another. They talked about their experiences all the time. You could go from room to room and hear them conversing about what had happened in the past. I was impressed. They had a lot in common even though they were from different economic brackets. They went from janitor, cook, up to professors. There were more men in this home, which was highly unusual. Some were more able to do things for themselves than were others. Most were pretty able to move around and take care of themselves. They all had private rooms. Three or four of us were there for three or four days. This was a different place.

There were a few homes that were religiously oriented that even brought the people closer together because they all had a common bond. I found that this was the case in both smaller and larger places. In the Jewish homes I visited the people seemed very close.

The following example suggests that ethnicity not only connects people through shared background and history but also can serve to increase sensitivity to the elderly through cultural beliefs that value old age.

In Florida, it was the Filipinos, in Maryland there was a Nepalese-run home. In these homes everyone was interacting with everyone else. This applies to the black run homes too. They were culturally oriented toward older folks. If this wasn't the case, you could walk into a home and everyone would be like robots; meaning the residents didn't really talk to each other. They would roll in and have their breakfast, not talk, then go sit and watch TV, then eat lunch, then take a nap.

Connections to the Facility

Congruence theories or models of person-environment fit have been developed to account for the ways in which variations in environmental features can affect different residents (e.g., Carp & Carp, 1984; Lawton, 1982, 1989; Moos & Lemke, 1985). The importance of matching residents with facilities is acknowledged by administrators, potential residents, and families. The observations of the evaluators illustrate the range of approaches taken by facilities when selecting a resident, the concerns of families and residents in selecting a facility, and the complexity involved in establishing one's life in a new place.

Selecting Residents. Owner-operators in smaller facilities and administrators or admission staff in larger facilities have the difficult task of determining whether a potential resident is a good match with a facility's policies and services. The evaluators noted a range of approaches to selecting residents. For example, some administrators are quite selective in deciding whom to admit. Beyond assessing the match between an individual's needs and the capacity of the staff to meet those needs, some facilities take into consideration how existing residents might react to new residents with certain problems.

The director of assisted living says that even though fifty people are on the waiting list for independent living, the residents there do not want more of what they call "demented residents."

The approach taken by this administrator is supported by empirical research showing that cognitively intact residents do not wish to share living spaces with those suffering from cognitive impairments (Kane et al., 1998; Teresi, Holmes & Monaco, 1993).

The process of selecting new residents can be complex, involving a long screening procedure or a trial period after admission. In one instance, a privately endowed facility required that residents seeking admission be reviewed by its board of directors to determine whether they met criteria established in the late 1800s. In another case, the administrator of a facility commented that if a person did not fit in after thirty days they would ask him or her to move to another facility. These examples suggest that facilities are selecting residents as much as residents are selecting facilities. However, in stark contrast to the complex rules governing the admission of residents in some facilities, an absence of rules is observed in other facilities.

> This facility takes those no one else will admit. Most of them are heavy duty psychiatric patients who had been homeless or on the street prior to moving there.

Selecting a Home. The theme of selecting a home emerged as an important topic, appearing in field journals, interviews with several of the evaluators, and debriefing sessions. The personal meanings and choices associated with moving into RC/AL facilities have received little research attention (Reed, Payton & Bond, 1998). If it is assumed that older people develop and maintain a sense of self through attachment to place, then relocation to a new place is a serious matter. As has been shown to be the case for relocation and institutionalization of the elderly in general (Brand & Smith, 1974), the impact on older persons relocating to residential-care settings may be mediated by their involvement in the relocation decision.

A study conducted by Nolan and associates (1996) showed that family members exercise a great deal of influence on the process of moving into a home, influencing its choice and location and precipitating the move. Another study, conducted by Allen, Hogg, and Peace (1992), found that crises and the urgency of an older person's need often determined the degree of choice that the elder was able to exercise. Central to evaluators' comments was the association of resident satisfaction with who made the choice to move and the immediacy associated with finding the home. On several occasions, evaluators reported that residents talked to them about who made the choice to move into the facility. Residents attributed their satisfaction to having made the choice to live there themselves. For example, one evaluator quotes a resident as stating, "I picked this place myself. I went around and looked at different places. I think that the people who are here of their own choice are happier than the ones whose families put them here."

As other studies note, urgency of need often determines the degree of choice that an older person might exercise in selecting and moving to a care facility. Need generated by a health crisis or cognitive declines places control in the hands of family members. For example, one evaluator noted an administrator commenting that waiting lists are irrelevant since the decision to move into a care facility is always a crisis.

> We don't have a waiting list. When people decide that mother needs a place to go, they take the first place available to them. It's usually an emergency, a crisis situation, so who is going to go on a waiting list?

Evaluators also report that both residents and their families lack information and knowledge essential to selecting a home. Some families may be overly influenced by the promises of marketing and "fancy" decor that overshadow elements of what life might really be like for the older person. One evaluator summarizes her experiences by stating:

> Families and consumers have a difficult time in trying to figure out what would be the best living situation when comparing facilities. Take for example small versus large facilities. They are very different types of environments with both positive and negative qualities. It depends on a person's physical needs and what other kinds of physical activities they expect. If you want lots of things to do, you would not want to go to a small home.

Finding a home can be complicated and unpredictable even when the choice is made by the older person. The following two examples illustrate how an individual's demographic characteristics (e.g., social class) and capacities (e.g., cognitive ability) influence adjustment and fit with other residents.

> One home had about six people who seemed quite content. And then there was one gentleman who had just come there who seemed out of it because he didn't fit in with this other group. The other people were very indigent and he seemed to be more well off, from a different class. It was sad for him that he couldn't communicate with them at all.

The VA suggested that he move to a warmer climate because he had this problem with his body temperature and circulation. So the social worker at the VA hospital placed him in a home in Plant City. He didn't like Plant City because it was too far from everything and he couldn't get around there. So he found a place on his own. He was the only person there not suffering from dementia. He had no socialization, no conversation with anybody except those staff who would give him some time.

Connections to the Community

The process of relocating from independent living to a residential-care setting has received little research attention. Although some studies have examined some aspects of the process, such as who makes the choice, very little attention has been given to the locational aspects of moving (Reed, Payton & Bond, 1998). Several researchers (Rowles, 1981; Wenger, 1990; Cuba & Hummon, 1993) address the important link between the dwelling environment of elderly persons and locality. Rowles (1981), for example, has discussed the notion of the "surveillance zone," the space that people can see from inside their homes. He notes that people attempt to arrange interior space to facilitate a link to others outside the home. On a similar theme, Wenger (1990) discusses the network of neighbors and friends that people build around their homes, a network that provides a sense of support and social identity. In addition, the type of dwelling, the type of neighborhood or community (e.g., rural town, urban ghetto), and the region have been shown to facilitate a sense of belonging and attachment between people and place (Cuba and Hummon, 1993).

The Location as a Facilitator. Corden and Wright (1993) argue that the location of a care home is important because it facilitates the maintenance of previous social networks and participation in valued activities. They also point out that little is known about the locational process of moving into a home and what constraints and opportunities exist. The comments of evaluators illustrate a range of ways that facility, staff, and resident connections with local communities might relate to quality of life. A shared history and identity with the local setting that preceded "resident" or "patient" status was observed as contributing to an ideal situation.

The residents grew up there. You'd ask them if family lived within an hour and they would tell you that everybody lives nearby. They would even say that their girlfriend lives there on the next hall. It seemed like such an ideal situation.

The home was in a small neighborhood sort of stuck in the city. The people living around it were neighbors. The operator had people living there that she grew up with. At lunch I sat on the porch and talked to one of them. She sat with me and she was quite happy to be there. Her sisters came, her neighbors came. They all went to the local church, that kind of thing.

What I mean by more personal care is that there is not as much turnover in staff because they are hiring local people. They seem to be a part of the community. Many of them have known these people since they were young children. This is especially so in the smaller towns and communities. It's an extension of the family.

Several evaluators commented on the dislocation from family, friends, and community caused by moving to another state to retire. Further differences are noted between rural and urban areas and connections with community.

I noted that few people living in urban facilities were actually from Florida and many were without family contacts. In the suburban and rural areas more of the residents had actually been born and raised there. They live in the home that was closest to where they were born, raised, lived, and worked.

Integrating into the Community. Both small and large homes achieve integration into their communities through planned activities between residents of the home and community groups. Regular church services involving residents of the facility and the community were held in some homes. In another setting, children from an organized day care program were brought to the facility to play on equipment installed specifically for that purpose. The following example illustrates how a large RC/AL facility connected with the local community.

The activities director told us about a relationship she developed with the Naval Academy midshipmen. She organized a prom-like party between the residents and midshipmen. The residents spent all day getting ready while the activity director's husband played old music for two hours before the midshipmen arrived, dressed in their uniforms. The residents were transformed to an earlier time. The dementia residents saw in the midshipmen their husbands and brothers. They became animated, got up and danced when they had previously been wheelchair fast. The change in the residents was unbelievable, they were so alive, flirting, and smiling.

Conclusion and Implications

Human beings are embedded in a web of social relationships, life experiences, and systems of personal meanings. These elements of personal identity and personhood are thought to underlie resident satisfaction and the quality of lived experience in long-term-care settings. Rubinstein (2000) argues strongly for a "person-centered" view of quality of life or of satisfaction, in which the constructs are embedded in cultural and ideological contexts linked to the person. From a qualitative perspective, the theme of connectedness, as discovered and reported by evaluators, begins to illustrate the nature and diversity of connections between residents, their care providers, and the places and locations where they live.

Connections between residents and their care providers are important to all people concerned with long-term care. Unlike the medical domains of hospitals and nursing homes, where people are admitted as patients and approached as patients, people moving to RC/AL seek nonmedical assistance in a setting more akin to home than institution. Within this context, the observations and comments of the evaluators reinforce the importance of staff's viewing residents as people rather than patients. Regardless of facility size, every effort should be made to facilitate primary relationships in which psychological and emotional needs are met and personal biography and identity supported. Although establishing close ties between residents and staff may be easier in smaller facilities, such ties can be fostered in large facilities with committed caregiving staff and supportive administrators.

There is a need to look more closely at the nature of connections from the residents' point of view. Little is known about the social and emotional connections between residents living in RC/AL settings. Qualitative studies suggest that quality of life is enhanced by close connections among residents, especially when instrumental assistance is provided, such as assistance with walking. Personal connections and exchanges of assistance can be facilitated by physical design and policies that counteract institutional features associated with hotel-like living quarters and dining arrangements. Moreover, as with life in general, shared characteristics and interests associated with common ethnicity or religious beliefs can facilitate a sense of belonging, identity, and community. Further research is needed to examine the extent to which moving into a RC/AL setting is an extension of a person's previous life rather than a departure from it. For example, does choosing a home that one "knows" contribute to satisfaction and quality of life? In what ways does shared or common locality among residents and staff create familiarity and social relations? To what extent do these connections with place and locality tangibly influence the lives of residents? And finally, in what ways can new, purpose-built assisted living facilities be integrated into local communities? The narratives provided by evaluators suggest that integration with locality exists among many established facilities and is attainable among new ones through conscious outreach efforts.

Perhaps the most striking feature of RC/AL is its diversity. A remarkably wide range of settings exist under this rubric. Settings vary in size; ownership; profit or not-for-profit status; religious or nonreligious affiliation; and urban, suburban, or rural location, to mention but a few. From the evaluators' viewpoint, diversity within RC/AL is one of its strengths, since, in its current state, it enlarges the potential of linking person (in terms of prior life circumstances, history, and preferences) with place. In this regard, until there are data to the contrary, every effort should be made to resist rules and regulations that homogenize RC/AL through a "one size fits all" formula.

References

Abt Associates. 1996. *Evaluation of the LTC Survey Process.* Report to the Health Care Financing Administration. Cambridge, MA: Abt Associates.

Allen, I., Hogg, D., & Peace, S. 1992. *Elderly People: Choice, Participation, and Satisfaction.* London: Policy Studies Institute.

Aller, L. J., & Van Ess Coeling, H. 1995. Quality of life: Its meaning to the long-term care resident. *Journal of Gerontological Nursing* 21:20–25.

Bernard, H. R. 1994. *Research Methods in Anthropology: Qualitative and Quantitative Approaches.* 2d ed. Thousand Oaks, CA: Sage.

Brand, F., & Smith, R. 1974. Life adjustment and relocation of the elderly. *Journal of Gerontology* 29:336–40.

Carp, F. M., & Carp, A. 1984. A complementary/congruence model of well-being or mental health for community elderly. In I. Altman, M. P. Lawton, & J. F. Wohlwill (eds.), *Elderly People and the Environment.* New York: Plenum.

Clark, P., & Bowling, A. 1990. Quality of everyday life in long stay institutions for the elderly: An observational study of long stay hospital and nursing home care. *Social Science and Medicine* 30:1201–10.

Cohn, J., & Sugar, J. A. 1991. Determinants of quality of life in institutions: Perceptions of frail older residents, staff, and families. In J. Birren, J. Luben, J. Rowe, & D. Deutchman (eds.), *The Concept and Measurement of Quality of Life in the Frail Elderly.* San Diego: Academic Press.

Corden, A., & Wright, K. 1993. Going into a home: Where can an elderly person choose? In T. Champion (ed.), *Population Matters.* London: Paul Chapman Publishing.

Cox, C., Kaeser, L., Montgomery, A., & Marion, I. 1991. Quality of life nursing care: An experimental trial in long-term care. *Journal of Gerontological Nursing* 17:6–11.

Cuba, L., & Hummon, D. M. 1993. A place to call home: Identification with dwelling, community, and region. *Sociological Quarterly* 34 (1): 11–31.

Donabedian, A. 1966. Evaluating the quality of medical care. *Milbank Memorial Fund Quarterly* 44:166–206.

Eckert, J. K., & Morgan, L. A. 2001. Quality in small residential care settings. In L. Noelker & Z. Harel (eds.), *Quality Long Term Care: Impact on Quality of Life.* New York: Springer.

Gilchrist, V. J. 1992. Key informant interviews. In B. F. Crabtree & W. L. Miller (eds.), *Doing Qualitative Research.* Research for Qualitative Methods for Primary Care, vol. 3. New York: Sage.

Johnson, C. L., & Grant, L. A. 1985. *The Nursing Home in American Society.* Baltimore: Johns Hopkins University Press.

Kahana, E. 1982. A congruence model of person-environment interaction. In M. P. Lawton, P. G. Windley, & T. O. Byerts (eds.), *Aging and the Environment: Theoretical Approaches.* New York: Springer.

Kane, R., Baker, M., Salmon, J., and Veazie, W. 1998. *Consumer Perspectives on Private versus Shared Accommodations in Assisted Living Settings.* Washington, DC: Public Policy Institute, American Association of Retired Persons.

Kayser-Jones, J. 1990. The environment and quality of life in long-term care institutions. *Nursing and Health Care* 10:121–30.

Lawton, M. P. 1982. Competence, environmental press, and the adaptation of older people. In M. P. Lawton, P. G. Windley, & T. O. Byerts (eds.), *Aging and the Environment: Theoretical Approaches.* New York: Springer.

————. 1989. Behavior-relevant ecological factors. In K. W. Schaie & C. Schoder (eds.), *Social Structure and Aging: Psychological Processes.* Hillsdale, NJ: Lawrence Erlbaum.

Moos, R. H. 1980. Specialized living environments for older people: A conceptual framework for evaluation. *Journal of Social Issues* 36 (2): 75–94.

Moos, R. H., & Lemke, S. 1985. Specialized living environments for older people. In J. E. Birren & K. W. Schaie (eds.), *Handbook of the Psychology of Aging*, 2d ed. New York: Van Nostrand Reinhold.

Morgan, L. A., Eckert, J. K., & Lyon, S. M. (eds.). 1995. *Small Board-and-Care Homes: Residential Care in Transition.* Baltimore: Johns Hopkins University Press.

Newcomer, R., Breuer, W., & Zhang, X. 1993. *Residents and the Appropriateness of Placement in Residential Care for the Elderly.* San Francisco: Institute for Health and Aging, University of California.

Nolan, M., Walker, G., Nolan, J., Williams, S., Poland, F., Curran, M., & Kent, B. C. 1996. Entry to care: Positive choice or *fait accompli*? Developing a more proactive nursing response to the needs of older people and their carers. *Journal of Advanced Nursing* 24 (2): 265–74.

Olson, M. 1965. *The Logic of Collective Action.* Cambridge: Harvard University Press.

Patrick, D. L., & Erickson, P. 1988. Assessing health-related quality in life for clinical decision making. In S. R. Walker and R. M. Rosser (eds.), *Quality of Life: Assessment and Application.* Lancaster, Eng.: MPT Press.

Reed, J., Payton, V. R., & Bond, S. 1998. The importance of place for older people moving into care homes. *Social Science and Nursing* 46 (7): 859- 67.

Reschovsky, J. D., & Ruchlin, H. S. 1993. Quality of board care homes serving low-income elderly: Structural and public policy correlates. *Journal of Applied Gerontology* 2:224–45.

Ross, M. 1990. Time-use in later life. *Journal of Advanced Nursing* 15:394–99.

Rowles, G. D. 1981. The surveillance zone as meaningful space to the aged. *Gerontologist* 21 (3): 304–11.

Rubinstein, R. L. 2000. Resident satisfaction, quality of life, and "lived experience" as domains to be assessed in long-term care. In J. Cohen-Mansfield (ed.), *Consumer Satisfaction in the Nursing Home.* New York: Springer.

Scolari, Sage Publications Software. 1997. *Qualitative Solutions and Research* (QSR NUD*IST). Thousand Oaks, CA: Sage.

Sherman, S. R., & Newman, E. S. 1988. *Foster Families for Adults: A Community Alternative in Long-Term Care.* New York: Columbia University Press.

Silverstone, B. 1978. The social, physical, and legal implications for adult foster care: A contrast with other models. In N. K. Haygood & R. E. Dunkle (eds.), *Perspective on Adult Foster Care*. Cleveland: Case Western Reserve University.

Teresi, J. A., Holmes, D., & Monaco, C. 1993. An evaluation of the effects of commingling cognitively and noncognitively impaired individuals in long-term care facilities. *Gerontologist* 33 (3): 350–58.

Wenger, G. C. 1990. The special role of friends and neighbors. *Journal of Aging Studies* 4 (2): 149–69.

III Future Directions in Assisted Living

14 Emerging Issues in Residential Care/ Assisted Living

Sheryl Zimmerman, Ph.D., Philip D. Sloane, M.D., M.P.H., and J. Kevin Eckert, Ph.D.

Many issues related to residential care/assisted living (RC/AL) have been raised throughout this book. This chapter compiles, summarizes, and expounds on some of the cross-cutting and pressing themes. The topics are not comprehensive and may not represent the most pressing concerns of all individuals, providers, or states. Nonetheless, these issues are highly pertinent for long-term care across the nation and do reflect the current state and future direction of RC/AL. When appropriate, reference is made to an earlier chapter or to data from the Collaborative Studies of Long-Term Care (CS-LTC, the four-state study of RC/AL on which part 2 of this book is based).

Definition of Assisted Living

The precise number of assisting living facilities and residents is uncertain because there is no uniformly accepted definition of assisted living nor any systematic way to count these facilities. In this book we chose to use the term *RC/AL* to reflect the fact that although the *assisted living* label is increasing in popularity, it alternately refers to a general social model of non-nursing-home residential care and to a very specific model of care that espouses specific philosophies (see chapter 1).

Broadly defined, *assisted living* is synonymous with *residential care;* it includes all settings for persons who can no longer live independently, who require assistance with activities of daily living (ADLs) but not the level of skilled nursing care provided in a nursing home. Within this broad definition, the actual use of the term *assisted living* varies widely in reference to state regulations and models of care. Depending on the state regulatory environment, assisted living includes options ranging from small, freestanding residential homes to single apartments within continuing-care retirement communities. Further variations emerge as states use

Medicaid Home and Community-Based Waivers and state sources of funding to explore whether assisted living can be a cost-effective alternative to nursing home care for some residents. Decentralized and state-driven, assisted living has no uniform model or organizational type within this broad definition.

Alternatively, assisted living can be conceptualized as a residential model with a clear philosophy that differentiates it from board and care and other residential care. Characteristics of assisted living that distinguish it from board and care include statements of philosophy emphasizing privacy, independence, decision making, and autonomy; an emphasis on apartment settings shared by resident choice; and provision or arrangement of nursing or other health-related services that allow facilities to admit or retain residents with specific needs. Complicating the matter of definition is that the term *assisted living* is used by facilities that do not necessarily subscribe to the philosophy, and it is not always used by facilities that do. In a recent national study of assisted living facilities, 28 percent did not identify themselves as assisted living facilities, even though in size, services, staffing, admission and discharge criteria, and resident characteristics they were similar to those that did use the term (Hawes, Rose & Phillips, 1999). Similarly, the data presented in this book from the CS-LTC (especially findings related to structure, process, and dementia care, in chapters 8, 9 and 11) demonstrate marked similarities and differences across settings.

In many states, considerable overlap exists between board-and-care and assisted living rules, and the terms may be used interchangeably. In some other states, assisted living is a distinct category with guidelines and regulations that distinguish it from other forms of supportive housing. Thus, assisted living has multiple meanings often reflecting different perspectives and approaches to regulation across states. Mollica notes that defining assisted living and differentiating it from other forms of residential care may be growing more difficult as state policymakers, regulators, and providers respond to the interests of local stakeholders. Given varying disabilities among their clientele and the fact that localities must be responsive to the needs of their population, a common definition of assisted living may not be feasible (Mollica, 1998) or necessarily desirable.

The Role of RC/AL in the Long-Term-Care System

Though the exact definition of *assisted living* is unclear, the types of residents who are served in these settings are very clear. The population served by RC/AL settings two decades ago was vastly different from that served today, and changes of a similar magnitude are likely to occur over the coming decades. In the ten years between 1983 and 1993, for example, residents became increasingly aged (64% in 1993 vs. 38% in 1983 were 75 and older), cognitively impaired (40% vs. 30%), incontinent (23% vs. 7%), and wheelchair dependent (15% vs. 3%); in addition a greater percentage required assistance with bathing (45% vs. 27%) and taking medications (75% vs. 43%) (Hawes et al., 1995). Assuming that no reports are forthcoming that put into question the ability of RC/AL settings to care for these persons, the percentage with these impairments can be expected to increase.

A central issue in RC/AL is its role in the long-term-care system. There are two differing perspectives on the role of RC/AL: the first is that it lies along the continuum from home care to nursing home care; the second is that it constitutes an approach and philosophy that can apply to all persons, regardless of their level-of-care need (Lewin-VHI, 1996). In some cases, RC/AL facilities provide care to residents who meet the level-of-care criteria for nursing homes (US GAO, 1999). There is some dynamic tension between RC/AL and the nursing home industry, with RC/AL facilities being increasingly viewed as competing with nursing homes for many of the same individuals. Furthermore, although reliable data on the subject are not plentiful, the notion is increasingly popular that RC/AL facilities may be able to serve certain individuals at a lower cost than do nursing homes. Less tension exists between the home health care industry and RC/AL, in part because the two services have had a fruitful symbiotic relationship. Nevertheless, the three big players in long-term care—home care, RC/AL, and nursing homes—all are in a dynamic state, with the populations served and services provided experiencing rapid change and variation across states and over time.

Relationship to Nursing Home Care

Data from the CS-LTC verify that RC/AL facilities serve a population that overlaps considerably with that of nursing homes. There is a tendency for the average resident of RC/AL facilities to be more independent and for nursing homes to serve a higher proportion of persons with impairment in multiple ADLs; however, both settings serve large proportions of persons with moderate cognitive and ADL impairment (see chapter 7). Thus, it is possible that RC/AL and nursing homes are indeed vying for the same prospective residents.

Furthermore, the CS-LTC data demonstrate that the RC/AL industry provides a diversity of distinct alternatives to nursing homes. All three types of RC/AL facilities in the CS-LTC exhibited certain distinct structural differences compared to nursing homes, two examples being facility size (table 6.4) and the proportion of private rooms (table 8.4). More striking, however, was the tremendous diversity across RC/AL facility types, such as in reference to owner involvement in the facility (8%–61%; see table 12.3) and the proportion of rooms with individualized heating controls (13%–82%; see table 8.4). Similar findings were noted regarding the process of care. Some features of RC/AL were consistently different from nursing homes, such as ADL admission policies and provision of selected formal activities (tables 9.5 and 9.10–9.12). Nevertheless, the differences across RC/AL facility types were often more striking than those between RC/AL and nursing homes, such as in relation to policy choice, clarity, and privacy (fig. 9.1).

Currently, several trends appear to be evident that distinguish RC/AL from nursing homes. RC/AL facilities are growing more rapidly than nursing homes. Many RC/AL facilities serve exclusively affluent individuals who pay privately, whereas most nursing homes have a mixture of individuals at different income levels. State Medicaid programs are beginning to make overtures to RC/AL homes, but Medicaid remains a major source of funding for nursing homes and a minor source of funding for RC/AL. The future role of RC/AL vis-à-vis nursing homes will hinge on the degree to which Medicaid programs choose to pay for RC/AL as an alternative to nursing homes and the extent to which research demonstrates differences in outcomes between the two settings.

Dementia Care

Two striking findings emerge from the CS-LTC data regarding the prevalence of dementia in RC/AL facilities. The first is that dementia is widely prevalent in these homes (table 11.2). The second is that the physically dependent population served in RC/AL facilities largely consists of individuals with dementia. As is indicated by table 7.5, between 6 and 11 percent of the residents in any type of CS-LTC facilities were both cognitively intact and dependent in three or more ADLs. In contrast, 9–11 percent of residents were cognitively impaired and dependent in three or more ADLs. Thus, "high acuity" care in RC/AL facilities is largely dementia care.

Data from the CS-LTC also indicate that RC/AL facilities offer a range of options for persons with dementia. Small homes tended to be more orienting and more homelike, whereas new-model homes tended to provide greater stimulation, better exit control, and more specialized units (see chapter 11). Process measures varied widely as well, but in general the data suggest that problems observed in nursing homes—such as high levels of psychotropic drug use and low resident participation in activities— are also present in RC/AL.

Some policymakers suggest that RC/AL facilities can provide equivalent or better care for dementia at a lower cost than nursing homes. Although there is preliminary support for this claim (Leon & Moyer, 1999), neither longitudinal outcome studies nor well-conducted cost analyses have been completed to verify it. Nevertheless, the future of RC/AL increasingly involves dementia care, and the needs of these persons should be acknowledged in facility design, staffing, program development, evaluation, and regulation.

Access and Availability

Income and Payment Source

Given the current status of Medicaid and Medicare reimbursement (see chapters 1 and 2), access and availability of RC/AL to economically disadvantaged and minority elderly persons is an important issue. Data from the CS-LTC suggest that access by economic status and race is different between RC/AL facilities and nursing homes and that it also differs by RC/AL facility type. It is important to learn whether and to what extent RC/AL constitutes a segregated system of care.

Recent growth in the RC/AL industry in the United States has been primarily aimed at well-to-do seniors (Meyer, 1998). Thus, it is not surprising that the new-model homes reported the lowest proportion of their revenues from public sources (13%), compared to other CS-LTC facility types (table 12.4). Somewhat surprising, however, is the fact that the proportion of public funding reported by older, large homes was not very different (19%). In contrast, small homes appeared to be more accessible for persons of low income; 33 percent of their revenues were reported to be from public sources. Even this rate, however, is considerably reduced in RC/AL compared to the same statistic for nursing homes: a recent report states that 68 percent of nursing home residents are on Medicaid (Kraus & Altman, 1998).

The current trend is for long-term care in the United States to be increasingly segregated by payment status, with nursing homes primarily serving a Medicaid clientele and RC/AL facilities serving those who can pay privately. This distinction is in contrast to northern European models, which have emphasized serving the broad range of community through the generous use of public revenues (see chapter 3). In this country such a solution appears quite unlikely, but a variety of states are experimenting with making Medicaid funds more available for persons in RC/AL. Most prominent among the states providing Medicaid support for persons in RC/AL is Oregon; however, other states have not been quick to follow suit. Most likely their reticence is due in part to states' concern that adding a new service area will strain their already-tight Medicaid budgets. Nonetheless, offering RC/AL to persons who cannot afford to pay is an important policy issue, because developing or maintaining a two-tiered system of long-term care is not a desired outcome. If the goal is to better serve all individuals, attempts to identify models of effective low-cost care should be continued, and states should be supported in their attempts to shift resources to a blend of service models.

Race and Ethnicity

Patterns of race and ethnicity in RC/AL facilities in the CS-LTC appear to parallel those of income. Thus, new-model homes served the fewest nonwhites (5%), traditional homes slightly more (8%), and small homes the most (15%) (table 7.1). Comparable resident-level data were not available on the proportion of nursing home residents in the four CS-LTC states; however, based on facility-level estimates from the operators of the CS-LTC nursing homes, that figure is estimated to be 25 percent. Thus, nursing homes appear to house significantly higher proportions of nonwhites (African Americans and others) than do RC/AL facilities. Within RC/AL, the fact that small homes served larger proportions of ethnic minorities may be an issue of economics—small homes have lower revenues (table 12.4). Other factors may also be operative. Small homes may be more able to serve distinct racial or ethnic subpopulations, such as African Americans, Hispanics, or certain religious groups because they can accommodate the primary culture. In addition, smaller homes may on average draw their residents from within a smaller radius; if this was the case, they would be more likely to reflect the neighborhood composition. Mutran and coauthors (chapter 5) found that ethnically segregated facilities exist, and Eckert, Zimmerman, and Morgan (chapter 13) found that shared religious and ethnic beliefs may support segregation. Certainly, better understanding of the degree and nature of segregation that exists in RC/AL will be important as the industry matures. If ethnic minorities are underserved, efforts to correct this deficiency should not merely foster integration; they should foster ethnic-sensitive models of care.

The Development of Knowledge

A survey of consumer preferences, concerns, and needs (Wilson, 1996) found that older people overwhelmingly prefer staying in their own homes, but if forced to move, 69 percent would rather move to a long-term-care facility than live in the home of relatives or friends. Among care facilities, older people greatly preferred small homes that provide care to a few people or apartment buildings that provide care services over moving into a nursing home. Thus, the report reaffirms consumers' interests in non-nursing-home RC/AL. As an increasing elderly population and consumer demand drive the growth of RC/AL, more and better information will be required with which consumers can make choices comparing different services, costs, and policies. Unfortunately, marketing material, admission contracts, and other facility information are often incomplete and sometimes vague or misleading; specific concern has been noted in reference to descriptions of the degree to which a particular facility can meet resident needs, for how long, and under what circumstances (US GAO, 1999). Consumers cannot make informed choices without full and complete disclosure, but there is no central source of information for RC/AL facilities. Though numerous checklists are available to help consumers learn which questions to ask, they may not know the most important questions to ask. For example, does staff experience matter more than facility service provision? The correct answer to this and other questions relates to personal preferences as well as to what constitutes quality care.

Information is needed for the growth and improvement of the RC/AL field, as well. For example, little is known about racial differences in the use and quality of RC/AL (see chapter 5). Also, recruiting and maintaining a sufficient and competent staff presents significant challenges; solutions to this crisis have been proposed, but their success has not been determined (see chapter 4). In another area, individual, facility, and community factors that are associated with aging in place have yet to be examined longitudinally, to determine whether and under what circumstances RC/AL facilities are able to provide care as resident needs increase (see chapter 10). Thus, the quantity and quality of information on RC/AL, though growing, is not keeping pace with the rapid expansion of the industry.

Regulation

A very important context in which the supply of knowledge is lagging is regulation of the industry. As the level of disability in RC/AL facilities has increased, so has the degree of regulatory oversight. Multiple influences have driven the expansion of regulation: the rapid growth of RC/AL, rising federal expenditures for disabled elderly persons in all settings, concerns about the limited governmental role in monitoring the quality of residential services, the emphasis on strengthening federal oversight of nursing home quality (which highlighted the lack of systematic information about RC/AL), and reports that residents were not receiving adequate care or protection from risks (US GAO, 1989, 1992a, 1992b; Hawes, Wildfire & Lux, 1993). As noted in chapter 1, as of 2000, twenty-nine states had RC/AL regulations and an additional twelve were drafting or revising assisted living or general board-and-care regulations (Mollica, 2000). Though not every state uses the term *RC/AL* or regulates RC/AL, virtually every state does regulate senior housing that has a service component (Murer, 1997).

The Scope and Impact of Regulation

Regulations set parameters for what is possible. They focus on requirements for the living unit, admission and retention standards, the level of services, administrator credentials, and staff training (Mollica, 1998). In general, the level of allowable service is increasing as policymakers recognize the higher level of care required as residents age in place and facilities strive to maintain occupancy rates. There is controversy as to the appropriate scope and content of RC/AL, however, and the extent to which RC/AL should be regulated. One point of view is that vulnerable residents require protection, limits should be placed on the level of frailty that can be served, and minimum standards must be established (Manard et al., 1992; Olson, 1994; Wilson, 1996; ALQC, 1998). Proponents of another perspective counter that regulations can subvert facility innovation and flexibility, impede resident autonomy and the ability to age in place, restrict the consumer-oriented focus of RC/AL, and result in a slide from homelike, efficient care to ponderous, expensive replicas of the nursing home (Buckwalter, Leibrock & Klein, 1996; Murer, 1997; Mollica, 1998). Chapter 3 presents an especially strong challenge to the benefits of regulation, by noting that it narrows flexibility, limits experimentation, and discourages creative approaches to care management. Furthermore, there is concern that regulations will tax the resources of small RC/AL facilities, resulting in their closure, and that the success of facilities therefore will be determined not by the quality of care but by regulatory and market pressures. As noted in chapter 7, small facilities serve a needy segment of the elderly population, and jeopardizing the future of these facilities is a cause for concern.

Related to these opposing viewpoints are indeterminate findings on the effects of regulation. Extensive regulation has been related to less use of psychotropic drugs and medications contraindicated for the elderly, more staff training, and greater availability of social aids and supportive devices. It has not been related to training requirements, the availability of licensed nurses, staff knowledge, facility cleanliness, prevalence of physical amenities, institutionalization of the environment, or satisfaction (Segal & Hwang, 1994; Hawes et al., 1995; Wildfire et al., 1997). If one were to draw from the CS-LTC data, it would appear that some regulatory efforts have achieved their aims; chapter 8 illustrates that nursing homes, long under federal regulation, are consistently superior to RC/AL in terms of safety, security, and the physical environment.

Negotiated Risk versus Consumer Protection

The concern over regulating RC/AL centers on how to impose regulations without unraveling the very fabric of the industry. RC/AL emphasizes self-governance; protection of resident rights, including the rights to make decisions about care and to take responsibility for risks that may result from those decisions; and the exercise of autonomy within the parameters of service provision. Chapter 1 introduced the concept of negotiated risk, the idea that residents have the right to make lifestyle decisions that may place them at risk of injury, for which providers might be held liable. The negotiated-risk process is one wherein preferences and assignment of liability are documented. Though it seems consistent with the mission of RC/AL, there is nonetheless concern that this concept could be abused because of the unequal bargaining positions of resident and provider and that it may be used to excuse providers from negligence (Wilson, 1996). It is not an easy matter to predict or define the risks associated with an activity, and it is even more difficult to create and adapt regulations that allow for risk and waive liability on an individual basis.

Accreditation

Related to regulation is accreditation, which is especially notable in that recent proposals have implications for staffing. The status of and perspectives related to solving the staffing crisis are addressed in chapter 4. Progress in this area will undoubtedly be emerging through the next decade. In spring 2000, both the Joint Commission for the Accreditation of Healthcare Organizations (JCAHO) and the Rehabilitation Accreditation Commission (CARF) finalized standards for accreditation of RC/AL facilities. JCAHO's standards on staffing are fairly general, requiring that staff be selected in a consistent and nondiscriminatory manner and that staff qualifications be appropriate for the level of resident need in the facility; ongoing training is also required. CARF's standards are only slightly more specific, requiring orientations and criminal background checks for all staff in addition to sufficient staffing levels and ongoing training. It remains to be seen how many RC/AL facilities will opt for accreditation and what effect the accreditation standards will have on care.

Quality

Although diversity is one of the characteristics of RC/AL—signaling an acute need for a careful and data-rich approach to regulation—and although the industry is already becoming increasingly regulated, there are few empirical data to guide the content of the emerging regulations. Consequently, there is concern that regulations are prematurely restricting residential options. Indeed, in regard to resident outcomes, many of the present regulatory structures do not appear to assure or promote quality and do not define the criteria to evaluate when RC/AL fails to meet residents' needs (Olson, 1994; ALQC, 1998; Meyer, 1998). The optimal approach would be to regulate select aspects of the structure and process of care that relate most strongly to resident outcomes.

Unfortunately, there are few comparative outcome data in this area, and even less is known regarding the relationship of the structure and process of care to resident quality of life. Nowhere in the evolution of the RC/AL movement has there been either a premeditated evaluative consideration of the cost-effectiveness and quality of care or an empirical evaluation of resident quality of life. It is only now, after RC/AL has taken form, that industry leaders are attending to internal quality evaluation and improvement and proposing rewards for high-quality outcomes (ALQC, 1998). Indeed, considering that the most recent U.S. General Accounting Office report (1999) found problems related to incorrect, incomplete, and misleading information provision; inadequate care; insufficient staffing; and medication errors, such oversight is warranted.

One deficit in this area is that most of the existing research has addressed the interests of regulatory bodies and policymakers. An understanding of quality of care and quality of life from the perspective of residents and their families is sorely lacking, and information is needed regarding consumer satisfaction. These measures of quality should be incorporated into RC/AL settings and could form the basis for consumer report cards and performance feedback systems.

Other deficits in knowledge relate to study design. Often, investigators have not studied outcomes directly; instead, they have examined relationships between structure and process and *assumed* that homes with certain features provide better care and better outcomes. Another difficulty with quality assessments in RC/AL is that the examinations to date have been cross-sectional in design, estimating quality by examining associations between resident well-being (or unmet need) and care provision. Data gathered in this manner suggest that less than one-half of residents have all needs met through RC/AL (Mor, Sherwood & Gutkin, 1986), that larger facilities and process components of care are related to well-being (Weihl, 1981; Namazi et al., 1989; Timko & Moos, 1989), and that cost savings can be achieved by substituting RC/AL for nursing home care (Leon & Moyer, 1999). These studies are limited in that the relationship of need to service provision and outcomes is undetermined, resident report tends to exclude those who are too cognitively impaired to respond for themselves (perhaps the most vulnerable segment of the population), samples are not random, the accuracy of respondent recall is uncertain, and cost data frequently are incomplete (e.g., omitting add-ons or home health care) or inadequately adjusted for differences in resident morbidity.

Because RC/AL is a new field of investigation, there are more questions than answers, and matters of definition are complex. For example, some components of RC/AL care, such as homelikeness, are not easy to define and measure: homelikeness means different things to different people, and its relative importance likely differs among residents. Also, though quality is determined with reference to outcomes, any one outcome may have multiple causes (for example, a fracture outcome may relate to resident status and environmental hazards, among other things), and what constitutes quality may differ depending on the outcome. For example, homelikeness may increase autonomy at the same time that it decreases safety and increases injury. Thus, the policy question arises: what matters more, autonomy or safety? This determination will differ across residents, and it also will differ within individuals over time, as they change and their health and functional status worsen and their needs for assistance increase (Zimmerman et al., 1997). Finally, it is worth noting that the provision of quality care assumes the existence of quality staff to provide such care; many providers and regulators are concerned that quality will suffer until progress is made in addressing the staffing crisis.

Conclusion

Residential care and assisted living are overlapping settings that are growing rapidly and have an indisputable but somewhat unclear position in the future of long-term care. Among the most pressing and controversial issues in this area are (1) the definition of assisted living and its relation to other forms of residential care, (2) the role of RC/AL vis-à-vis nursing homes, (3) the current lack of access for persons of low income, (4) questions about access and quality for minorities, (5) how, for whom, and toward what outcomes RC/AL facilities should provide dementia care, (6) the definition and measurement of quality of care, (7) the need for a qualified and stable workforce, (8) the role, scope, and impact of regulation, and (9) the degree to which principles such as autonomy and negotiated risk can be accommodated in the face of increasing regulation.

Despite the uncertainties underlying the future of RC/AL, there is no doubt that this form of long-term care will continue to grow and flourish. The challenges are many, but the impending boom in this nation's elderly population underscores the importance of shaping the growth of this industry. Improvements in the field will require the contributions of creative providers, sensitive regulators, and dedicated researchers. Comparisons across types of care settings (such as those explored in this book), examination of international models, and a focus on resident outcomes will be crucial. Hopefully, the future of RC/AL will be guided in a manner that provides equal access to high-quality care for all elderly persons and that spearheads improvements in the quality of residential care for all disabled persons.

References

Assisted Living Quality Coalition. 1998. *Assisted Living Quality Initiative: Building a Structure That Promotes Quality.* Washington, DC: Assisted Living Quality Coalition.

Buckwalter, K., Leibrock, C., & Klein, P. 1996. Residential care for persons with dementia: Are codes and regulations protective or counter-productive? *Journal of Gerontological Nursing* 22:43–47.

Hawes, C., Mor, V., Wildfire, J., Lux, L., Green, R., Iannacchione, V., & Phillips, C. D. 1995. *Executive Summary: Analysis of the Effects of Regulation on the Quality of Care in Board and Care Homes.* Research Triangle Park, NC: Research Triangle Institute.

Hawes, C., Rose, M., & Phillips, C. D. 1999. *A National Study of Assisted Living for the Frail Elderly: Executive Summary: Results of a National Survey of Facilities.* Beachwood, OH: Meyers Research Institute.

Hawes, C., Wildfire, J. B., & Lux, L. J. 1993. *The Regulation of Board and Care Homes: Results of a Survey in the 50 States and the District of Columbia: National Summary.* Washington, DC: American Association of Retired Persons.

Krauss, N. A., & Altman, B. M. 1998. *Characteristics of Nursing Home Residents, 1996.* MEPS Research Findings no. 5. AHCPR pub. no. 99-0006. Rockville, MD: Agency for Health Care Policy and Research, U.S. Department of Health and Human Services.

Leon, J., & Moyer, D. 1999. Potential cost savings in residential care for Alzheimer's disease patients. *Gerontologist* 39:440–49.

330 S. Zimmerman, P. D. Sloane, and J. K. Eckert

Lewin-VHI. 1996. *National Study of Assisted Living for the Frail Elderly: Literature Review Update.* Contract no. HHS-1-94-0024. U.S. Department of Health and Human Services, Washington, DC.

Manard, B. B., Atman, W., Bray, N., Kane, L., & Zeuschner, A. 1992. *Policy Synthesis on Assisted Living for the Frail Elderly.* Washington, DC: U.S. Department of Health and Human Services, Office of the Assistant Secretary for Planning and Evaluation.

Meyer, H. 1998. The bottom line on assisted living. *Hospitals and Health Networks,* July 20, 22–25.

Mollica, R. L. 1998. *State Assisted Living Policy, 1998.* Portland, ME: National Academy for State Health Policy.

———. 2000. *State Assisted Living Policy, 2000.* Portland, ME: National Academy for State Health Policy.

Mor, V., Sherwood, S., & Gutkin, C. E. 1986. A national study of residential care for the aged. *Gerontologist* 26:405–17.

Murer, M. 1997. Assisted living: The regulatory outlook. *Nursing Homes* 46:24–28.

Namazi, K. H., Eckert, J. K., Kahana, E., & Lyon, S. 1989. Psychological well-being of elderly board and care home residents. *Gerontologist* 29:511–16.

Olson, S. R. 1994. Linking services to standards. *Provider* (January): 51–53.

Segal, S. P., & Hwang, S. D. 1994. Licensure of sheltered care facilities: Does it assure quality? *Social Work* 39:124–31.

Timko, C., & Moos, R. H. 1989. Choice, control, and adaptation among elderly residents of sheltered care settings. *Journal of Applied Social Psychology* 19:636–55.

U.S. Congress, General Accounting Office. 1989. *Insufficient Assurances that Residents' Needs Are Identified and Met.* Washington, DC: Government Printing Office.

———. 1992a. *Board and Care Homes: Elderly at Risk from Mishandled Medications.* Report to House Subcommittee on Health and Long-Term Care. Washington, DC: Government Printing Office.

———. 1992b. *Drug Use and Misuse in America's Board and Care Homes: Failure in Public Policy.* Report to House Select Committee on Aging. Washington, DC: Government Printing Office.

———. 1999. *Assisted Living: Quality of Care and Consumer Protection Issues in Four States.* Report to Congressional Requesters. Washington, DC: Government Printing Office.

Weihl, H. 1981. On the relationship between the size of residential institutions and the well-being of residents. *Gerontologist* 21:247–50.

Wildfire, J. B., Hawes, C., Mor, V., Lux, L., & Brown, I. 1997. The effect of regulation on the quality of care in board and care homes. *Generations* 21:25–29.

Wilson, K. 1996. *Assisted Living: Reconceptualizing Regulations to Meet Consumers' Needs and Preferences.* Washington, DC: Public Policy Institute, American Association of Retired Persons.

Zimmerman, S. I., Sloane, P. D., Gruber-Baldini, A., Calkins, M., Leon, J., Magaziner, J., & Hebel, J. R. 1997. The philosophy of special care in Alzheimer's special care units. *Journal of Mental Health and Aging* 3:169–81.

Index

abuse, elder, 26, 75, 83
activities: availability of, 200, 202, 204, 206, 209–16, 283, 286; and community integration, 308–9; and dementia care, 24, 259, 260, 265, 266, 321; group, 63, 65, 187; mental, 25, 65, 67; physical, 65–67; productive, 65–67, 72; social, 200, 204, 211; staff for, 25, 286, 287; structured, 162–63
activities of daily living (ADL), 3–4, 152–54; and admission-and-retention policies, 215, 217, 225; and aging in place, 226, 230–33, 235; assessment of, 126; assistance with, 5n2, 159, 254, 317; and dementia, 252, 253, 266; and HMOs, 38; and impaired functioning, 164, 201–2; instrumental (IADL), 101–4, 146; measurement of, 124, 127; and nursing home care, 320; personal, 5n2, 73, 184, 205; and physical therapy, 67; and race, 92, 101–4; and resident characteristics, 166–67, 207
ADA (Americans with Disabilities Act), 73
adaptability, 73–74
ADL. See activities of daily living
admission-and-retention policies, 23, 304–7, 320; and ADL, 215, 217, 225; and dementia, 24, 258, 262; and process of care, 199, 201, 202, 217; and resident agreements, 19–21; and retention models, 225

adult-care homes, 5n2, 247; attitudes toward, 99–100; diversity in, 96, 111, 310; and race, 94, 96–100, 106–10; willingness to use, 101–6. See also board-and-care homes
adult day care, 44, 69, 72, 211, 212
African Americans, 92–112, 149–50, 166; attitudes toward RC/AL of, 95, 99–106, 111–12
age: and diversity, 62–63; and impairment, 152, 180; of residents, 148–49, 165–66, 169
aging in place, vii, 57, 144, 163, 224–40, 324; and ADL, 226, 230–33, 235; alternatives to, 43; and assisted living philosophy, 2, 15, 227; and available services, 23, 226; and behavior problems, 233, 235; community-level factors in, 225–26, 228–30, 234–39; and corporations, 227–30; defined, 224; facility-level factors in, 74, 226–29, 234–38; and family, 10, 226; individual-level factors in, 228, 230–35, 239; and medical needs, 231, 233–34, 236; and public support, 145, 231, 233, 236, 237; and regulations, 4, 9, 11, 21, 225, 237–39, 325
Alabama, 12, 18, 81
Alaska, 12, 18
alcohol abuse, 205, 206, 233, 237. See also behavior problems
Allen, I., 305
Aller, L. J., 301